Traumatic Brain Injury

Editors

PAUL M. VESPA
DANIEL HIRT
GEOFFREY T. MANLEY

NEUROSURGERY CLINICS OF NORTH AMERICA

www.neurosurgery.theclinics.com

Consulting Editors
RUSSELL LONSER
DANIEL K. RESNICK

October 2016 • Volume 27 • Number 4

ELSEVIER

1600 John F. Kennedy Boulevard • Suite 1800 • Philadelphia, Pennsylvania, 19103-2899

http://www.theclinics.com

NEUROSURGERY CLINICS OF NORTH AMERICA Volume 27, Number 4
October 2016 ISSN 1042-3680, ISBN-13: 978-0-323-46319-5

Editor: Jennifer Flynn-Briggs
Developmental Editor: Colleen Viola

Neurosurgery Clinics of North America (ISSN 1042-3680) is published quarterly by Elsevier Inc., 360 Park Avenue South, New York, NY 10010-1710. Months of issue are January, April, July, and October. Business and Editorial Offices: 1600 John F. Kennedy Blvd., Suite 1800, Philadelphia, PA 19103-2899. Customer Service Office: 11830 Westline Industrial Drive, St. Louis, MO 63146. Periodicals postage paid at New York, NY, and additional mailing offices. Subscription prices are $385.00 per year (US individuals), $639.00 per year (US institutions), $415.00 per year (Canadian individuals), $794.00 per year (Canadian institutions), $495.00 per year (international individuals), $794.00 per year (international institutions), $100.00 per year (US students), and $255.00 per year (international and Canadian students). International air speed delivery is included in all *Clinics* subscription prices. All prices are subject to change without notice. **POSTMASTER:** Send address changes to *Neurosurgery Clinics of North America*, Elsevier Periodicals Customer Service, 11830 Westline Industrial Drive, St. Louis, MO 63146. **Customer Service: 1-800-654-2452 (US and Canada). From outside the US and Canada, call: 1-314-453-7041. Fax: 1-314-453-5170. E-mail: JournalsCustomerService-usa@elsevier.com (for print support) and journalsonlinesupport-usa@elsevier.com (for online support).**

Reprints. For copies of 100 or more, of articles in this publication, please contact the Commercial Reprints Department, Elsevier Inc., 360 Park Avenue South, New York, NY 10010-1710. Tel. 212-633-3874; Fax: 212-633-3820; E-mail: reprints@elsevier.com.

Neurosurgery Clinics of North America is covered in *MEDLINE/PubMed (Index Medicus)*, *EMBASE/Excerpta Medica*, and *Current Contents/Clinical Medicine (CC/CM)*.

Contributors

CONSULTING EDITORS

RUSSELL LONSER, MD
Professor and Chair, Department of
Neurological Surgery, The Ohio State
University Wexner Medical Center,
Columbus, Ohio

DANIEL K. RESNICK, MD, MS
Professor and Vice Chairman; Program
Director, Department of Neurosurgery,
University of Wisconsin School of Medicine
and Public Health, Madison, Wisconsin

EDITORS

PAUL M. VESPA, MD, FCCM
Division of Neurocritical Care, Department of
Neurosurgery, Ronald Reagan UCLA Medical
Center, David Geffen School of Medicine at
University of California, Los Angeles, Los
Angeles, California

DANIEL HIRT, MD
UCLA Brain Injury Research Center;
Department of Neurosurgery, David Geffen
School of Medicine at University of California,
Los Angeles, Los Angeles, California

GEOFFREY T. MANLEY, MD, PhD
Brain and Spinal Injury Center, San Francisco
General Hospital; Professor; Vice Chairman,
Department of Neurological Surgery, University
of California, San Francisco, San Francisco,
California

AUTHORS

HADIE ADAMS, MD
Division of Neurosurgery, Department of
Clinical Neurosciences, Addenbrooke's
Hospital, University of Cambridge, Cambridge,
United Kingdom

AMINUL I. AHMED, MA (Cantab), MD, PhD
Clinical Lecturer, Clinical Experimental
Sciences, University Hospitals Southampton,
University of Southampton, Southampton,
United Kingdom; International Research
Fellow, Miami Project to Cure Paralysis,
University of Miami, Miami, Florida

MICHAEL L. ALOSCO, PhD
Department of Neurology; CTE Program,
Alzheimer's Disease Center, Boston University
School of Medicine, Boston, Massachusetts

DANIEL BRAAS, PhD
Department of Molecular and Medical
Pharmacology, David Geffen School of

Medicine at University of California, Los
Angeles; UCLA Metabolomics Center,
University of California, Los Angeles, Los
Angeles, California

MANUEL M. BUITRAGO BLANCO, MD, PhD
Division of Neurocritical Care, Department of
Neurosurgery, University of California, Los
Angeles, Los Angeles, California

M. ROSS BULLOCK, MD, PhD
Director and Professor, Neurotrauma,
Department of Neurosurgery, Miller School of
Medicine, Lois Pope Life Center, University of
Miami, Miami, Florida

RAMON DIAZ-ARRASTIA, MD, PhD
Center for Neuroscience and Regenerative
Medicine, Uniformed Services University
of the Health Sciences, Rockville,
Maryland

W. DALTON DIETRICH, PhD
Scientific Director and Professor, Miami
Project to Cure Paralysis, Lois Pope Life
Center, University of Miami, Miami, Florida

ALISA GEAN, MD
Professor Emeritus, Department of Radiology,
San Francisco General Hospital, Adjunct
Professor Emeritus of Neurology and
Neurosurgery, University of California, San
Francisco, San Francisco, California

CHRISTOPHER C. GIZA, MD
Professor, Division of Pediatric Neurology,
Department of Neurosurgery, Mattel Children's
Hospital-UCLA, University of California, Los
Angeles, Los Angeles, California

THOMAS C. GLENN, PhD
UCLA Brain Injury Research Center;
Department of Neurosurgery, David Geffen
School of Medicine at University of California,
Los Angeles, Los Angeles, California

GREGORY W.J. HAWRYLUK, MD, PhD
Assistant Professor; Director of Neurosurgical
Critical Care, Department of Neurosurgery,
University of Utah, Salt Lake City, Utah

DANIEL HIRT, MD
UCLA Brain Injury Research Center;
Department of Neurosurgery, David Geffen
School of Medicine at University of California,
Los Angeles, Los Angeles, California

BERTRAND R. HUBER, MD, PhD
Department of Pathology and Laboratory
Medicine, VA Boston Healthcare System;
Department of Neurology, Boston University
School of Medicine, Boston, Massachusetts

PETER J. HUTCHINSON, FRCS SN, PhD
Division of Neurosurgery, Department of
Clinical Neurosciences, Addenbrooke's
Hospital, University of Cambridge, Cambridge,
United Kingdom

JOSHUA KAMINS, MD
Fellow, Department of Neurology, University of
California, Los Angeles, Los Angeles, California

ANGELOS G. KOLIAS, MRCS
Division of Neurosurgery, Department of
Clinical Neurosciences, Addenbrooke's
Hospital, University of Cambridge, Cambridge,
United Kingdom

CHRISTOS LAZARIDIS, MD
Division of Neurocritical Care, Department of
Neurology, Baylor College of Medicine Medical
Center, Baylor College of Medicine, Houston,
Texas

GEOFFREY T. MANLEY, MD, PhD
Brain and Spinal Injury Center, San Francisco
General Hospital; Professor; Vice Chairman,
Department of Neurological Surgery, University
of California, San Francisco, San Francisco,
California

MELISSA J. McGINN, PhD
Assistant Professor, Department of Anatomy
and Neurobiology, Medical College of Virginia
Campus of Virginia Commonwealth University,
Richmond, Virginia

ANN C. McKEE, MD
Department of Pathology and Laboratory
Medicine, VA Boston Healthcare System;
CTE Program, Alzheimer's Disease Center;
Department of Neurology and Pathology,
Boston University School of Medicine,
Boston, Massachusetts

DANIEL MINTER, BS
Department of Neurological Surgery, University
of California, San Francisco, San Francisco,
California

CHRISTOPHER A. MUTCH, MD, PhD
Clinical Neuroradiology Fellow, Department
of Radiology, University of California, San
Francisco, San Francisco, California

JOHN T. POVLISHOCK, PhD
Professor and Chair, Department of Anatomy
and Neurobiology, Medical College of Virginia
Campus of Virginia Commonwealth University,
Richmond, Virginia

GIYARPURAM N. PRASHANT, MD
Division of Neurocritical Care, Department of
Neurosurgery, University of California, Los
Angeles, Los Angeles, California

CLAUDIA S. ROBERTSON, MD
Department of Neurosurgery, Baylor College of
Medicine, Houston, Texas

JASON F. TALBOTT, MD, PhD
Assistant Professor, Department of Radiology,
San Francisco General Hospital, University of
California, San Francisco, San Francisco,
California

PAUL M. VESPA, MD, FCCM
Division of Neurocritical Care, Department of
Neurosurgery, Ronald Reagan UCLA Medical
Center, David Geffen School of Medicine at
University of California, Los Angeles, Los
Angeles, California

ETHAN A. WINKLER, MD, PhD
Brain and Spinal Injury Center, San Francisco
General Hospital; Department of Neurological
Surgery, University of California, San
Francisco, San Francisco, California

STEPHANIE M. WOLAHAN, PhD
UCLA Brain Injury Research Center;
Department of Neurosurgery, David
Geffen School of Medicine at University
of California, Los Angeles, Los Angeles,
California

JOHN K. YUE, BA
Brain and Spinal Injury Center, San
Francisco General Hospital; Department
of Neurological Surgery, University of
California, San Francisco, San Francisco,
California

LARA L. ZIMMERMANN, MD
Department of Neurosurgery, Ronald
Reagan UCLA Medical Center, Los Angeles,
California

JASON F. TALBOTT, MD, PhD
Assistant Professor, Department of Radiology, San Francisco General Hospital, University of California, San Francisco, San Francisco, California

PAUL M. VESPA, MD, FCCM
Division of Neurocritical Care, Department of Neurosurgery, Ronald Reagan UCLA Medical Center, David Geffen School of Medicine at University of California, Los Angeles, Los Angeles, California

ETHAN A. WINKLER, MD, PhD
Brain and Spinal Injury Center, San Francisco General Hospital, Department of Neurological Surgery, University of California, San Francisco, California

STEPHANIE M. WOLAHAN, PhD
UCLA Brain Injury Research Center, Department of Neurosurgery, David Geffen School of Medicine at University of California, Los Angeles, Los Angeles, California

JOHN K. YUE, BA
Brain and Spinal Injury Center, San Francisco General Hospital, Department of Neurological Surgery, University of California, San Francisco, California

LARA L. ZIMMERMANN, MD
Department of Neurosurgery, Ronald Reagan UCLA Medical Center, Los Angeles, California

Contents

Traumatic brain injury (TBI) is the greatest cause of death and severe disability in young adults; its incidence is increasing in the elderly and in the developing world. Outcome from severe TBI has improved dramatically as a result of advancements in trauma systems and supportive critical care, however we remain without a therapeutic which acts directly to attenuate brain injury. Recognition of secondary injury and its molecular mediators has raised hopes for such targeted treatments. Unfortunately, over 30 late-phase clinical trials investigating promising agents have failed to translate a therapeutic for clinical use. Numerous explanations for this failure have been postulated and are reviewed here. With this historical context we review ongoing research and anticipated future trends which are armed with lessons from past trials, new scientific advances, and improved research infrastructure and funding. There is great hope that these new efforts will finally lead to an effective therapeutic for TBI as well as better clinical management strategies.

This article provides a concise overview, at the structural and functional level, of those changes evoked by traumatic brain injury across the spectrum of the disease. Using data derived from animals and humans, the pathogenesis of focal versus diffuse brain damage is presented for consideration of its overall implications for morbidity. Emphasis is placed on contusion and its potential expansion in concert with diffuse changes primarily assessed at the axonal level. Concomitant involvement of neuroexcitation and its role in global and focal metabolic changes is considered. Lastly, the influence of premorbid factors including age, genetics, and socioeconomic background is discussed.

Traumatic brain injury (TBI) is a major cause of morbidity and mortality worldwide. Imaging plays an important role in the evaluation, diagnosis, and triage of patients with TBI. Recent studies suggest that it also helps predict patient outcomes. TBI consists of multiple pathoanatomic entities. This article reviews the current state of TBI imaging including its indications, benefits and limitations of the modalities, imaging protocols, and imaging findings for each of these pathoanatomic entities. Also briefly surveyed are advanced imaging techniques, which include several promising areas of TBI research.

Chronic traumatic encephalopathy (CTE) is a distinctive neurodegenerative disease that occurs as a result of repetitive head impacts. CTE can only be diagnosed by postmortem neuropathologic examination of brain tissue. CTE is a unique disorder with a pathognomonic lesion that can be reliably distinguished from other neurodegenerative diseases. CTE is associated with violent behaviors, explosivity, loss of control, depression, suicide, memory loss and cognitive changes. There is increasing evidence that CTE affects amateur athletes as well as professional athletes and military veterans. CTE has become a major public health concern.

NEUROSURGERY CLINICS OF NORTH AMERICA

RELATED INTEREST

Critical Care Nursing Clinics of North America, June 2013 (Vol. 25, Issue 2)
Traumatic Brain Injury: Pathophysiology, Monitoring, and Mechanism-Based Care
Richard B. Arbour, *Editor*

THE CLINICS ARE AVAILABLE ONLINE!
Access your subscription at:
www.theclinics.com

Erratum

In the July issue (Volume 27, number 3), for the article "Measurement of Trigeminal Neuralgia Pain: Penn Facial Pain Scale," Sukhmeet K. Sandhu's name was erroneously omitted from the author list. The correct author list should be Sukhmeet K. Sandhu and John Y.K. Lee, and the correct article reference is Sandhu SK, Lee JYK. Measurement of Trigeminal Neuralgia Pain: Penn Facial Pain Scale. Neurosurg Clin N Am. 2016 Jul;27(3):327-36.

Neurosurg Clin N Am 27 (2016) xiii
http://dx.doi.org/10.1016/j.nec.2016.08.009
1042-3680/16/$ – see front matter © 2016 Elsevier Inc. All rights reserved.

Erratum

Preface
Advances in Neurotrauma Research

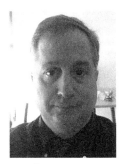

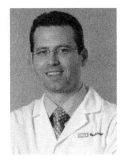

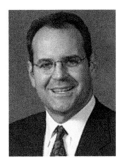

Paul M. Vespa, MD   Daniel Hirt, MD   Geoffrey T. Manley,
                                                        MD, PhD

Editors

Traumatic brain injury continues to be the cause of significant morbidity and mortality in the United States and presents numerous challenges, during the acute as well as the long-term care of these patients. Therefore, the idea to collaborate and publish an issue on Neurotrauma was inspired by the complexity of this disease process and the tremendous advances in all aspects of the care of these patients.

Advances in imaging have resulted in significant improvements in outcome, by providing efficiency in diagnoses and prognosis. In one of the early articles on imaging modalities, new techniques in MRI are discussed that have yielded insight not only into the structural but also into the metabolic changes following traumatic brain injury.

Metabolic alterations following brain injury have become more and more of a focus in recent studies investigating new treatment targets. The preservation of vulnerable cells within the penumbra of the injury site remains a major therapy goal in the intensive care unit during the acute stage of recovery. Understanding the metabolic changes following injury is crucial to salvage these cells and provide the brain-injured patient with the best possible chance for a good recovery from this devastating disease. Individualized patient care has gained enormous momentum throughout many disease processes, including cancer, diabetes, and heart disease. Based on decades of research, traumatic brain injury is no different,

and the vast variability between patients has continued to make the acute care phase extraordinarily challenging. It is therefore important to further delineate the metabolic changes following traumatic brain injury and find ways to identify individual metabolic profiles and biomarkers within this profile that can be manipulated to improve outcome. Different aspects of the metabolic profile and alterations of the injured brain are discussed, and possible target therapies are presented.

We then conclude this journey into the advances in Neurotrauma with a detailed look at the long-term concerns and sequelae of traumatic brain injury as well as possible postacute care treatment strategies. And so, with a comprehensive look at the past, present, and future of traumatic brain injury research, this issue on Neurotrauma delivers a complete overview of the advances in all aspects of the brain-injured patient's treatment paradigm.

Paul M. Vespa, MD
Department of Neurosurgery
David Geffen School of Medicine at UCLA
Box 957436, RRUMC 6236
Los Angeles, CA 90095-7436, USA

Daniel Hirt, MD
Department of Neurosurgery
David Geffen School of Medicine at UCLA
465 Wasserman, 300 Stein Plaza
Los Angeles, CA 90095-6901, USA

Neurosurg Clin N Am 27 (2016) xv–xvi
http://dx.doi.org/10.1016/j.nec.2016.08.008
1042-3680/16/© 2016 Published by Elsevier Inc.

neurosurgery.theclinics.com

Geoffrey T. Manley, MD, PhD
Department of Neurological Surgery
University of California, San Francisco
505 Parnassus Avenue, Room M779
San Francisco, CA 94143-0112, USA

E-mail addresses:
PVespa@mednet.ucla.edu (P.M. Vespa)
DHirt@mednet.ucla.edu (D. Hirt)
ManleyG@neurosurg.ucsf.edu (G.T. Manley)

Past, Present, and Future of Traumatic Brain Injury Research

Gregory W.J. Hawryluk, MD, PhD[a], M. Ross Bullock, MD, PhD[b],*

KEYWORDS

- Traumatic brain injury (TBI) • Research • Secondary injury • Clinical trials • Trends • History
- Big data

KEY POINTS

- Traumatic brain injury (TBI) is the greatest cause of death and severe disability in young adults; its incidence is increasing in the elderly and in the developing world.
- Mortality rates have decreased from more than 80% for severe TBI in the 1940s to about 20% currently in well-resourced hospitals, largely as a result of improvements in trauma systems and supportive critical care.
- Recognition of secondary injury and secondary insults has led to novel basic science and clinical approaches aimed at improving outcomes from TBI.
- Over 30 late-phase clinical trials have failed to translate a therapeutic agent for clinical use and numerous explanations for this failure have been postulated.
- New research is armed with lessons from past trials, new scientific advances, as well as improved research infrastructure and funding; there is great hope that an effective therapeutic for TBI will be translated to clinical use in the coming years.

INTRODUCTION

Traumatic brain injury (TBI) of any severity has the potential to devastate the lives of patients over minutes or hours. An intracranial hematoma can transform an active life to a vegetative state, death, or severe disability more dramatically than almost any other consequence of trauma. The evolution of trauma care systems, rapid delivery of imaging, neurocritical care, and rehabilitation has improved outcomes.[1] In contrast, despite 8 decades of research aimed at developing targeted "neuroprotective" drug therapies for severe TBI, none has been successfully translated. Although the same holds true for occlusive stroke, multiple sclerosis has, in contrast, been transformed by new drugs.[2] TBI scientists have revealed many pathologic molecular processes that cause progressive brain damage after the initial injury, suggesting a therapeutic window and multiple potential drug targets. Paralleling this basic science advancement is recognition of the methodologic shortcomings of the approximately 35 phase III TBI trials undertaken to date, which likely contributed to their failure.[3] There is thus great optimism that victims of TBI may soon benefit from novel and efficacious therapeutics that have been long elusive. In this article, we aim to provide an overview of TBI research to date, both successes and failures, with a particular focus on putative reasons for the failure to translate preclinical findings into clinical trial success (**Table 1**).

[a] Department of Neurosurgery, University of Utah, 175 North Medical Drive East, Salt Lake City, UT 84132, USA;
[b] Neurotrauma, Department of Neurosurgery, Miller School of Medicine, Lois Pope LIFE Center, University of Miami, 1095 NW 14th Terrace, Miami, FL 33136, USA
* Corresponding author.
E-mail address: rbullock@med.miami.edu

Neurosurg Clin N Am 27 (2016) 375–396
http://dx.doi.org/10.1016/j.nec.2016.05.002
1042-3680/16/© 2016 Elsevier Inc. All rights reserved.

Table 1
Themes in the advancement of the traumatic brain injury field: past, present, and future

	Basic Science Advancement	Advance in Clinical Management	Major Research Efforts
Past	Recognition of secondary injury and secondary insults	Birth of clinical practice guidelines and efforts to standardize care; treatment thresholds for physiologic parameters (ICP, CPP, P_{CO_2}, etc)	Numerous clinical trials of neuroprotective agents
Present	Introspection relating to trial failures of the past; increased focus on mild/repetitive TBI, chronic traumatic encephalopathy; increasingly robust preclinical data (Operation Brain Trauma Therapy); cell therapies and early regenerative medicine strategies	Recognition of the importance of cerebrovascular autoregulation; the IMPACT model and improved prognostication; development of common data elements; maturation and expansion of guidelines efforts; scrutiny of the role of conventional treatment (ICP monitoring and decompressive craniectomy)	Novel trial and analytical methodologies (more sensitive statistics, comparative effectiveness research)
Future	Novel neuroprotectants and regeneration-stimulating agents	Shift from routine implementation of guidelines to "personalized medicine" accounting for patients' unique physiology and physiologic states	Big data in research efforts and in care of individual patients, improved classification scheme for TBI; greater use of genomic and proteomic data; studies of combinations of agents; more sensitive outcome measures

Abbreviations: CPP, cerebral perfusion pressure; ICP, intracranial pressure; TBI, traumatic brain injury.

EPIDEMIOLOGY

TBI is changing demographically. Economic growth in developing nations such as Brazil, China, and India has led to an increase in motor vehicle use and a significant increase in TBI in these countries.[4,5] Additionally, in the United States, Europe, and Japan an increasing proportion of TBI is being seen in the elderly as a result of falls.[6] TBI remains, however, the leading cause of death in young adults under the age of 45 in the United States and is believed to cost society more than $60 billion annually.[7] Fortunately, only 10% of the 500,000 people admitted to hospital for TBI each year sustain a severe injury.[8] One-third who sustain severe TBI die and survivors frequently have lasting deficits of motor, sensory, and cognitive functions.[8] Despite the increase in incidence, the outcome after TBI is improving though these outcomes depend on the quality of care provided.[1,5] An analysis of survival in placebo groups in major head injury trials has noted progressive improvement since the mid 1980s: contemporary mortality rates are now less than one-half of what they were 3 decades ago.[9]

Almost one-third of Americans will sustain a mild TBI, or concussion in their lifetime, and increasing evidence suggests that cumulative concussions, or concussion in vulnerable individuals may progress to dementia, a potential future public health and "social engineering" dilemma of massive proportions, that is covered elsewhere in this issue. Likewise, penetrating TBI owing to gunshot and explosive shrapnel injuries has increased significantly in the United States.

TRAUMATIC BRAIN INJURY RESEARCH METRICS

Meaningful TBI outcomes and demographic research was not possible until the advent of the Glasgow Coma Scale (GCS) in 1974.[10] This scale is now one of the most commonly used clinical metrics in all of medicine because it provides an objective means of assessing neurologic function across the spectrum of brain function (albeit with little usefulness in mild TBI) and facilitates communication and comparison of patients across centers. The TBI research field was further assisted by the additional publication of the Glasgow Outcome Scale (GOS) in 1976,[11] which provides a standardized means out assessing outcome from TBI. Since these publications, the volume of published TBI research has shown an exponential increase over time (**Fig. 1**). More than 4000 papers on the subject are now published annually.

In a recent analysis of the top 100 citations in neurosurgical journals, 4 TBI papers made the list (**Table 2**).[12–15] "Citation classics" are defined as papers cited more than 400 times and 14 TBI papers have made the bar (**Table 3**).[10,13–24] Indeed, the 2 most cited works in the history of neurosurgery are—not surprisingly—the GCS[10] and the GOS.[16] All of these papers represent major advances in TBI and provided the impetus for TBI to become the first major area in clinical neuroscience to provide evidence-based guidelines for care,[25] and emphasize that systems of care maybe more powerful than "the Holy Grail" of phase III controlled clinical trials in improving outcomes. Nevertheless, it is clear that the GOS, a relatively coarse, subjective metric of functional outcome may lack sufficient sensitivity as the ideal "primary outcome measure" in clinical trials. Major new initiatives (the Transforming Research and Clinical Knowledge in Traumatic Brain Injury [TRACK-TBI] and Collaborative European Neuro-Trauma Effectiveness Research in TBI [Center-TBI] studies) are under way to address this issue, as we will describe.

SECONDARY INJURY AND TARGETS FOR PHARMACOLOGIC TRIALS IN TRAUMATIC BRAIN INJURY

Familiarity with the concept of secondary injury is key to understanding the central dilemma and failures of pharmacologic trials in TBI. Established dogma holds that the damage done at the moment of impact to the brain and spinal cord (known as primary injury) cannot be reversed by any drug treatment. A subsequent cascade of cell death events leads to astrocytic hypertrophy and demolition of destroyed neurons (associated with tissue swelling and high intracranial pressure [ICP]), which sets the stage for regeneration, recovery, and repair. Secondary injury is classically thought to be a cascade of interrelated molecular processes that occur in a delayed fashion after the initial (or primary) injury to cause progressive delayed damage to the central nervous system, which may therefore be preventable if a therapy can be delivered to the intracellular molecular target before the damaging cascade is set in progress. Secondary injury is considered distinct from secondary insults, which are events occurring at the level of the whole patient that exacerbate the injury such as hypoxia, hypotension, and fever; mitigating secondary insults is the focus of supportive intensive care. Although the delayed nature of secondary injury makes it attractive for therapeutic targeting, no such agent has been translated successfully. This simplistic view is increasingly being refuted, because primary and secondary injury are intertwined: the "classic example" of diffuse axonal injury, long held to be an instantaneous mechanical axotomy, has now been shown to be a delayed, biochemically induced process, occurring over hours to days,

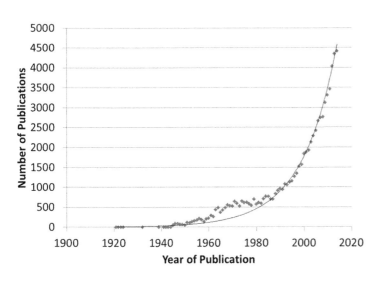

Fig. 1. Number of "traumatic brain injury" citations by year: the search term "traumatic brain injury" was searched in Pubmed (www. pubmed.com) and the number of publications documented in the database by year between 1900 and 2014 are presented graphically.

Table 2
Traumatic brain injury publications among the 100 most cited works in neurosurgery journals

Citation Rank	Reference
16	Katayama Y, Becker DP, Tamura T, et al. Massive increases in extracellular potassium and the indiscriminate release of glutamate following concussive brain injury. J Neurosurg 1990;73:889–900.[12]
17	Rimel RW, Giordani B, Barth JT, et al. Disability caused by minor head injury. Neurosurgery 1981;9: 221–8; 553.[13]
18	Becker DP, Miller JD, Ward JD, et al. The outcome from severe head injury with early diagnosis and intensive management. J Neurosurg 1977;47:491–502.[14]
22	Obrist WD, Langfitt TW, Jaggi JL, et al. Cerebral blood flow and metabolism in comatose patients with acute head injury. Relationship to intracranial hypertension. J Neurosurg 1984;61:241–53.[15]

Adapted from Ponce FA, Lozano AM. Highly cited works in neurosurgery. Part I: the 100 top-cited papers in neurosurgical journals. J Neurosurg 2010;112:225.

which can be mitigated effectively in the laboratory by drugs and hypothermia.[26,27] Herein we review select secondary injury mediators and experimental therapeutics that have targeted them (**Table 4**). In the future, cell replacement therapies will increasingly aim to exploit natural tissue regeneration cues that are set up by the injury. These are believed to guide implanted cells to differentiate along neuronal lines and to extend processes along anatomic pathways serving to enhance the delayed natural recovery that can occur for years after human severe TBI (see below).

Excitotoxicity

Excitotoxicity has been identified as one of the most important and earliest occurring secondary injury mediators; attempts have been made to antagonize this pathway in several clinical trials for TBI.[28–30] Milliseconds after impact, extracellular levels of the excitatory neurotransmitter glutamate increase rapidly as a result of mechanical shearing forces to synaptic vesicles and ion channels themselves. Accordingly, glutamate levels

increase by 100- to 1000-fold in the synaptic cleft, and extracellular fluid in the first 24 hours after injury.[28] Glutamate may remain markedly elevated for as long as 7 days after injury.[28] Glutamate binds to N-methyl-D-aspartate (NMDA), alpha-amino-3-hydroxy-5-methyl-4-isoxazole propionic acid, and kainate receptors, opens more ion channels, allows calcium entry, and plays a major role in triggering cell death through excessive excitatory neurotransmission. Opening of glutamate receptor-associated ion channels increases intracellular calcium, which in turn destroys mitochondrial enzymes and causes failure of energy-dependent transporters owing to insufficient ATP to drive the ATPase Na/K–dependent transporter.[31] This in turn causes the cytotoxic early cell swelling (buffered by astrocytes) seen as the universal indicator of bad outcome: the "dark brain" seen on early computed tomography (CT) scans of patients with the most severe TBI. Excitotoxicity can cause the death of neurons and possibly oligodendrocytes as will be discussed.[32] NMDA receptor antagonism has been convincingly shown to reduce glutamate toxicity in both in vitro and in vivo laboratory TBI models.[33]

Numerous glutamate antagonists have been explored in human clinical trials, although none have demonstrated sufficient safety and efficacy to convince "big pharma" to deploy the many millions needed to further develop these compounds for TBI. Selfotel is a competitive glutamate antagonist and was the first glutamate antagonist to go into phase III trials after an extensive preclinical evaluation process.[8,34] Magnesium acts as a noncompetitive NMDA receptor antagonist by physiologically blocking the NMDA receptor ion channel and as an intracellular calcium antagonist.[35–37] Magnesium administration showed promise in animal models of TBI, but unfortunately 5-day infusions of magnesium administered to humans within 8 hours of moderate or severe TBI showed no neuroprotective effect in a phase III, single-center study.[38] Aptiganel (Cerestat) is a use-dependent noncompetitive glutamate antagonist that binds receptor only when it is activated by high concentrations of glutamate.[8] Aptiganel was studied in a large human trial; however, the results of this trial have never been published and are presumed to be negative.[8] The most recently completed trial of a glutamate antagonist was with a "second-generation" NR2B-selective NMDA antagonist, CP 101-606.[39] Unfortunately, even though the outcome was 7% to 11% better in males in the treated group over placebo, Pfizer elected to not develop the compound further, even with support from the National Institutes of Health (NIH), for unknown internal reasons.[39]

Table 3
Traumatic brain injury citation classics

Citation Rank	Reference[a]
1	Jennett B, Bond M. Assessment of outcome after severe brain-damage. Lancet 1975; 1:480–4.[16]
2	Teasdale G, Jennett B. Assessment of coma and impaired consciousness. A practical scale. Lancet 1974;2:81–4.[10]
32	Chesnut RM, Marshall LF, Klauber MR, et al. The role of secondary brain injury in determining outcome from severe head injury. J Trauma 1993;34:216–22.[17]
34	Marion DW, Penrod LE, Kelsey SF, et al. Treatment of traumatic brain injury with moderate hypothermia. N Engl J Med 1997;336:540–6.[18]
48	Rimel RW, Giordani B, Barth JT, et al. Disability caused by minor head injury. Neurosurgery 1981;9:221–8.[13]
49	Becker DP, Miller JD, Ward JD, et al. The outcome from severe head injury with early diagnosis and intensive management. J Neurosurg 1977;47:491–502.[14]
55	Obrist WD, Langfitt TW, Jaggi JL, et al. Cerebral blood flow and metabolism in comatose patients with acute head injury. Relationship to intracranial hypertension. J Neurosurg 1984;61:241–53.[15]
73	Clifton GL, Miller ER, Choi SC, et al. Lack of effect of induction of hypothermia after acute brain injury. N Engl J Med 2001;344:556–63.[19]
86	Levin HS, Mattis S, Ruff RM, et al. Neurobehavioral outcome following minor head injury: a three-center study. J Neurosurg 1987;66:234–43.[20]
89	Adams JH, Graham DI, Murray LS, et al. Diffuse axonal injury due to nonmissile head injury in humans: an analysis of 45 cases. Ann Neurol 1982;12:557–63.[21]
92	Rosner MJ, Rosner SD, Johnson AH. Cerebral perfusion pressure: management protocol and clinical results. J Neurosurg 1995;83:949–62.[22]
93	Muizelaar JP, Marmarou A, Ward JD, et al. Adverse effects of prolonged hyperventilation in patients with severe head injury: a randomized clinical trial. J Neurosurg 1991;75: 731–9.[173]
95	Miller JD, Becker DP, Ward JD, et al. Significance of intracranial hypertension in severe head injury. J Neurosurg 1977;47:503–16.[23]
104	Rappaport M, Hall KM, Hopkins K, et al. Disability rating scale for severe head trauma: coma to community. Arch Phys Med Rehabil 1982;63:118–23.[24]

[a] Studies which have been cited at least 400 times are considered citation classics.
Adapted from Ponce FA, Lozano, AM. Highly cited works in neurosurgery. Part I: the 100 top-cited papers in neurosurgical journals. J Neurosurg 2010;112:223–2.

Intracellular Calcium

Intracellular calcium dysregulation is a central common pathway for enzyme and particularly mitochondrial death and dysfunction in secondary brain injury of many types. Excessive intracellular calcium activates injurious enzymes such as calpains, which degrade the cytoskeleton. Hypercalcemia additionally causes mitochondrial dysfunction, exacerbates excitotoxicity (as glutamate release is calcium dependent), and triggers free radical production, which can culminate in cell death.[40,41] The degradation of spectrin, an important constituent of the cytoskeleton, generates measureable levels of breakdown products in serum, which are currently being explored as a biomarker of brain injury.[42]

Among calcium channel antagonists, nimodipine has been the most investigated in TBI. A series of 4 HIT (head injury trial) trials investigated the efficacy of nimodipine in TBI; however, none demonstrated robust benefit.[43–45] There has, however, been suggested benefit in the subgroup of patients with traumatic subarachnoid hemorrhage.[46] A study of SNX-111, another Ca^{++} antagonist, was suspended when the treatment group demonstrated higher mortality than placebo.[8] With all these calcium antagonists, the central issue has been achieving adequate rapid delivery of the drug to the neuronal calcium channels or

Table 4
Completed neuroprotective trials in Traumatic brain injury, 1980 to 2015

Agent	Year	n	Status	Result
Calcium antagonism				
Nimodipine[174] (HIT I)	1991	351	Completed	Negative
Nimodipine[44] (HIT II)	1994	852	Completed	Negative (overall)
Nimodipine[46] (HIT III)	1996	123	Completed	Positive
SNX-111	1998	237	Terminated, unpublished	Harmful
Nimodipine (HIT IV)	1999	592	Completed, unpublished	Negative
Antiinflammatory agent				
High-dose dexamethasone[175]	1983	161	Completed	Negative
Dexamthasone[176]	1986	130	Completed	Negative
Tromethamine[177]	1993	149	Completed	Negative (Overall)
Dexamethasone[178]	1994	300	Completed	Negative
Triamcinolone[179]	1995	396	Completed	Negative
Deltibant (Bradycor)[82]	1999	139	Terminated	Negative
Methylprednisolone[148]	2005	10,008	Terminated	Harmful
Glutamate antagonism				
Eliprodil	1995	452	Completed	Negative
Selfotel[34]	1999	693	Terminated	Negative
D-CPP-ene Saphir	1997	924	Completed, unpublished	Negative
Aptiganel (Cerestat)	1997	532	Terminated, unpublished	Negative
CP 101–606[180]	2005	404	Completed	11% better outcome in males
Magnesium sulfate[38]	2007	499	Completed	Harmful
Free-radical scavenging				
Tirilizad (Upjohn)	1994	1155	Terminated, unpublished	Negative
PEG-SOD[74]	1996	1562	Completed	Negative
Hypothermia				
Hypothermia[181]	2001	392	Halted	Negative
Mild hypothermia[182]	2003	396	Completed	Positive
Mild hypothermia[183]	2006	215	Completed	Positive
Management strategy				
Hyperbaric oxygen[184]	1992	168	Completed	Positive
CBF-directed management[185]	1999	189	Completed	Positive
Decompressive craniectomy[186]	2003	230	Completed	Positive
Hypertonic saline[187]	2004	229	Completed	Negative
Decompressive craniectomy[188]	2005	468	Completed	Positive
Neuroprotective, multiple mechanisms				
Dexanabinol[189]	2006	861	Completed	Negative
Progesterone[190]	2008	159	Completed	Positive
Progesterone[85]	2013	882	Terminated	Negative

Included studies involved at least 100 patients 15 years of age or older with moderate or severe traumatic brain injury. Studies from Cruz et al were removed because they are suspected to be products of academic misconduct.

Abbreviations: CBF, cerebral blood flow; HIT, head injury trial; PEG-SOD, polyethylene glycol-superoxide dismutase.

Adapted from Maas AI, Roozenbeek B, Manley GT. Clinical trials in traumatic brain injury: past experience and current developments. Neurotherapeutics 7, 117–18.

intracellular sites of action after intravenous infusion.

Ischemia and Mitochondrial Dysfunction

Hypoxic–ischemic damage is believed to be a central factor in the delayed damage that occurs after TBI evidenced by the high frequency of the classical ischemic neuronal damage pathologic findings seen at autopsy, including pyknosis, necrosis, and loss of nuclear definition.[47] It is now known that such changes can also be produced by contusion, vascular occlusion, seizures, and meningitis. Because a continuous supply of oxygen is, of course, critical to the electron transport chain and energy generation in mitochondria, cellular energy failure is an inevitable consequence of hypoxia. This results in failure of energy-dependent ionic pumps and ionic dysregulation.[48–50] Accumulation of sodium within the cell, for instance, leads to cytotoxic edema from the resulting influx of water.[51] Calcium overload induces opening of the mitochondrial permeability transition pore, which compromises the electrochemical gradient required to generate ATP and further compromises the ability of the cells to maintain ionic homeostasis.[52–56] This translates to the loss of grey–white definition, and dark brain seen after cardiac arrest, and the severest forms of TBI. Milder degrees of oxygen delivery impairment can in turn lead to cell death by necrosis or apoptosis.[53–55]

After a human case report of a much better than expected outcome in a patient with severe TBI who had been given cyclosporin A (CsA) for a transplant,[56] this immunosuppressant has been investigated for putative additional neuroprotective properties. It was subsequently discovered that CsA prevents mitochondria from accumulating calcium during cellular ischemia and inhibits mitochondrial permeability transition pore opening.[57–60] CsA has since shown promise in numerous preclinical studies[59,61–65] as well as a small phase II prospective randomized placebo-controlled human trial. This human study did not demonstrate improvement in neurologic outcome, although CsA seemed to be safe to administer to the severe TBI population.[66] Several similar drugs are currently being investigated that are believed to have the neuroprotective properties of CsA without its immunosuppressive effects.[67]

Free Radical-Mediated Injury

Free radicals are highly reactive molecules because they bear a free electron in their outer shell. Free radicals are generated by mitochondria in hypoxic conditions and they damage cellular membranes and intracellular molecules contributing to the death of both neurons and glia.[68] Antioxidant molecules that neutralize free radicals thus have a strong theoretic basis for efficacy after TBI. Numerous endogenous and synthetic antioxidants have been investigated for this purpose.[69–72] Noteworthy trials investigated antioxidants including polyethylene glycol-superoxide dismutase (PEG-SOD) and tirilizad (Upjohn). PEG-SOD, also known as pegorgotein, showed benefit in a phase II trial.[73] In a phase III, trial 2 doses were compared with placebo.[74] Nonsignificant benefit was observed; however, the agent has not been studied further. The tirilizad study was completed but showed no effect, as was also seen in a large spinal cord injury trial.[75] Tempol, a modern antioxidant with apparent rapid bioavailability, has not been approved by the US Food and Drug Administration (FDA) for human intravenous use, but has shown benefit in laboratory TBI studies.[76]

Drugs Acting on Neuroinflammation

The inflammatory process after TBI is highly complex, much less studied, and involves numerous cellular and noncellular mediators.[77–79] Some aspects of the inflammatory response clearly exacerbate secondary injury, and others contribute in beneficial ways such as phagocytosis to remove cellular debris and enhance the local microenvironment for regenerative growth.[78] Steroids were among the first drugs tried for TBI, and were used commonly in the management of head injury in the past. The landmark Corticosteroid Randomisation After Significant Head Injury (CRASH) trials, however, have clearly shown that nonselective antiinflammatories (eg methylprednisolone, dexamethasone) are clearly harmful after TBI, because of higher pneumonia incidence and deaths owing to noncranial complications, such as infection.[80,81] Numerous antiinflammatory drugs have been studied in human TBI trials. A prospective, randomized trial studying deltibant (Bradycor), a bradykinin antagonist, was halted when concerns were identified in a concurrent animal study.[8,82]

CLINICAL TRIAL DESIGN: THE FAILURE TO TRANSLATE

Since the advent of the GCS and GOS, there have been 28 large phase III studies for TBI with an additional 6 trials unpublished,[3,8,83,84] some of which were discussed previously. No therapeutic agent has as yet demonstrated sufficient benefit to satisfy the FDA allowing translation to clinical use for human TBI. Elsewhere in the world, however, unproven "neutraceuticals" are in common use as neuroprotectants, for most TBI patients

(Nootropil, for example). Pessimism surrounding these failures has led to a decrease in TBI studies since the mid 1990s.[3] The recent closure of the Progesterone for the Treatment of Traumatic Brain Injury III (ProTECT III) trial for futility has been a particular blow to the field because this study was supported by better trial design and supportive preclinical data.[85] TBI research has accordingly shifted away from the study of neuro-protective drugs to therapeutic strategies such as hypothermia or decompressive craniectomy.[3]

These trial failures caused the neurotrauma community to enter a period of introspection, similar to that seen in the stroke field.[86] One of the first signs of this was a 2000 National Institute of Neurological Disorders and Stroke workshop that was convened to try to prevent repeating mistakes of the past.[8] Numerous reasons for these failures have been proposed and are reviewed herein.[40,83,87]

Limitations of Animal Models

The path to clinical translation for most investigational drugs for TBI begins in preclinical animal models. Rats have been used most frequently and common experimental models include fluid percussion, controlled cortical impact, and weight drop.[88] The frequent benefit seen in these models and the corresponding failure in humans has been a focus of the TBI community's introspection. The relevance of these models has been questioned: patients with severe TBI are by definition comatose yet experimental animals modelling these injuries are not injured to the point of requiring critical care or mechanical ventilation,[8,89] with very rare exceptions.[90] Moreover, rats are lissencephalic with axial, cylindrically constructed 2-g brains very different in structure compared with the "pendulum-like" arrangement of the much larger 1200-g human brain/craniospinal axis. Many agents have only been tested in a single experimental model of TBI, and few have been tested in large animal models.[89] In some cases, experimental drugs were not tested at clinically relevant time points such as aptiganel, which was never tested later than 15 minutes after insult in the animal model.[89,91] Moreover, few studied agents have had studies performed to demonstrate any blood–brain barrier penetration.[89,91] It is also possible that certain mechanisms of secondary injury are more problematic in certain TBI subtypes.[92] For instance, contusional brain injury has been shown to differ from diffuse axonal injury, because the former has a more marked inflammatory response, and is often characterized by focal lesion progression.[3] It is also possible that multiple mechanisms of secondary injury must be targeted concurrently to achieve benefit.[83,93] Such "synergistic" or multiple agent preclinical studies, which would be helpful in making these determinations, are ongoing and will help to inform which patients are most likely to benefit from particular combinations of drugs.[87]

Heterogeneity of the Traumatic Brain Injury Population and Sample Size Insufficiency

The tremendous heterogeneity of the human TBI population is often blamed for the failure to translate therapeutics.[92] Multiple pathoanatomic lesions typically coexist in TBI such as extraaxial hematomas (subdural and epidural), brain contusion and diffuse axonal injury. Moreover, TBI and the brain have been described as the most complex injury to the most complex structure in the known universe and the same injury processes can have markedly different consequences when only slightly different in location. Increasing the complexity further are other systemic injuries, shock, medical comorbidities, time to presentation to hospital, intoxications, and genetics.[84] There are also noteworthy center effects related to practice variation, population coverage, age and injury mix, and treatment protocols that are an important issue in multicenter trials. The variability inherent to human patients[19,89] is thus in stark contrast with homogenous animal models,[91] and requires that trials be performed in "ecologically appropriate" locations. For example, the recent Benchmark Evidence from South American Trials: Treatment of Intracranial Pressure (BEST-TRIP) trial of ICP monitoring in Bolivian/Ecuadorian neurosurgical centers with no prior experience of ICP monitoring, unsurprisingly showed no benefit for use of ICP monitors, because the observation of high ICP went untreated for a mean period of about 20 hours, in marked contrast with most US and European TBI studies.[94]

As heterogeneity increases, the sample size needed to demonstrate a clinical effect, it is now generally believed that the great majority of trials in TBI have been grossly underpowered. Indeed, Dickinson and colleagues[95] demonstrated that out of 203 human TBI trials none was large enough to reliably detect a 5% absolute reduction in the risk of death or disability, and only 8 were large enough to detect an absolute reduction of 10%. Especially problematic is that statistical power depends on every patient in a study having the potential to have their outcome changed by an intervention. When a simple "good/bad" outcome dichotomy is used, many patients studied in TBI trials are incapable of changing their outcome because they are either too well or too injured to be influenced by a therapeutic, because none have the "magic bullet" effect sizes seen with antibiotics, for example. This has led contemporary studies to explore more sensitive statistical approaches to analyze clinical trials (see below). The CRASH megatrial used the alternate approach of accruing an extremely large sample size (approximately 20,000) in a very simple trial design, to compensate for heterogeneity[80,89] however, this approach is very resource intensive.

Questionable Research Findings

There is growing concern that many published scientific findings are not readily reproducible.[96] There are many potential explanations for this such as differences in experimental skill or technique, type I error, and biased experimentation or data interpretation. Some of the most high-profile journals now heavily scrutinize submissions to minimize problems with falsified or biased data, but the necessary resources are not widely available. To help safeguard against such problems and to increase the chances of an agent being successful in humans, verification of positive findings in a second independent laboratory has been recommended.[91] The stroke field has developed the Stroke Therapy Academic Industry Roundtable (STAIR) criteria, which set a very rigorous set of standards that must be met before an attempt at human translation (**Box 1**).[97] The TBI field has instituted the Operation Brain Trauma Treatment (OBTT) preclinical studies, funded by the Department of Defense, to address this issue.[98]

RECENT PROGRESS
Lessons from the International Mission on Prognosis and Clinical Trial Design

The International Mission on Prognosis and Clinical Trial Design (IMPACT) sought to explore the reasons behind the failure of translational research in the TBI field and made a number of additional important contributions.[99,100] IMPACT was an international initiative that saw the merger of individual patient data from 8 randomized TBI trials and 3 prospective observational studies for a total of nearly 10,000 patients.[84,101] In its second phase, the IMPACT database was further expanded to 44,073 patients by incorporating data from the CRASH trial and other databases.

IMPACT's first achievement was to advance significantly our understanding of TBI prognostication based on variables that can be measured early after presentation to the hospital. The *Journal of*

Box 1
Criteria to be met before initiating clinical trials in acute stroke (Stroke Therapy Academic Industry Roundtable Committee)

- Preclinical results should be independently replicated in at least 2 laboratories.
- Studies should be carried out in a blinded, randomized fashion.
- Studies should be conducted on male as well as female animals.
- Behavioral studies should be performed for an extended period after insult.
- It is reasonable to explore drugs that show promise in rats, subsequently in primate models.
- The route of administration should be carefully considered as many putative treatments might not easily cross the blood–brain barrier.
- Careful toxicologic studies in several species, including both intact animals and animals with experimental insult are indicated.
- Careful dose–response studies are necessary.
- The time window of opportunity for treatment is an important variable in preclinical models.

Adapted from Stroke Therapy Academic Industry Roundtable (STAIR). Recommendations for standards regarding preclinical neuroprotective and restorative drug development 1999;30(12):2752–8.

Neurotrauma published this work as a supplemental issue in 2007. The prognostic value of demographic information,[102] such as the GCS and pupil reactivity,[103] injury mechanism,[104] secondary insults,[105] admission blood pressure,[106] CT imaging characteristics,[106] and admission laboratory values[106] were included. They found that worse outcome correlated most strongly with age, GCS motor score, pupil response, and CT characteristics, including the Marshall CT classification and traumatic subarachnoid hemorrhage.[107] Other important prognostic factors included hypotension, hypoxia, the eye and verbal components of the GCS, glucose, platelets, and hemoglobin. The authors used multivariate analyses and came up with 3 prognostic models, which are accessible online at www.tbi-impact. org. These prognostic models have been repeatedly validated and explain from 75% to 83% of the observed variance in patient outcomes.[108–115]

Importantly, these publications demonstrated that there are no true prognostic thresholds. One of the most influential thresholds in the field had been one published in the Brain Trauma Foundation's (BTF) Prognosis Guidelines. Age over 65 was reported to be associated with worse outcome.[116] As a result, many neurosurgeons would routinely recommend palliative approaches in patients older than 65. The IMPACT publications instead show complex continuous relationships between studies variables and outcome without any clear thresholds.

Statistical modelling completed with the IMPACT database led to important recommendations regarding means of increasing trial efficiency and statistical power. Their findings demonstrated that broad inclusion criteria with subsequent covariate adjustment for prespecified variables reduces sample size requirements by 25% or more and speeds trial recruitment.[91,117] An additional benefit is improved generalizability of the results.[91]

IMPACT also advanced the notion of a "sliding dichotomy" and proportional odds modelling as being superior to the traditional approach of dichotomization of the GOS into good and bad outcomes. Statistical power calculations assume that every patient's a priori risk of unfavorable outcome is approximately 50%. The reality is that many patients are incapable of converting from a bad to a good outcome because they are either too seriously or too mildly injured. Indeed, approximately one-third of patients in the IMPACT database had an extreme prognosis (ie, prognostic risk estimate of more than 80% or <20% for unfavorable outcome). In the sliding dichotomy model each patient is compared with his or her predicted outcome.[91] In other words, the sliding dichotomy seeks to detect 'better than expected outcome' based on a robust prediction model. The IMPACT study also concluded that proportional odds statistical analysis is superior to the dichotomized analysis.[91] The proportional odds model considers every way that an ordinal scale can be dichotomized and thus takes into account changes across the whole spectrum of the GOS. The proportional odds model assumes that the treatment effect is the same across the breadth of the outcome measure; however, it is a robust approach even when the assumption is violated.[91] IMPACT found that the proportional odds model consistently performed a bit better than the sliding dichotomy and that the combination of covariate adjustment and proportional odds model analysis led to a remarkable 40% increase in statistical power.[91]

IMPACT has also facilitated several other advances. It has informed the importance of center effects relevant to the conduct of multicenter clinical trials. Clinical trials have demonstrated important differences in outcome between centers that are greater than what can be accounted for by differences in patient characteristics.[118] This has helped to support the notion of comparative effectiveness research. Indeed, the NIH currently views this approach as a cost-effective alternative to randomized controlled trials and is encouraging studies of this nature. The IMPACT study also facilitates the measurement of quality of health care delivery. Hospitals have traditionally used gross measures of mortality for quality control, which is suboptimal in the TBI population, where vegetative or very severely disabled survival is arguably worse than death.[91] The IMPACT database now allows hospitals to judge the quality of care they provide by comparing the observed with the expected outcome for each patient they treat. This approach should serve to reduce confounds inherent to population differences between hospitals. Comparing actual patient outcomes with those predicted by the IMPACT model is now advocated by the American College of Surgeons.[119]

In combining the datasets that comprise the IMPACT database, the investigators recognized substantive differences in how variables were being defined and scored. Overcoming this was perhaps the greatest success of IMPACT and it led to an effort to standardize the definition and collection of variables in TBI studies. The result is the NIH-supported "common data-elements"[83,91] (also described at www.tbi-impact.org). This important effort will increase the comparability of trials in the future, and will additionally make pooling of patient data more facile.

The lessons learned from the IMPACT study have very important implications for future TBI research. In particular, they have offered new hope to a field looking to move forward on the heels of numerous failed trials. Perhaps most interesting is the possibility that the component historical trials of the IMPACT study might be reanalyzed with the more powerful statistical methods recommended by the authors. The discovery that a potentially beneficial therapy that was previously overlooked could be a major advance for the TBI field.

Role of Clinical Practice and "Evidence-Based" Guidelines in Traumatic Brain Injury

Another key advance for the TBI field has been the development of guidelines. Although relatively little high-quality evidence exists to guide management decisions relevant to severe TBI, the TBI field, led by the BTF, has been one of the first fields of medicine to produce high quality guidelines that have been widely used. Also noteworthy are the number of guidelines which the BTF has produced. Three editions of the "Guidelines for the Management of Severe TBI" have been published,[25,120,121] and a fourth edition is anticipated soon. Two editions each of the "Guidelines for the Pre-Hospital Management of Severe TBI"[122,123] and "Guidelines for the Acute Medical Management of Severe TBI in Infants, Children and Adolescents" have been published.[124,125] A single edition of each of the "Surgical Guidelines for the Management of Severe TBI,"[126] "Guidelines for the Field Management of Combat-Related Head Trauma,"[127] and "Early Indicators of Prognosis in Severe TBI"[128] have been published. Guidelines for the management of penetrating TBI have also been published independent of the BTF[129]; a recent attempt to revise these guidelines found insufficient new data to justify an update.

The TBI guidelines have been widely adopted in at least 16 countries and have been widely translated and modified for local conditions in countries like China, Colombia, and Estonia. Numerous publications suggest that using these guidelines improves outcome and reduces health care costs.[130–132] The recommendations contained within these documents are not meant to be indiscriminately applied to all patients, but instead serve as a starting point for individualizing and "benchmarking" care. This is particularly important to consider in an era of increasingly personalized medicine. Many experts in the field would now contend that the overall approach to a patient changes based on, for instance, autoregulatory status. The BTF guidelines are thus an excellent resource, but must be uniquely adapted to each patient to provide optimal care.

Recently, 2 new sources of guidance for the management of TBI have appeared. The Neurocritical Care Society has begun producing guidelines.[133] Unfortunately these differ from the BTFs guidelines in some important ways; for instance, they recommend a brain oxygen treatment threshold on 20 mm Hg instead of the 15 mm Hg threshold currently recommended by the BTF.[134] The American College of Surgeons recently produced a practical set of consensus statements on the management of TBI patients, which incorporates all the recommendations of the neurosurgically driven BTF guidelines, but included important teaching principles on the use of the GCS, resuscitation, and integration of TBI care within care of the injured patient in general.[119]

Definition and Classification

It was recently felt necessary to convene a group of experts to redefine TBI[135] in light of new advances in concussion research and awareness that even mild concussion—when cumulative—may be harmful to the brain. In 2010, the Demographics and Clinical Assessment Working Group of the International and Interagency Initiative toward Common Data Elements for Research on Traumatic Brain Injury and Psychological Health defined TBI as "an alteration in brain function, or other evidence of brain pathology, caused by an external force" where the alteration in brain function consists of any period of loss of, or a decreased level of consciousness, any anterograde or retrograde amnesia, neurologic deficits or any alteration in mental state at the time of the injury.[135] Blast injury, mild TBI, confounding effects of intoxication, and delayed presentation of symptoms were recognized as challenges to a simple definition. An agreed-upon definition of TBI is, of course, an important first step in clinical research efforts and particularly in efforts to subclassify TBI.

There are additional ongoing efforts to develop a more sensible classification system for TBI than one based merely on severity.[136] The extreme complexity of the brain and the multitude of ways in which it can be injured are substantial impediments to such a classification scheme. A consensus conference was convened in 2007 to address this important challenge, with the goal being to develop a classification system that would provide a rational approach for targeted TBI therapies.[92,136] A better classification system is a goal of a major international effort currently underway (TRACK-TBI and CENTER-TBI).

Concussion or Mild Traumatic Brain Injury

Recently, there has been increased recognition of the significance of mild traumatic brain injury and concussion. Repetitive impacts have also been recognized as deleterious and the term chronic traumatic encephalopathy has become widely known by physicians and the lay public alike.[137] Recent years have seen numerous reports of professional players with a history of physical play reporting debility in later life and several suicides have been reported. There have been high-profile settlements and increased attention to preventing and treating concussion in both professional and amateur athletes. Fortunately, there has been a substantial increase in research related to concussion, which after all is the most common form of brain injury. Moreover, we have learned that outcomes from mild TBI and concussion are worse than had been thought.[138] TBI has been associated with an increased rate of dementia and a recent study has clarified that the pathologic changes in the brain are similar to those seen in Alzheimer's disease, but distinct in their distribution.[139] Persistently elevated levels of inflammatory indicators have been noted long after TBI and this has been postulated to link the injury to the progressive neurologic decline; however, this theory remains to be proven.[140] Progress is badly needed in this realm of TBI, because much remains to be learned about the science and clinical care of these injuries.[141,142] Indeed, a recent effort to generate concussion guidelines found insufficient evidence available.[143] This aspect is more fully covered in another article in this issue.

RECENT PITFALLS AND CHALLENGES

Two recent high-profile TBI clinical trials might be considered setbacks for the field. Decompressive craniectomy has been used clinically to treat the worst severe TBI patients—usually with high ICP—for decades. Two prospective randomized trials were established recently in an effort to definitively determine the role for this procedure. The Early Decompressive Craniectomy in Patients With Severe Traumatic Brain Injury (DECRA) trial was recently completed and published.[144] The 155 patients enrolled in DECRA had diffuse brain swelling and ICP elevation to values of less than 20 mm Hg for more than 15 minutes within a 1-hour period that were refractory to first tier therapies. The patients were randomized to bifrontal decompressive craniectomy or an initial period of further medical management. The results demonstrated that those undergoing early decompression had worse outcomes at 6 months after injury as measured by the Extended GOS (GOS-E). A baseline imbalance in preoperative pupillary reactivity was felt by some to account for this finding and indeed after multivariate adjustment the associated P value suggesting harm increased just above the .05 threshold for significance. It is our opinion that DECRA was a well-conducted study with valid findings; however, the unique nature of the inclusion criteria and frontal decompressive surgery limit the extent to which these findings can be extrapolated. Most TBI experts continue to perform decompressive craniectomies, although some are slower to perform these as a result of DECRA's findings. The Randomised Evaluation of Surgery with Craniectomy for Uncontrollable Elevation of ICP (RESCUEicp) trial is a second prospective randomized study that recently completed enrollment. This trial investigates a more common population of patients with abnormal CT imaging, to include contusions and unilateral swelling. The results of this trial are eagerly awaited.

A second recently published high-profile trial was a randomized controlled trial of ICP monitoring, the BEST-TRIP trial.[94] This study was performed in Latin America because it was felt ICP monitoring was already the standard of care in North America. This trial randomized 324 patients to ICP-directed therapy or intensive management based on physical examination and imaging. The study found a trend to improved outcomes in those who underwent ICP monitoring 2 weeks after injury, but was negative overall. It demonstrated that ICP-directed management was associated with fewer days in intensive care, but patients in this group did experience more decubitus ulcers. Of importance, in the ICP-monitored group the period of increased ICP was far in excess of that reported in any other trials. An editorial accompanying the report of the BEST-TRIP trial concluded that "stupor, coma, posturing, and dilatation of the pupils indicate compression of the midbrain, and according to this study they are very suitable observations to use in directing treatment."[145]

Most TBI experts would strongly disagree, including the lead author of the trial report. Most continue to feel that ICP monitoring is an essential component of the care of most severe TBI patients. Indeed, one must know the ICP to know the cerebral perfusion pressure. Stronger evidence supports cerebral perfusion pressure–directed therapy than that which supports ICP-directed therapy.[146,147]

Although TBI experts argue that neither of these trials should lead to substantial changes in practice, there is no question that they have at least partly undermined the role of the neurosurgeon in the care of TBI patients as decompressive craniectomy and ICP monitor placement have been 2 of the most important interventions that neurosurgeons have offered TBI patients. These studies have furthered the need for introspection in the field and serve to challenge and inspire a new generation of TBI researchers to question every tenet of the TBI field.

FUTURE DIRECTIONS

Over the last 5 years, US congressional mandates and Department of Defense funding together with NIH-funded major initiatives such as TRACK-TBI have provided more opportunities for TBI research than ever before. With a strong need for more data across the breadth of the field, the only research limitations relate to motivation, manpower, and resources. Many important new efforts are underway that offer hope for the future. Indeed, annual funding for translational TBI research is now approximately $70 million from the NIH.[4]

Big Data

Advances in computing and analytical approaches are making the analysis of very large datasets increasingly commonplace. Such large datasets are being built in dementia/Alzheimer's disease, military medicine (the Millenium cohort study) and many other areas of medicine. They are believed to be particularly helpful in the neurotrauma field, because they have the potential to overcome important challenges such as patient heterogeneity. The CRASH[148] and IMPACT[84] databases were perhaps the first examples of "big data" in the TBI field and indeed both have made extremely important contributions. There is thus hope that such additional studies may yield findings of similar importance.

Even a busy neurotrauma center will accrue approximately 50 severe TBI patients per year.[149] It is thus impossible for a single center to accrue enough patients for a meaningful study within a reasonable period of time, and they certainly cannot generate "big data."

TRACK-TBI and CENTER-TBI are sister studies ongoing in North America and Europe, respectively, that promise to generate "big data" in the future. These trials were conceived after the establishment of the International Initiative for Traumatic Brain Injury in 2011 by the European Commission, the Canadian Institutes of Health Research, and the NIH. The goal of this organization has been to generate big data through a broad international collaboration in hopes of succeeding where smaller studies have failed. These studies will work together to gather a large volume of demographic, imaging, genetic, and proteomic information from TBI patients similar, but much greater in scale than the now historic Traumatic Coma Database. An improved classification scheme and a precision medicine approach to TBI will hopefully be just 2 important advances to come from this work. Hopefully, other clinical trial networks of the past such as the American and European Brain Injury Consortia will continue to function and support advancement of the TBI field through clinical trials.

New Therapeutic Frontiers

There remains great optimism that advances in molecular biology will innovate the care of TBI patients. Progress is being made in the search for biomarkers of TBI. Experimental therapeutics continue to be investigated in varied preclinical

models of central nervous system insult. It should be remembered that a novel agent demonstrating benefit in stroke or spinal cord injury may also have usefulness in TBI. Experimental small molecule therapeutics can be broadly classified as neuroprotective, those effecting neural repair or regeneration, and those that improve function in residual tissue or organ—"disease modification" in the jargon of big pharma.

A biomarker, or perhaps a series of biomarkers,[150] would ideally detect brain injury in patients with minor TBI that might otherwise be missed[151] and provide prognostic information that might assist in resource planning across the spectrum of severity. Such a marker would ideally be measurable in the blood,[152] although measurements in CSF obtained from an external ventricular drain would also be acceptable, albeit only of usefulness in severe TBI. The ideal TBI biomarker has yet to be defined much less discovered and validated, but promising leads are being studied.[153] Attention so far has focused on proteins known to be specific to neurons and glia such as glial fibrillary acidic protein[150,154] found in astrocytes and neuron specific enolase[155] found in neurons. Promising data also exist for spectrin breakdown products,[156] which are a product of calpain degradation, as discussed. No biomarker to date has demonstrated sufficient usefulness for "FDA-approved" human application, although S100B is in universal clinical use in Scandinavian countries to select mild TBI patients for serial CT scanning and in-hospital observation.[157] Interest has also been shown in use of novel MRI sequences, such as fluid-attenuated inversion recovery, to diagnose diffuse axonal injury, in particular, with better sensitivity.

Drug Studies

Although there continue to be many studies exploring small molecules in preclinical studies of acute TBI, there are relatively few ongoing human studies involving small molecules. The CRASH-3 trial is exploring a putative role of the procoagulant tranexamic acid in TBI (NCT01402882). It builds on a phase II study that found a decrease in death owing to hemorrhage, especially when administered early after TBI.[158] According to the trial website, more than 4000 patients have been enrolled in the study so far. Other agents currently being studied are human growth hormone (NCT00957671), minocycline (NCT01058395), CsA (NCT01825044), lactate (NCT01573507), nerve growth factor (NCT01212679), and NNZ-2566 (an antiinflammatory, NCT00805818).

A larger group of studies are exploring management strategies for acute TBI patients.

Hypothermia continues to be an area of interest. A new study (HypOthermia for Patients requiring Evacuation of Subdural Hematoma [HOPES]) will examine a novel cooling regimen in a population restricted to those with acute subdural hematomas (NCT02064959). Focal brain cooling is also being increasingly explored.[159,160] Brain oxygen monitoring was recently subject to a phase II randomized controlled study (NCT00974259) and a phase III is being initiated. Hyperbaric oxygen is also an active area of study (NCT02407028, NCT00594503, NCT01847755).

Cell Therapies

Cellular transplantation strategies have generated tremendous interest among patients, scientists, and clinicians alike. Many different cellular substrates have been investigated in preclinical studies of neurotrauma, including neural precursor cells, bone marrow stromal cells, Schwann cells, olfactory ensheathing cells, and autologous activated macrophages.[161] For almost all of these, the mesenchymal origin cells have been delivered intravenously, with the huge limitations that less than 5% of cells pass though the "lung filter" and almost none actually remain in the brain. Most authorities also agree that mesenchymal origin cells cannot differentiate into neurons, so they are assumed to function rather in a trophic "helper cell" role. Several human clinical trials of cellular transplantation strategies are currently ongoing for patients with spinal cord injury. To our knowledge, only 2 such human trials are currently ongoing in victims of TBI. Both involve bone marrow stromal cell transplantation. One is being conducted in India (NCT02028104), and the other is a pediatric trial being performed in Texas (NCT01851083). Nevertheless, direct intraparenchymal stereotactic injection of fetal origin stem cells has been performed in human stroke (China) and has yielded many tantalizing results in laboratory studies. If efficacy for such procedures can be shown, these procedures may dramatically expand the role of neurosurgery in the future, and allow us to bring regenerative therapies to the most severely affected TBI patients.

Recent work in the spinal cord injury field has sought to objectively grade the strength of preclinical research and to identify priorities for human translation.[162] The TBI field has made a similar effort. Establishing research priorities in TBI was the goal of the Conemaugh International Brain Injury Symposium[163] as well as an NIH consensus conference.[164] Work that seeks to advance the recommendations that have stemmed from these conferences should be viewed as a top priority for researchers and for funding agencies.

New Methodology

It will be imperative for new trials to heed the lessons garnered from failures of the past and from the IMPACT and TRACK-TBI studies. New trials must use new methodologies more likely to demonstrate the benefit of a truly efficacious therapy. Preclinical screening must be more rigorous to exclude profit-driven, biased studies, and must demand multiple verifications of results before clinical trial planning. As discussed, cost-effective alternatives to randomized controlled trials such as comparative effectiveness research are likely to be increasingly important in the future.

Combination of Agents

Given the numerous molecular processes that cause secondary injury, it is possible that single agents targeting a single pathway will be insufficient to achieve neuroprotection. Indeed, a combinatorial approach similar to the one being successfully used in the treatment of HIV[83,165,166] may be needed. In 2008, a symposium was convened to address this issue.[83] This meeting discussed promising strategies, inherent methodologic challenges, and potential solutions to these challenges. The group felt that combination therapies should affect multiple targets, produce synergistic effects on a single target, increase distribution and half-life or decrease toxicity of other agents, target sequential stages of injury, or focus on either novel therapeutics or previously tested drugs in combinations.[83]

Fortunately, the FDA has formal regulations related to testing coadministered therapeutics. The experimental design will be extremely difficult, and will likely need to assess the contributions of each agent to the therapeutic effect and must demonstrate that the combination is better than with either alone.[83] It is important to consider that pharmacokinetics and pharmacodynamics of applied therapeutics may be altered when combined,[83] which mandates careful testing. Unfortunately, powering multiple pairwise comparisons requires a larger than normal sample size, which must be considered.[83]

Alternate Trial Designs

In addition to the comparative effectiveness studies already discussed, it is probable that new trial designs will be increasingly used in early phase studies. Traditional studies that are designed to detect the benefit of a therapeutic are termed superiority trials. In the future equivalence, noninferiority or futility trials may be used more often. In these studies, a lower threshold difference for success is set. In a futility trial, a treatment group is compared with a predetermined, clinically meaningful threshold instead of with a control group, in which the mean outcome may not be known with certainty.[83] Equivalence trials set out to demonstrate that 2 therapeutics differ in their effects by no more than a specific amount. Noninferiority trials instead aim to show that an experimental treatment is not worse than a control. Most medical device studies are run on this basis in the European Union and North America. A problem with these alternate designs is that a well-executed clinical trial that correctly demonstrates the treatments to be similar cannot be easily distinguished from a poorly executed trial that fails to find a true difference.[167] Such trials are, in our opinion, most likely to be used for studies of management strategies or novel devices as opposed to trials of putative neuroprotective agents. Given the difficulty in translating neuroprotective therapeutics to date, it is probable that superiority trials will continue to be mandated in the early phase trials of these agents as a suggestion of efficacy will likely be required to garner funding for expensive late-phase trials.

Outcome Measures

The development of more sensitive outcome measures must be an important part of future TBI research. The dichotomized GOS (death, vegetative state, or severe disability vs moderate disability or good recovery) is now generally accepted to be insensitive, as discussed elsewhere in this paper.[83,91,149] This is particularly true for subtle deficits in memory, executive function, and affect, which are the consequence of mild and moderate TBI and produce significant disability.[91,168] This problem is made worse by GOS misclassification,[169] which may reduce power and effect size.[169–171] Future studies must use surrogate endpoints such as imaging biomarkers or neuropsychological measures cautiously. For instance, ICP improvement is a common surrogate that does not necessarily correlate with improved outcome.[19,172]

The FDA has hitherto mandated that the primary outcome measure should be a functional outcome measure in drug trials. A surrogate outcome measure may not be used as the primary outcome in a drug trial until it has been validated against functional outcome measures. Quality of life has become an increasingly important outcome throughout medicine.[83] Outcome measures such as the Disability Rating Scale, the American Brain Injury Consortium Neuropsychological Test Battery, the Functional Independence Measure, the Delta Score, and the Health Utility Index[89] are a selection of contemporary measures that may be advantageous to use in the TBI population. Undoubtedly, future trials will combine multiple outcome measures as all have their inherent strengths and weaknesses. Indeed, composite outcome measures have been used in recent high-profile TBI studies.[38,94]

SUMMARY

It is clear that TBI research cannot repeat the mistakes of the past. Fortunately, the vast array of new mechanistic knowledge gained from the laboratory, the lessons of past trials, and massive injections of new research funding have produced a more opportunity filled environment for TBI research than ever before. It is hoped that young neurosurgeons will take their place in this progression, and that their new ideas will combine with the laboratory science to advance the TBI field and meaningfully improve outcomes for TBI patients. "Big data" approaches might be the needed solution to TBI heterogeneity and has already yielded important advances.[101,148] Finally, it is tantalizing to consider that we may have already overlooked a truly efficacious therapy. A reanalysis of completed TBI trials with more sensitive methodologies has been shown to be possible by IMPACT. This would seem to be an obvious starting point for the next generation of clinical TBI researchers to begin.

REFERENCES

1. Stein SC, Georgoff P, Meghan S, et al. Relationship of aggressive monitoring and treatment to improved outcomes in severe traumatic brain injury. J Neurosurg 2010;112:1105–12.
2. Tanasescu R, Ionete C, Chou IJ, et al. Advances in the treatment of relapsing-remitting multiple sclerosis. Biomed J 2014;37:41–9.
3. Maas AI, Roozenbeek B, Manley GT. Clinical trials in traumatic brain injury: past experience and current developments. Neurotherapeutics 2010;7:115–26.
4. Vink R, Bullock MR. Traumatic brain injury: therapeutic challenges and new directions. Neurotherapeutics 2010;7:1–2.
5. Georgoff P, Meghan S, Mirza K, et al. Geographic variation in outcomes from severe traumatic brain injury. World Neurosurg 2010;74:331–45.
6. Harvey LA, Close JC. Traumatic brain injury in older adults: characteristics, causes and consequences. Injury 2012;43:1821–6.

7. Finkelstein EA, Corso PS, Miller TR. The incidence and economic burden of injuries in the United States. New York: Oxford University Press; 2006.

8. Narayan RK, Michel ME, Ansell B, et al. Clinical trials in head injury. J Neurotrauma 2002;19:503–57.

9. Bullock R. Mortality rates of placebo groups in severe traumatic brain injury trials. Trauma Care 1997;7:16–7.

10. Teasdale G, Jennett B. Assessment of coma and impaired consciousness. A practical scale. Lancet 1974;2:81–4.

11. Jennett B, Teasdale G, Braakman R, et al. Predicting outcome in individual patients after severe head injury. Lancet 1976;1:1031–4.

12. Katayama Y, Becker DP, Tamura T, et al. Massive increases in extracellular potassium and the indiscriminate release of glutamate following concussive brain injury. J Neurosurg 1990;73:889–900.

13. Rimel RW, Giordani B, Barth JT, et al. Disability caused by minor head injury. Neurosurgery 1981;9:221–8.

14. Becker DP, Miller JD, Ward JD, et al. The outcome from severe head injury with early diagnosis and intensive management. J Neurosurg 1977;47:491–502.

15. Obrist WD, Langfitt TW, Jaggi JL, et al. Cerebral blood flow and metabolism in comatose patients with acute head injury. Relationship to intracranial hypertension. J Neurosurg 1984;61:241–53.

16. Jennett B, Bond M. Assessment of outcome after severe brain damage. Lancet 1975;1:480–4.

17. Chesnut RM, Marshall LF, Klauber MR, et al. The role of secondary brain injury in determining outcome from severe head injury. J Trauma 1993;34:216–22.

18. Marion DW, Penrod LE, Kelsey SF, et al. Treatment of traumatic brain injury with moderate hypothermia. N Engl J Med 1997;336:540–6.

19. Clifton GL, Miller ER, Choi SC, et al. Lack of effect of induction of hypothermia after acute brain injury. N Engl J Med 2001;344:556–63.

20. Levin HS, Mattis S, Ruff RM, et al. Neurobehavioral outcome following minor head injury: a three-center study. J Neurosurg 1987;66:234–43.

21. Adams JH, Graham DI, Murray LS, et al. Diffuse axonal injury due to nonmissile head injury in humans: an analysis of 45 cases. Ann Neurol 1982;12:557–63.

22. Rosner MJ, Rosner SD, Johnson AH. Cerebral perfusion pressure: management protocol and clinical results. J Neurosurg 1995;83:949–62.

23. Miller JD, Becker DP, Ward JD, et al. Significance of intracranial hypertension in severe head injury. J Neurosurg 1977;47:503–16.

24. Rappaport M, Hall KM, Hopkins K, et al. Disability rating scale for severe head trauma: coma to community. Arch Phys Med Rehabil 1982;63:118–23.

25. Bullock R, Chesnut RM, Clifton G, et al. Guidelines for the management of severe head injury. Brain Trauma Foundation. Eur J Emerg Med 1996;3:109–27.

26. Johnson VE, Stewart W, Smith DH. Axonal pathology in traumatic brain injury. Exp Neurol 2013;246:35–43.

27. Li XY, Feng DF. Diffuse axonal injury: novel insights into detection and treatment. J Clin Neurosci 2009;16:614–9.

28. Bullock R, Zauner A, Woodward JJ, et al. Factors affecting excitatory amino acid release following severe human head injury. J Neurosurg 1998;89:507–18.

29. Rothman SM, Olney JW. Glutamate and the pathophysiology of hypoxic–ischemic brain damage. Ann Neurol 1986;19:105–11.

30. Zauner A, Bullock R. The role of excitatory amino acids in severe brain trauma: opportunities for therapy: a review. J Neurotrauma 1995;12:547–54.

31. Lipton SA, Rosenberg PA. Excitatory amino acids as a final common pathway for neurologic disorders. N Engl J Med 1994;330:613–22.

32. Park E, Velumian AA, Fehlings MG. The role of excitotoxicity in secondary mechanisms of spinal cord injury: a review with an emphasis on the implications for white matter degeneration. J Neurotrauma 2004;21:754–74.

33. Tymianski M. Emerging mechanisms of disrupted cellular signaling in brain ischemia. Nat Neurosci 2011;14:1369–73.

34. Morris GF, Bullock R, Marshall SB, et al. Failure of the competitive N-methyl-D-aspartate antagonist Selfotel (CGS 19755) in the treatment of severe head injury: results of two phase III clinical trials. The Selfotel Investigators. J Neurosurg 1999;91:737–43.

35. Fawcett WJ, Haxby EJ, Male DA. Magnesium: physiology and pharmacology. Br J Anaesth 1999;83:302–20.

36. Muir JK, Raghupathi R, Emery DL, et al. Postinjury magnesium treatment attenuates traumatic brain injury-induced cortical induction of p53 mRNA in rats. Exp Neurol 1999;159:584–93.

37. Heath DL, Vink R. Magnesium sulphate improves neurologic outcome following severe closed head injury in rats. Neurosci Lett 1997;228:175–8.

38. Temkin NR, Anderson GD, Winn HR, et al. Magnesium sulfate for neuroprotection after traumatic brain injury: a randomised controlled trial. Lancet Neurol 2007;6:29–38.

39. Merchant RE, Bullock MR, Carmack CA, et al. A double-blind, placebo-controlled study of the safety, tolerability and pharmacokinetics of CP-101,606 in patients with a mild or moderate traumatic brain injury. Ann N Y Acad Sci 1999;890:42–50.

40. Reinert MM, Bullock R. Clinical trials in head injury. Neurol Res 1999;21:330–8.

41. Schanne FA, Kane AB, Young EE, et al. Calcium dependence of toxic cell death: a final common pathway. Science 1979;206:700–2.

42. Czogalla A, Sikorski AF. Spectrin and calpain: a 'target' and a 'sniper' in the pathology of neuronal cells. Cell Mol Life Sci 2005;62:1913–24.

43. Teasdale G, Bailey I, Bell A, et al. A randomized trial of nimodipine in severe head injury: HIT I. British/Finnish Co-operative Head Injury Trial Group. J Neurotrauma 1992;9(Suppl 2):S545–50.

44. A multicenter trial of the efficacy of nimodipine on outcome after severe head injury. The European Study Group on Nimodipine in Severe Head Injury. J Neurosurg 1994;80:797–804.

45. Murray GD, Teasdale GM, Schmitz H. Nimodipine in traumatic subarachnoid haemorrhage: a re-analysis of the HIT I and HIT II trials. Acta Neurochir (Wien) 1996;138:1163–7.

46. Harders A, Kakarieka A, Braakman R. Traumatic subarachnoid hemorrhage and its treatment with nimodipine. German tSAH Study Group. J Neurosurg 1996;85:82–9.

47. Graham DI. The pathology of brain ischaemia and possibilities for therapeutic intervention. Br J Anaesth 1985;57:3–17.

48. Ankarcrona M, Dypbukt JM, Bonfoco E, et al. Glutamate-induced neuronal death: a succession of necrosis or apoptosis depending on mitochondrial function. Neuron 1995;15:961–73.

49. Xiong Y, Gu Q, Peterson PL, et al. Mitochondrial dysfunction and calcium perturbation induced by traumatic brain injury. J Neurotrauma 1997; 14:23–34.

50. Clausen T, Zauner A, Levasseur JE, et al. Induced mitochondrial failure in the feline brain: implications for understanding acute post-traumatic metabolic events. Brain Res 2001;908:35–48.

51. Bullock R, Maxwell WL, Graham DI, et al. Glial swelling following human cerebral contusion: an ultrastructural study. J Neurol Neurosurg Psychiatr 1991;54:427–34.

52. Clausen T, Bullock R. Medical treatment and neuroprotection in traumatic brain injury. Curr Pharm Des 2001;7:1517–32.

53. Sullivan PG, Rabchevsky AG, Waldmeier PC, et al. Mitochondrial permeability transition in CNS trauma: cause or effect of neuronal cell death? J Neurosci Res 2005;79:231–9.

54. Lifshitz J, Sullivan PG, Hovda DA, et al. Mitochondrial damage and dysfunction in traumatic brain injury. Mitochondrion 2004;4:705–13.

55. Starkov AA, Chinopoulos C, Fiskum G. Mitochondrial calcium and oxidative stress as mediators of ischemic brain injury. Cell Calcium 2004;36: 257–64.

56. Gogarten W, Van Aken H, Moskopp D, et al. A case of severe cerebral trauma in a patient under chronic treatment with cyclosporine A. J Neurosurg Anesthesiol 1998;10:101–5.

57. Crompton M. The mitochondrial permeability transition pore and its role in cell death. Biochem J 1999;341(Pt 2):233–49.

58. Mazzeo AT, Beat A, Singh A, et al. The role of mitochondrial transition pore, and its modulation, in traumatic brain injury and delayed neurodegeneration after TBI. Exp Neurol 2009;218:363–70.

59. Okonkwo DO, Povlishock JT. An intrathecal bolus of cyclosporin A before injury preserves mitochondrial integrity and attenuates axonal disruption in traumatic brain injury. J Cereb Blood Flow Metab 1999;19:443–51.

60. Okonkwo DO, Melon DE, Pellicane AJ, et al. Dose-response of cyclosporin A in attenuating traumatic axonal injury in rat. Neuroreport 2003; 14:463–6.

61. Verweij BH, Muizelaar JP, Vinas FC, et al. Mitochondrial dysfunction after experimental and human brain injury and its possible reversal with a selective N-type calcium channel antagonist (SNX-111). Neurol Res 1997;19:334–9.

62. Buki A, Okonkwo DO, Povlishock JT. Postinjury cyclosporin A administration limits axonal damage and disconnection in traumatic brain injury. J Neurotrauma 1999;16:511–21.

63. Alessandri B, Rice AC, Levasseur J, et al. Cyclosporin A improves brain tissue oxygen consumption and learning/memory performance after lateral fluid percussion injury in rats. J Neurotrauma 2002;19:829–41.

64. Sullivan PG, Thompson MB, Scheff SW. Cyclosporin A attenuates acute mitochondrial dysfunction following traumatic brain injury. Exp Neurol 1999;160:226–34.

65. Sullivan PG, Thompson M, Scheff SW. Continuous infusion of cyclosporin A postinjury significantly ameliorates cortical damage following traumatic brain injury. Exp Neurol 2000;161:631–7.

66. Mazzeo AT, Brophy GM, Gilman CB, et al. Safety and tolerability of cyclosporin a in severe traumatic brain injury patients: results from a prospective randomized trial. J Neurotrauma 2009; 26:2195–206.

67. McEwen ML, Sullivan PG, Springer JE. Pretreatment with the cyclosporin derivative, NIM811, improves the function of synaptic mitochondria following spinal cord contusion in rats. J Neurotrauma 2007;24:613–24.

68. Xiong Y, Rabchevsky AG, Hall ED. Role of peroxynitrite in secondary oxidative damage after spinal cord injury. J Neurochem 2007;100:639–49.

69. Hillard VH, Peng H, Zhang Y, et al. Tempol, a nitroxide antioxidant, improves locomotor and

histological outcomes after spinal cord contusion in rats. J Neurotrauma 2004;21:1405–14.

70. Scott GS, Cuzzocrea S, Genovese T, et al. Uric acid protects against secondary damage after spinal cord injury. Proc Natl Acad Sci U S A 2005;102:3483–8.

71. Fehlings MG. Summary statement: the use of methylprednisolone in acute spinal cord injury. Spine (Phila Pa 1976) 2001;26:S55.

72. Kwon BK, Tetzlaff W, Grauer JN, et al. Pathophysiology and pharmacologic treatment of acute spinal cord injury. Spine J 2004;4:451–64.

73. Muizelaar JP, Marmarou A, Young HF, et al. Improving the outcome of severe head injury with the oxygen radical scavenger polyethylene glycol-conjugated superoxide dismutase: a phase II trial. J Neurosurg 1993;78:375–82.

74. Young B, Runge JW, Waxman KS, et al. Effects of pegorgotein on neurologic outcome of patients with severe head injury. A multicenter, randomized controlled trial. JAMA 1996;276:538–43.

75. Marshall LF, Maas AI, Marshall SB, et al. A multicenter trial on the efficacy of using tirilazad mesylate in cases of head injury. J Neurosurg 1998;89:519–25.

76. Rak R, Chao DL, Pluta RM, et al. Neuroprotection by the stable nitroxide Tempol during reperfusion in a rat model of transient focal ischemia. J Neurosurg 2000;92:646–51.

77. Donnelly DJ, Popovich PG. Inflammation and its role in neuroprotection, axonal regeneration and functional recovery after spinal cord injury. Exp Neurol 2008;209:378–88.

78. Fleming JC, Norenberg MD, Ramsay DA, et al. The cellular inflammatory response in human spinal cords after injury. Brain 2006;129:3249–69.

79. Popovich PG, Wei P, Stokes BT. Cellular inflammatory response after spinal cord injury in Sprague-Dawley and Lewis rats. J Comp Neurol 1997;377:443–64.

80. Ghajar J, Hesdorffer DC. Steroids CRASH out of head-injury treatment. Lancet Neurol 2004;3:708.

81. Bratton SL, Chestnut RM, Ghajar J, et al. Guidelines for the management of severe traumatic brain injury. XV. Steroids. J Neurotrauma 2007;24(Suppl 1):S91–5.

82. Marmarou A, Nichols J, Burgess J, et al. Effects of the bradykinin antagonist Bradycor (deltibant, CP-1027) in severe traumatic brain injury: results of a multi-center, randomized, placebo-controlled trial. American Brain Injury Consortium Study Group. J Neurotrauma 1999;16:431–44.

83. Margulies S, Hicks R. Combination therapies for traumatic brain injury: prospective considerations. J Neurotrauma 2009;26:925–39.

84. Maas AI, Marmarou A, Murray GD, et al. Prognosis and clinical trial design in traumatic brain injury: the IMPACT study. J Neurotrauma 2007;24:232–8.

85. Wright DW, Yeatts SD, Silbergleit R, et al, NETT Investigators. Very early administration of progesterone for acute traumatic brain injury. N Engl J Med 2014;371:2457–66.

86. O'Collins VE, Macleod MR, Donnan GA, et al. 1,026 experimental treatments in acute stroke. Ann Neurol 2006;59:467–77.

87. Doppenberg EM, Choi SC, Bullock R. Clinical trials in traumatic brain injury: lessons for the future. J Neurosurg Anesthesiol 2004;16:87–94.

88. Povlishock JT, Hayes RL, Michel ME, et al. Workshop on animal models of traumatic brain injury. J Neurotrauma 1994;11:723–32.

89. Tolias CM, Bullock MR. Critical appraisal of neuroprotection trials in head injury: what have we learned? NeuroRx 2004;1:71–9.

90. Smith DH, Nonaka M, Miller R, et al. Immediate coma following inertial brain injury dependent on axonal damage in the brainstem. J Neurosurg 2000;93:315–22.

91. Maas AI, Steyerberg EW, Marmarou A, et al. IMPACT recommendations for improving the design and analysis of clinical trials in moderate to severe traumatic brain injury. Neurotherapeutics 2010;7:127–34.

92. Saatman KE, Duhaime AC, Bullock R, et al. Classification of traumatic brain injury for targeted therapies. J Neurotrauma 2008;25:719–38.

93. Faden AI. Neuroprotection and traumatic brain injury: the search continues. Arch Neurol 2001;58:1553–5.

94. Chesnut RM, Temkin N, Carney N, et al, Global Neurotrauma Research Group. A trial of intracranial-pressure monitoring in traumatic brain injury. N Engl J Med 2012;367:2471–81.

95. Dickinson K, Bunn F, Wentz R, et al. Size and quality of randomised controlled trials in head injury: review of published studies. BMJ 2000;320:1308–11.

96. Laine C, Goodman SN, Griswold ME, et al. Reproducible research: moving toward research the public can really trust. Ann Intern Med 2007;146:450–3.

97. Stroke Therapy Academic Industry Roundtable (STAIR). Recommendations for standards regarding preclinical neuroprotective and restorative drug development. Stroke 1999;30:2752–8.

98. Kochanek PM, Bramlett HM, Dixon CE, et al. Operation brain trauma therapy: approach to modeling, therapy evaluation, drug selection, and biomarker assessments for a Multicenter Pre-Clinical Drug Screening Consortium for acute therapies in severe traumatic brain injury. J Neurotrauma 2015;33(6):513–22.

99. Roozenbeek B, Maas AI, Lingsma HF, et al. Baseline characteristics and statistical power in randomized controlled trials: selection, prognostic

targeting, or covariate adjustment? Crit Care Med 2009;37:2683–90.

100. Maas AI, Murray GD, Roozenbeek B, et al, International Mission on Prognosis Analysis of Clinical Trials in Traumatic Brain Injury (IMPACT) Study Group. Advancing care for traumatic brain injury: findings from the IMPACT studies and perspectives on future research. Lancet Neurol 2013;12: 1200–10.

101. Marmarou A, Lu J, Butcher I, et al. IMPACT database of traumatic brain injury: design and description. J Neurotrauma 2007;24:239–50.

102. Mushkudiani NA, Engel DC, Steyerberg EW, et al. Prognostic value of demographic characteristics in traumatic brain injury: results from the IMPACT study. J Neurotrauma 2007;24:259–69.

103. Marmarou A, Lu J, Butcher I, et al. Prognostic value of the Glasgow Coma Scale and pupil reactivity in traumatic brain injury assessed pre-hospital and on enrollment: an IMPACT analysis. J Neurotrauma 2007;24:270–80.

104. Butcher I, McHugh GS, Lu J, et al. Prognostic value of cause of injury in traumatic brain injury: results from the IMPACT study. J Neurotrauma 2007;24: 281–6.

105. McHugh GS, Engel DC, Butcher I, et al. Prognostic value of secondary insults in traumatic brain injury: results from the IMPACT study. J Neurotrauma 2007;24:287–93.

106. Butcher I, Maas AI, Lu J, et al. Prognostic value of admission blood pressure in traumatic brain injury: results from the IMPACT study. J Neurotrauma 2007;24:294–302.

107. Murray GD, Butcher I, McHugh GS, et al. Multivariable prognostic analysis in traumatic brain injury: results from the IMPACT study. J Neurotrauma 2007;24:329–37.

108. Wong GK, Teoh J, Yeung J, et al. Outcomes of traumatic brain injury in Hong Kong: validation with the TRISS, CRASH, and IMPACT models. J Clin Neurosci 2013;20:1693–6.

109. Maas AI, Lingsma HF, Roozenbeek B. Predicting outcome after traumatic brain injury. Handb Clin Neurol 2015;128:455–74.

110. Raj R, Siironen J, Kivisaari R, et al. External validation of the international mission for prognosis and analysis of clinical trials model and the role of markers of coagulation. Neurosurgery 2013;73: 305–11 [discussion: 311].

111. Lingsma H, Andriessen TM, Haitsema I, et al. Prognosis in moderate and severe traumatic brain injury: external validation of the IMPACT models and the role of extracranial injuries. J Trauma Acute Care Surg 2013;74:639–46.

112. Roozenbeek B, Lingsma HF, Lecky FE, et al, International Mission on Prognosis Analysis of Clinical Trials in Traumatic Brain Injury (IMPACT) Study Group, Corticosteroid Randomisation After Significant Head Injury (CRASH) Trial Collaborators, Trauma Audit and Research Network (TARN). Prediction of outcome after moderate and severe traumatic brain injury: external validation of the International Mission on Prognosis and Analysis of Clinical Trials (IMPACT) and Corticoid Randomisation After Significant Head injury (CRASH) prognostic models. Crit Care Med 2012;40:1609–17.

113. Roozenbeek B, Chiu YL, Lingsma HF, et al. Predicting 14-day mortality after severe traumatic brain injury: application of the IMPACT models in the Brain Trauma Foundation TBI-trac(R) New York State database. J Neurotrauma 2012;29:1306–12.

114. Panczykowski DM, Puccio AM, Scruggs BJ, et al. Prospective independent validation of IMPACT modeling as a prognostic tool in severe traumatic brain injury. J Neurotrauma 2012;29:47–52.

115. Yeoman P, Pattani H, Silcocks P, et al. Validation of the IMPACT outcome prediction score using the Nottingham Head Injury Register dataset. J Trauma 2011;71:387–92.

116. The Brain Trauma Foundation. The American Association of Neurological Surgeons. The Joint Section on Neurotrauma and Critical Care. Age. J Neurotrauma 2000;17(6–7):573–81.

117. Machado SG, Murray GD, Teasdale GM. Evaluation of designs for clinical trials of neuroprotective agents in head injury. European Brain Injury Consortium. J Neurotrauma 1999;16:1131–8.

118. Gelpke GJ, Braakman R, Habbema JD, et al. Comparison of outcome in two series of patients with severe head injuries. J Neurosurg 1983;59:745–50.

119. American College of Surgeons. Best practices in the management of traumatic brain injury. Chicago: American College of Surgeons; 2015.

120. Brain Trauma Foundation, American Association of Neurological Surgeons, Congress of Neurological Surgeons, et al. Guidelines for the management of severe traumatic brain injury. Methods. J Neurotrauma 2007;24(Suppl 1):S3–6.

121. The Brain Trauma Foundation. The American Association of Neurological Surgeons. The Joint Section on Neurotrauma and Critical Care. Initial management. J Neurotrauma 2000;17:463–9.

122. Badjatia N, Carney N, Crocco TJ, et al, Brain Trauma Foundation, BTF Center for Guidelines Management. Guidelines for prehospital management of traumatic brain injury 2nd edition. Prehosp Emerg Care 2008;12(Suppl 1):S1–52.

123. Gabriel EJ, Ghajar J, Jagoda A, et al. Guidelines for prehospital management of traumatic brain injury. J Neurotrauma 2002;19:111–74.

124. Kochanek PM, Carney N, Adelson PD, et al, American Academy of Pediatrics-Section on Neurological Surgery, American Association of Neurological Surgeons/Congress of Neurological

Surgeons, Child Neurology Society, European Society of Pediatric and Neonatal Intensive Care, Neurocritical Care Society, Pediatric Neurocritical Care Research Group, Society of Critical Care Medicine, Paediatric Intensive Care Society UK, Society for Neuroscience in Anesthesiology and Critical Care, World Federation of Pediatric Intensive and Critical Care Societies. Guidelines for the acute medical management of severe traumatic brain injury in infants, children, and adolescents–second edition. Pediatr Crit Care Med 2012;13(Suppl 1):S1–82.

125. Adelson PD, Bratton SL, Carney NA, et al, American Association for Surgery of Trauma, Child Neurology Society, International Society for Pediatric Neurosurgery, International Trauma Anesthesia and Critical Care Society, Society of Critical Care Medicine, World Federation of Pediatric Intensive and Critical Care Societies. Guidelines for the acute medical management of severe traumatic brain injury in infants, children, and adolescents. Chapter 1: Introduction. Pediatr Crit Care Med 2003;4:S2–4.

126. Bullock MR, Povlishock JT. Guidelines for the management of severe traumatic brain injury. Editor's Commentary. J Neurotrauma 2007;24(Suppl 1):2. p preceding S1.

127. Brain Trauma Foundation. Guidelines for the field management of combat related head trauma. New York: Brain Trauma Foundation; 2005.

128. The Brain Trauma Foundation. The American Association of Neurological Surgeons. The Joint Section on Neurotrauma and Critical Care. Methodology. J Neurotrauma 2000;17:561–2.

129. Part 1: Guidelines for the management of penetrating brain injury. Introduction and methodology. J Trauma 2001;51:S3–6.

130. Palmer S, Bader MK, Qureshi A, et al. The impact on outcomes in a community hospital setting of using the AANS traumatic brain injury guidelines. Americans Associations for Neurologic Surgeons. J Trauma 2001;50:657–64.

131. Talving P, Karamanos E, Teixeira PG, et al. Intracranial pressure monitoring in severe head injury: compliance with Brain Trauma Foundation guidelines and effect on outcomes: a prospective study. J Neurosurg 2013;119:1248–54.

132. Faul M, Wald MM, Rutland-Brown W, et al. Using a cost-benefit analysis to estimate outcomes of a clinical treatment guideline: testing the Brain Trauma Foundation guidelines for the treatment of severe traumatic brain injury. J Trauma 2007;63:1271–8.

133. Committee, N.G. NCS Guidelines. 2015. Available at: http://www.neurocriticalcare.org/education-training/ncs-guidelines.

134. Bratton SL, Chestnut RM, Ghajar J, et al. Guidelines for the management of severe traumatic brain injury. X. Brain oxygen monitoring and thresholds. J Neurotrauma 2007;24(Suppl 1):S65–70.

135. Menon DK, Schwab K, Wright DW, et al, Demographics and Clinical Assessment Working Group of the International and Interagency Initiative toward Common Data Elements for Research on Traumatic Brain Injury and Psychological Health. Position statement: definition of traumatic brain injury. Arch Phys Med Rehabil 2010;91:1637–40.

136. Hawryluk GW, Manley GT. Classification of traumatic brain injury: past, present, and future. Handb Clin Neurol 2015;127:15–21.

137. Stein TD, Alvarez VE, McKee AC. Chronic traumatic encephalopathy: a spectrum of neuropathological changes following repetitive brain trauma in athletes and military personnel. Alzheimers Res Ther 2014;6:4.

138. Levin HS, Diaz-Arrastia RR. Diagnosis, prognosis, and clinical management of mild traumatic brain injury. Lancet Neurol 2015;14:506–17.

139. Shively S, Scher AI, Perl DP, et al. Dementia resulting from traumatic brain injury: what is the pathology? Arch Neurol 2012;69:1245–51.

140. Giunta B, Obregon D, Velisetty R, et al. The immunology of traumatic brain injury: a prime target for Alzheimer's disease prevention. J Neuroinflammation 2012;9:185.

141. Craton N, Leslie O. Time to re-think the Zurich Guidelines? A critique on the consensus statement on concussion in sport: the 4th International Conference on Concussion in Sport, held in Zurich, November 2012. Clin J Sport Med 2014;24:93–5.

142. McCrory P, Meeuwisse WH, Aubry M, et al. Consensus statement on concussion in sport: the 4th International Conference on Concussion in Sport, Zurich, November 2012. J Athl Train 2013;48:554–75.

143. Carney N, Ghajar J, Jagoda A, et al. Concussion guidelines step 1: systematic review of prevalent indicators. Neurosurgery 2014;75(Suppl 1):S3–15.

144. Cooper DJ, Rosenfeld JV, Murray L, et al, DECRA Trial Investigators, Australian and New Zealand Intensive Care Society Clinical Trials Group. Decompressive craniectomy in diffuse traumatic brain injury. N Engl J Med 2011;364:1493–502.

145. Ropper AH. Brain in a box. N Engl J Med 2012;367:2539–41.

146. Mehta A, Kochanek PM, Tyler-Kabara E, et al. Relationship of intracranial pressure and cerebral perfusion pressure with outcome in young children after severe traumatic brain injury. Dev Neurosci 2010;32:413–9.

147. Young JS, Blow O, Turrentine F, et al. Is there an upper limit of intracranial pressure in patients with severe head injury if cerebral perfusion pressure is maintained? Neurosurg Focus 2003;15:E2.

148. Edwards P, Arango M, Balica L, et al. Final results of MRC CRASH, a randomised placebo-controlled trial of intravenous corticosteroid in adults with head injury-outcomes at 6 months. Lancet 2005;365: 1957–9.

149. Choi SC, Bullock R. Design and statistical issues in multicenter trials of severe head injury. Neurol Res 2001;23:190–2.

150. Diaz-Arrastia R, Wang KK, Papa L, et al. Acute biomarkers of traumatic brain injury: relationship between plasma levels of ubiquitin C-terminal hydrolase-L1 and glial fibrillary acidic protein. J Neurotrauma 2014;31:19–25.

151. Mondello S, Schmid K, Berger RP, et al. The challenge of mild traumatic brain injury: role of biochemical markers in diagnosis of brain damage. Med Res Rev 2014;34:503–31.

152. Neher MD, Keene CN, Rich MC, et al. Serum biomarkers for traumatic brain injury. South Med J 2014;107:248–55.

153. Zetterberg H, Blennow K. Fluid markers of traumatic brain injury. Mol Cell Neurosci 2015;66: 99–102.

154. Okonkwo DO, Yue JK, Puccio AM, et al, Transforming Research and Clinical Knowledge in Traumatic Brain Injury (TRACK-TBI) Investigators. GFAP-BDP as an acute diagnostic marker in traumatic brain injury: results from the prospective transforming research and clinical knowledge in traumatic brain injury study. J Neurotrauma 2013;30:1490–7.

155. Cheng F, Yuan Q, Yang J, et al. The prognostic value of serum neuron-specific enolase in traumatic brain injury: systematic review and meta-analysis. PLoS one 2014;9:e106680.

156. Yokobori S, Hosein K, Burks S, et al. Biomarkers for the clinical differential diagnosis in traumatic brain injury–a systematic review. CNS Neurosci Ther 2013;19:556–65.

157. Daoud H, Alharfi I, Alhelali I, et al. Brain injury biomarkers as outcome predictors in pediatric severe traumatic brain injury. Neurocrit Care 2014; 20:427–35.

158. CRASH-2 Collaborators, Intracranial Bleeding Study. Effect of tranexamic acid in traumatic brain injury: a nested randomised, placebo controlled trial (CRASH-2 Intracranial Bleeding Study). BMJ 2011;343:d3795.

159. Liu WG, Qiu WS, Zhang Y, et al. Effects of selective brain cooling in patients with severe traumatic brain injury: a preliminary study. J Int Med Res 2006;34:58–64.

160. Qiu W, Shen H, Zhang Y, et al. Noninvasive selective brain cooling by head and neck cooling is protective in severe traumatic brain injury. J Clin Neurosci 2006;13:995–1000.

161. Hawryluk GW, Rowland J, Kwon BK, et al. Protection and repair of the injured spinal cord: a review of completed, ongoing, and planned clinical trials for acute spinal cord injury. Neurosurg Focus 2008;25:E14.

162. Kwon BK, Okon EB, Tsai E, et al. A grading system to evaluate objectively the strength of pre-clinical data of acute neuroprotective therapies for clinical translation in spinal cord injury. J Neurotrauma 2011;28:1525–43.

163. Zitnay GA, Zitnay KM, Povlishock JT, et al. Traumatic brain injury research priorities: the Conemaugh International Brain Injury Symposium. J Neurotrauma 2008;25:1135–52.

164. D'Onofrio G, Jauch E, Jagoda A, et al. NIH Roundtable on Opportunities to Advance Research on neurologic and psychiatric emergencies. Ann Emerg Med 2010;56:551–64.

165. Harrington M, Carpenter CC. Hit HIV-1 hard, but only when necessary. Lancet 2000;355:2147–52.

166. May MT, Sterne JA, Costagliola D, et al. HIV treatment response and prognosis in Europe and North America in the first decade of highly active antiretroviral therapy: a collaborative analysis. Lancet 2006;368:451–8.

167. Snapinn SM. Noninferiority trials. Curr Control Trials Cardiovasc Med 2000;1:19–21.

168. McCauley SR, Levin HS, Vanier M, et al. The neurobehavioural rating scale-revised: sensitivity and validity in closed head injury assessment. J Neurol Neurosurg Psychiatr 2001;71:643–51.

169. Choi SC, Clifton GL, Marmarou A, et al. Misclassification and treatment effect on primary outcome measures in clinical trials of severe neurotrauma. J Neurotrauma 2002,19:17–22.

170. Lu J, Murray GD, Steyerberg EW, et al. Effects of Glasgow Outcome Scale misclassification on traumatic brain injury clinical trials. J Neurotrauma 2008;25:641–51.

171. Wilson JT, Slieker FJ, Legrand V, et al. Observer variation in the assessment of outcome in traumatic brain injury: experience from a multicenter, international randomized clinical trial. Neurosurgery 2007; 61:123–8 [discussion: 128–9].

172. Struchen MA, Hannay HJ, Contant CF, et al. The relation between acute physiological variables and outcome on the Glasgow Outcome Scale and Disability Rating Scale following severe traumatic brain injury. J Neurotrauma 2001;18: 115–25.

173. Muizelaar JP, Marmarou A, Ward JD, et al. Adverse effects of prolonged hyperventilation in patients with severe head injury: a randomized clinical trial. J Neurosurg 1991;75:731–9.

174. Bailey I, Bell A, Gray J, et al. A trial of the effect of nimodipine on outcome after head injury. Acta Neurochir (Wien) 1991;110:97–105.

175. Braakman R, Schouten HJ, Blaauw-van Dishoeck M, et al. Megadose steroids in severe

head injury. Results of a prospective double-blind clinical trial. J Neurosurg 1983;58:326–30.

176. Dearden NM, Gibson JS, McDowall DG, et al. Effect of high-dose dexamethasone on outcome from severe head injury. J Neurosurg 1986;64: 81–8.

177. Wolf AL, Levi L, Marmarou A, et al. Effect of THAM upon outcome in severe head injury: a randomized prospective clinical trial. J Neurosurg 1993;78:54–9.

178. Gaab MR, Trost HA, Alcantara A, et al. "Ultrahigh" dexamethasone in acute brain injury. Results from a prospective randomized double-blind multicenter trial (GUDHIS). German Ultrahigh Dexamethasone Head Injury Study Group. Zentralbl Neurochir 1994;55:135–43.

179. Grumme T, Baethmann A, Kolodziejczyk D. Treatment of patients with severe head injury by triamconolone: a prospective, controlled multicenter clinical trial of 396 cases. Res Exp Med (Berl) 1995;195:217–29.

180. Yurkewicz L, Weaver J, Bullock MR, et al. The effect of the selective NMDA receptor antagonist traxoprodil in the treatment of traumatic brain injury. J Neurotrauma 2005;22:1428–43.

181. Clifton GL, Choi SC, Miller ER, et al. Intercenter variance in clinical trials of head trauma–experience of the National Acute Brain Injury Study: Hypothermia. J Neurosurg 2001;95:751–5.

182. Zhi D, Zhang S, Lin X. Study on therapeutic mechanism and clinical effect of mild hypothermia in patients with severe head injury. Surg Neurol 2003;59: 381–5.

183. Jiang JY, Xu W, Li WP, et al. Effect of long-term mild hypothermia or short-term mild hypothermia on outcome of patients with severe traumatic brain injury. J Cereb Blood Flow Metab 2006;26:771–6.

184. Rockswold GL, Ford SE, Anderson DC, et al. Results of a prospective randomized trial for treatment of severely brain-injured patients with hyperbaric oxygen. J Neurosurg 1992;76:929–34.

185. Robertson CS, Valadka AB, Hannay HJ, et al. Prevention of secondary ischemic insults after severe head injury. Crit Care Med 1999;27:2086–95.

186. Lu LQ, Jiang JY, Yu MK, et al. Standard large trauma craniotomy for severe traumatic brain injury. Chin J Traumatol 2003;6:302–4.

187. Cooper DJ, Myles PS, McDermott FT, et al. Prehospital hypertonic saline resuscitation of patients with hypotension and severe traumatic brain injury: a randomized controlled trial. JAMA 2004;291: 1350–7.

188. Jiang JY, Xu W, Li WP, et al. Efficacy of standard trauma craniectomy for refractory intracranial hypertension with severe traumatic brain injury: a multicenter, prospective, randomized controlled study. J Neurotrauma 2005;22:623–8.

189. Maas AI, Murray G, Henney H 3rd, et al. Efficacy and safety of dexanabinol in severe traumatic brain injury: results of a phase III randomised, placebo-controlled, clinical trial. Lancet Neurol 2006;5:38–45.

190. Xiao G, Wei J, Yan W, et al. Improved outcomes from the administration of progesterone for patients with acute severe traumatic brain injury: a randomized controlled trial. Crit Care 2008;12:R61.

Pathophysiology of Traumatic Brain Injury

Melissa J. McGinn, PhD, John T. Povlishock, PhD*

KEYWORDS

- Focal and diffuse damage • Diffuse axonal injury • Neuronal circuit disruption
- Altered neuronal and vascular responses • Influence of comorbid factors

KEY POINTS

- Traumatic brain injury (TBI) remains one of the most complex diseases in the most complex of all organs in the body.
- The causes of TBI are many and varied and include penetrating and nonpenetrating injuries that, based on their overall level of severity, can evoke different degrees of morbidity, typically framed within the context of the Glasgow Coma Scale (GCS) score.
- In considering the pathobiology of TBI across the spectrum of the disease ranging from mild through severe, it is common to discuss this disease within the context of focal versus diffuse change, with the inference that these events typically occur in isolation, with each following a unique footprint of pathophysiologic change.

Traumatic brain injury (TBI) remains one of the most complex diseases known in the most complex of all organs in the body. The causes of TBI are many and varied and include penetrating and nonpenetrating injuries that, based on their overall level of severity, can evoke different degrees of morbidity, typically framed within the context of the Glasgow Coma Scale (GCS) score.[1] Although imperfect, the GCS helps, together with other biologic factors, to frame the degree of injury evoked by the traumatic event, thereby providing information of diagnostic and prognostic value. Although historically it was assumed that all patients with a similar GCS had sustained comparable forms of central nervous system (CNS) injury, more recent studies and consensus conferences have illustrated the inaccuracy of such assumptions, explaining in part why overreliance of the GCS has confounded many clinical studies and related trials.[2] In light of this, more recent studies have focused on patient pathoanatomic features to allow for more meaningful comparisons between patients groups.[2] In considering the pathobiology of TBI across the spectrum of the disease ranging from mild through severe, it is common to discuss this disease within the context of focal versus diffuse change, with the inference that these events typically occur in isolation, with each following a unique footprint of pathophysiologic change. Although this premise is overly simplistic and dismisses that most severe and moderate forms of injury involve combinations of focal and diffuse injury, this categorization does help frame key concepts regarding brain injury.[3] Accordingly, its usage is maintained in the current text. Additionally, for simplification this consideration of pathobiology of injury is confined to nonpenetrating TBIs.

FOCAL TRAUMATIC BRAIN INJURY

Focal injuries are consistent features of most forms of severe and moderate injury following change within the intra-axial and extra-axial

The authors declare that they have no conflict of interest.
Department of Anatomy and Neurobiology, Medical College of Virginia Campus of Virginia Commonwealth University, 1101 East Marshall Street, Room 12-048, Richmond, VA 23298-0709, USA
* Corresponding author.
E-mail address: john.povlishock@vcuhealth.org

neurosurgery.theclinics.com

compartments. Subdural and epidural hematomas are the result of mechanical deformation and different forms of vascular disruption that can exert morbidity by ensuing brain compression, with recent literature suggesting that subdural hematomas can also exert damaging local responses related to focal ischemia, reperfusion injury, vasogenic edema, and reduced cerebral blood flow.[4] Contusional changes most commonly involve the frontal and temporal lobes, although other loci can be involved via the generation of coup, directly beneath the site of impact, versus countercoup, directly opposite the site of impact, lesions. Contusions are typically hemorrhagic lesions that began within the cortex and are most common at the crests of the cerebral gyri, and advance into the subcortical white matter in the more severe forms of injury. Despite this primary cortical predilection, in some cases contusions can develop at the grey/white interface with subsequent expansion into the overlying grey matter. The presence of hemorrhage within the contusion gives rise to local edema and ischemic change, which leads to tissue destruction, neuronal necrosis, and ultimately cavitation with surrounding reactive gliosis. In some cases, continued hemorrhagic progression or expansion of the contusion in the pericontusional zones has been observed.

Although historically this hemorrhagic progression was postulated to occur secondary to coagulopathy, other contemporary studies suggest that other causative factors are at work. Recently, Kurland and colleagues[5] have shown that the cerebral vasculature is mechanosensitive, with the likelihood that mechanosensitive endothelial cells are activated in the penumbra, which does not experience the destructive forces occurring within the contusional core itself. In this scenario, the contusional penumbra experiences endothelial mechanosensitive activation of two transcription factors, specificity protein 1 and nuclear factor-B.[5] These factors play a key role in the regulation of sulfonylurea receptor 1, which forms the regulatory subunit of the NC_{Ca-ATP} channel. This subunit has been implicated in vascular dysfunction and/or damage, leading to endothelial necrosis.[5]

Irrespective of the contusion's origin and expansion, the morbidity associated with these collective contusional changes is a direct function of their location, size, depth, and potential for bilateral brain involvement. Thus, large bilateral lesions exert considerably more morbidity than seen in isolated lesions, which unless involving homologous cortical domains may exert little to no morbidity.[3] Because of their bloody constituents, focal lesions are readily identified with routine imaging, such as computed tomography, although recent biomarker discovery has shown the utility for blood biomarkers, such as glial fibrillary acidic protein, and its breakdown products in recognizing ultraearly, the presence of contusion even in injury of relatively minor severity.[6–8] The assumption is that the contusion also evokes glial cell damage and the subsequent release of glial fibrillary specific protein, which is detected in the systemic circulation. Although such biomarkers do not replace the need for routine imaging, they may be of ultimate value in prescreening patients sustaining milder forms of injury, which may require more advanced imaging to detect modest contusional damage that would negatively impact outcome.[9]

DIFFUSE TRAUMATIC BRAIN INJURY

By definition, diffuse injury is more scattered, and is not linked to a specific focus of destructive tissue damage. Rather, it shows a more widespread distribution wherein damaged structures are scattered among other intact/unaltered neuronal and vascular components. To date, in animals and humans, diffuse injuries have been shown to potentially involve diffuse neuronal damage, microvascular change, and axonal perturbation and disconnection.[10,11] The understanding of the pathogenesis of neuronal and microvascular change, however, is somewhat limited and focuses on the potential that the mechanical forces of injury elicit various forms of membrane change leading to ionic dysregulation and/or altered permeability that in turn evokes lethal and sublethal damage. In the context of diffuse and focal neuronal cell death, multiple cell death pathways have been identified[12]; however, their overall prevalence in the context of diffuse TBI and their overall implications for morbidity remain a matter of controversy.

In contrast to the incomplete appreciation clinicians have of the pathophysiology of diffuse neuronal and microvascular change, understanding of scattered axonal injury is much more complete and its implications for animal and patient morbidity are better understood. Since the groundbreaking work of Adams and others in the postmortem examination of brain-injured humans, it is now appreciated that scattered or diffuse axonal injury (DAI) is a consistent component of most forms of TBI and a key contributor to TBI-induced morbidity.[13,14] Although first described in the corpus callosum, subcortical white matter, fornix, and varied brainstem white matter systems, it is now well recognized that DAI may occur at numerous brain sites involving white and grey matter. Based on early pathologic analysis using silver salts, the occurrence of DAI was confirmed in humans by the finding of axonal spheroids, with the belief that the axons were immediately severed at the time of injury leading to retraction and expulsion of a ball of axoplasm.[13,15] More contemporary studies exploring these issues in animals and humans suggested that this is not the case. Rather, they demonstrated that the course of injury focally perturbed the axonal membrane leading to a cascade of calcium-mediated events that impair axonal transport resulting in progressive focal axonal swelling and disconnection.[16–20] With disconnection the distal, detached axonal projections then undergo target deafferentation and synaptic loss, together with generalized wallerian degeneration.[21,22] From this perspective, DAI is conceptualized as a disease of disconnection, which has led many to consider TBI as a disorder of diffuse circuit disruption, disrupting excitatory and inhibitory networks (discussed later).

Although traditionally, the identification of DAI has relied on postmortem examination to confirm the presence of axonal spheroids either through the use of silver salts or antibodies to amyloid precursor protein, the last decade has witnessed an explosive growth in the ability of advanced imaging techniques to identify this pathology. Specifically, use of MRI, incorporating diffusion-weighted imaging and/or susceptibility-weighted imaging has allowed clinicians to better appreciate the potential for the occurrence of DAI and its distribution in an injured brain.[9,23–25] Although these techniques have not been fully characterized and controversy persists regarding their overall ability to recognize specific features of DAI, they do represent important noninvasive diagnostic approaches.

Although the previous discussion suggests that all DAI is characterized by a progression of changes that ultimately lead to axonal swelling and disconnection, it is also important to note that other recent studies have shown that the forces of injury can also evoke damage to other axonal populations that show no evidence of swelling but rather, show evidence of cytoskeletal collapse and rapid destructive and degradative processes.[26] This finding suggests that reliance on markers of axonal swelling alone underestimates the overall burden of axonal injury. Furthermore, it was also initially assumed that these axonal events occurred exclusively in large tract myelinated axons; however, it is now well recognized that unmyelinated axons are preferentially vulnerable to the forces of injury and thus, may be more important players in the pathobiology and morbidity of injury.[27] Collectively, these findings illustrate the importance of DAI while also speaking to its heterogeneity and biologic complexity.

Of further interest, in the context of DAI, is that it can be identified in humans and animals across the spectrum of TBI, ranging from mild to severe. Although overall numbers and anatomic loci involved are reduced in the milder forms of injury, this does not imply that this axonal injury is innocuous and without biologic consequence. Rather, recent findings in animals and humans suggest that such limited injury in the grey and white matter can trigger an imbalance of the brain's excitatory and inhibitory networks thereby leading to dysfunction.[28–32] Thus, in a sense TBI is a disease of brain network/circuit dysfunction where increasing injury severity leads to increasing circuit disruption followed by increased morbidity.

FUNCTIONAL CHANGES EVOKED BY TRAUMATIC BRAIN INJURY

There is a growing appreciation that the pathobiologic response to injury is also characterized by widespread functional changes involving the intact cerebral microcirculation and intact neuronal circuitry. Although these functional changes have been best described in the milder forms of TBI, there is compelling evidence that suggests that they also occur with injuries of increased severity. On the vascular front, it is well recognized that more severe forms of head injury are associated with a loss of cerebrovascular autoregulation where cerebral blood flow becomes directly pressure passive dependent on the systemic blood pressure to elicit either hyperperfusion or hypoperfusion.[33,34] Importantly, these disturbances in autoregulation occur in the absence of overt structural damage in the cerebral conductance vessels and thus reflect a direct functional response to the traumatic episode.

In addition to these autoregulatory disturbances, other more subtle vascular changes can occur and these have been identified across the spectrum of injury ranging from mild through severe.[35,36] Multiple experimental and more limited clinical studies have confirmed that although intact, many arterioles and arteries exhibit impaired vasoreactivity to normal physiologic challenges involving endothelial-dependent and smooth muscle–dependent processes.[37–40] Such abnormal vascular responses to normal endothelial-dependent pathways and smooth muscle responsivity have been described in the acute phases postinjury and in the more chronic phases at which time substantial neurologic recovery occurs. The biologic implications of such impaired vascular reactivity are not well appreciated. However, it is postulated that these impaired responses could contribute to continued morbidity, should the injured brain sustain a posttraumatic, secondary insult involving hypotension, hypoxia, and/or other vascular response factors.

In addition to the recognition of widespread functional vascular change following TBI, there is now compelling evidence of a series of complex neuronal functional changes that impact posttraumatic neurologic function and subsequent recovery.[41,42] These changes seem to be more subtle and reversible in the milder forms of injury wherein little overt structural damage is observed within the brain parenchyma. Comparably, although more pronounced in the more severe forms of injury wherein overt structural damage is identified, these functional changes may also be significant players in the ensuing continued brain dysfunction/morbidity.

Although the understanding of the electrophysiologic responses of the brain to various forms of injury is in its infancy, there is now compelling evidence that the traumatic episode can, at multiple levels, trigger changes in excitation and inhibition involving glutaminergic and GABAergic function.[42] This elicits an imbalance of the normal excitation and inhibition needed to control brain function and support cognition.[32] In animal mild TBI, there is compelling evidence that many intact, undamaged neurons within the neocortex become hyperexcitable within days postinjury, contributing to brain dysfunction. Similarly, within the hippocampal domains, a large number of electrophysiologic studies using slice preparations have shown comparable posttraumatic changes in hippocampal circuits where, once again, TBI can affect excitatory and inhibitory synaptic transmission, giving rise to dysfunctional hippocampal circuits.[43]

Although there is some variance in the general physiologic findings across studies, with some showing posttraumatic decrease in excitability in the hippocampal area CA1, others have shown in in vivo preparations increased excitability, which may be a function of in vivo versus in vitro differences and other technical confounds.[44] Nevertheless, there is compelling evidence that these parameters do change over time postinjury. Collectively these data suggest that the imbalance of excitation and inhibition can contribute to disequilibrium with catastrophic consequences for CNS circuits that underlie cognitive function and other high level cortical activities.[42] Although most of these observations have been made with hippocampal slices and neocortical whole cell patch clamp analyses, other more direct physiologic assessments have also shown evidence of functional change, which directly relates to initial morbidity and potential recovery. Reeves and colleagues[27] have recently shown that following TBI,

there is a marked suppression of compound action potentials in the myelinated and unmyelinated fiber populations within the corpus callosum. Although in the animal model assessed there was evidence of limited structural change within the callosal myelinated and unmyelinated fiber populations, the overall degree of this damage did not significantly complicate data analysis. In these studies, Reeves and colleagues[27] showed in the early posttraumatic period a significant suppression of myelinated and unmyelinated fiber compound action potential generation. Over time postinjury, however, the compound action potentials showed a virtually complete recovery in the assumed nonaxotomized myelinated fiber population, whereas the unmyelinated fibers exhibited persistent and enduring compound action potential suppression.

Collectively, these findings reinforce the concept of electrophysiologic change following injury, showing in some cases there is significant recovery, whereas in others there is enduring change. How all of these findings relate to those events occurring in humans with TBI remains to be determined, yet their very occurrence and characterization suggests a complex series of functional changes involving neocortical, cortical, and intercortical circuitry that can contribute to a multilevel platform of circuit disruption.

EXCITOTOXICITY AND IONIC FLUX

Occurring in concert with and contributing to the evolution of the previously described focal and diffuse abnormalities is a host of generalized changes that serve to further perpetuate the progression of TBI pathophysiology. Such perturbations, which include widespread neuroexcitation, ionic flux, and neurometabolic change, among other sequelae, are diverse and as with all other features of TBI, are influenced by the nature and severity of the injury. Excessive excitatory amino acid signaling is recognized as a key factor in the cascade of pathophysiologic events that follow TBI. A rapid, transient increase in extracellular glutamate has been described within minutes following insult to the brain, the magnitude and duration of which have been shown to correlate to injury severity.[45–50] This acute increase in extracellular glutamate levels in the injured brain has been attributed to the excessive release of glutamate from presynaptic nerve terminals of depolarized neurons, leakage of glutamate from neuronal and glial (mainly astrocytic) cells exhibiting damaged/perturbed membranes, or the extravasation of glutamate through a disrupted blood-brain barrier (BBB).[51,52] Also contributing to heightened glutamate levels within the synaptic cleft are alterations in astrocytic glutamate reuptake mechanisms, either caused by the functional impairment of astrocytes (resulting from mechanical injury or energy depletion) or by the downregulation and/or decreased activity of astrocytic glutamate transporters (ie, GLAST, GLT-1).[53–55]

The acute interstitial glutamate surge, which has been observed in experimental and clinical TBI settings, triggers the unregulated and excessive stimulation of glutamate receptors (particularly N-methyl-D-aspartate receptors), leading to ionic dysregulation in the form of massive accumulations in extracellular [K+] and the influx of Na^+ and Ca^{2+} through glutamate receptor-gated ion channels.[45,56,57] Furthermore, the release of Ca^{2+} from intracellular stores (ie, endoplasmic reticulum) together with the activation of voltage gated calcium channels results in the additional accumulation of free intracellular Ca^{2+}. This ionic flux induces a state of metabolic crisis, ultimately approaching energy failure, as the brain attempts to restore ionic homeostasis via increased activity of ATP-dependent ion pumps (discussed later). The increased intracellular Ca^{2+} concentrations that result from excessive glutamate signaling also induce cellular damage through a variety of additional mechanisms, including (1) the activation of destructive calcium-dependent proteases (ie, calpains and caspases), (2) the generation of damaging reactive oxygen and nitrogen species, and (3) mitochondrial impairment (caused by Ca^{2+} overload) and mitochondrial permeability transition pore formation, leading to apoptotic events.[58–60] Such processes have been described in the context of the focal and diffuse somatic, axonal, and vascular changes described previously, operant at varying degrees along the spectrum from mild to severe TBI. For example, in the context of TBI-induced cell death, it is posited that more modest increases in cell intracellular free Ca^{2+} levels will drive the cellular machinery toward apoptosis, whereas excessive glutamate receptor activation with markedly enhanced Ca^{2+} levels promote necrotic events.

METABOLIC CHANGE

In concert with the previously described changes in excitotoxicity and ionic flux, metabolic change occurs following TBI of all severities; with regional, multifocal, and/or global abnormalities in metabolism likely occurring as a consequence of the injury-induced circuit disruption and network destabilization described previously. A crucial event that triggers some metabolic dysfunction is the increase in the release of excitatory amino acids, particularly glutamate, into the extracellular milieu following injury.[45,61–63] The ionic flux that results from the dramatic, yet brief rise in extracellular glutamate concentrations induces marked increases in cerebral glucose use (and consequent accumulation of extracellular lactate), presumably to promote the re-establishment of ionic homeostasis in the face of evolving neuropathologic change.[61,64] Following this brief period of hyperglycolysis in the acute phase (ie, first few days postinjury in humans), a global reduction in glycolysis occurs, persisting until recovery, which in humans can range from weeks to months postinjury.[65–69] The clinical course of recovery typically parallels the restoration of normal brain glucose use.

The ability to detect and monitor the ongoing metabolic changes associated with TBI has been made possible by PET, in vivo microdialysis (MD), and proton magnetic resonance spectroscopy (discussed elsewhere in this issue). MD monitoring of the brain interstitial fluid and PET functional imaging studies have revealed the hypermetabolic/hypometabolic temporal sequence described previously, characterized by acute increases in glucose metabolism (with a concomitant decline in extracellular glucose) localized predominantly within the contusion and pericontusional regions within the involved hemisphere, with more global, uniform declines in (glucose and oxygen) metabolism occurring at later time points postinjury.[65–68,70,71] A similar sequence and time course in the period of metabolic depression (approximately 2 to 4 weeks) is observed irrespective of injury severity, which has been speculated to relate either to the duration of posttraumatic confusion and posttraumatic amnesia in moderate to severe diffusely injured patients or to the less overt cognitive effects associated with a more mild diffuse injury.[3,72] Alternatively, differences in glucose compartmentalization in mild versus severe TBI may be a factor.

The declining levels of extracellular glucose that characterize the MD pattern seen during the acute hypermetabolic period following injury are often paralleled by elevations in microdialysate lactate levels, suggesting a shift to anaerobic glycolysis.[73,74] Elevated brain lactate levels gradually normalize after a few days in those who survive the traumatic episode, but remain heightened 5- to 10-fold over basal levels in fatal TBI.[75] Although studies have validated glucose metabolism–related microdialysate measurements against established indices of oxygen metabolism and cerebral blood flow (ie, jugular venous oxygen saturation, partial pressure of oxygen in brain tissue, or PET measurements) in severely injured patients with TBI exhibiting confirmed ischemic episodes, several recent MD studies have suggested that ischemia may be a less common phenomenon in TBI than previously assumed and that increased lactate/pyruvate ratios seen in patients with TBI may alternatively indicate either limited glucose supply or impairment of the glycolytic pathway machinery (ie, mitochondrial damage) as opposed to an overt lack of oxygen.[76–79] In patients with severe TBI, the previously described nonischemic excitotoxicity and metabolic crisis are associated with spreading depolarizations (cortical spreading depressions), which are pathologic waves of depolarization of neurons and astrocytes that propagate through the cerebral gray matter, suppressing synaptic activity as they do so.[80] Spreading depolarizations have been recently described following experimental and clinical TBI, where they are thought to contribute to ongoing ionic dysregulation and energy crisis, and have been linked to poor outcome.[81–83]

NEUROINFLAMMATION

Although traditionally considered a site of "immunologic privilege" because of the lack of a lymphatic system and the presence of a relatively impermeable BBB to activated immune/inflammatory cells, it is now recognized that the CNS does not constitute an immunoprivileged system but rather, that the brain exhibits the classic hallmarks of inflammation following TBI.[84] The inflammatory response of the brain to traumatic insult is multifactorial, encompassing the activation of resident CNS immune cells and the cerebral infiltration of peripheral immune cells (by way of an altered BBB), both of which mediate inflammatory processes through a variety inflammatory cytokines, chemokines, adhesion molecules, reactive oxygen and nitrogen species, and complement factors, among others. Occurring concurrently and as a consequence of these inflammatory events is the formation of cerebral edema, subsequent brain swelling, and increased intracranial pressure, all of which contribute to unfavorable outcome following TBI.

Although inflammatory events are evoked in response to focal and diffuse TBI, the sequelae of posttraumatic inflammation has predominately been characterized in the context of focal insult. The primary tissue damage (somatic and axonal) induced by mechanical insult to the brain triggers inflammation through the release of intracellular and intra-axonal contents, extravasated blood products, and increased free radical production/oxidative stress, among other factors.[85,86] In response to these perturbations in tissue homeostasis, the local activation of CNS microglia occurs.[87–89] In addition to the scavenging and phagocytosis of cellular debris, these resident immune surveillance cells also mediate inflammation through the production of various inflammatory cytokines, proteases, and reactive free radical species.[90–92] Over and above this acute microglial response to injury, several recent studies have shown that microglia can maintain a primed, or proinflammatory profile for weeks to months after the acute effects of injury have dissipated.[93] It is surmised that this primed and possibly hyperreactive microglial phenotype can potentially set the stage for more progressive degenerative change and chronic patient morbidity, along with an increased vulnerability to subsequent insult.

Concomitant with the local microglial inflammatory response is the cerebral infiltration and accumulation of peripheral immune cells via their extravasation across a BBB exhibiting increased permeability caused by mechanical disruption or vascular dilatation and leakage mediated by vasoactive inflammatory molecules.[94–97] The recruitment of peripheral immune cells to the injured brain is further promoted by vascular endothelial changes (ie, the cytokine-induced upregulation of adhesion molecules, such as intercellular adhesion molecule-1) and the release of chemokines by resident CNS cells.[98–100] The infiltrating peripheral immune cells most associated with TBI-induced inflammation include neutrophils and macrophages/monocytes, both of which have been shown to mediate early inflammatory events via the release of various inflammatory cytokines, proteases, free radicals, and other inflammatory mediators (leukotrienes and prostaglandins) in addition to phagocytosing cellular and/or axotomy-related debris. The sequence of events associated with the cerebral infiltration of peripheral immune cells in response to a focal/contusive TBI involves early neutrophilic recruitment within the first 24 hours postinjury followed by the delayed recruitment of macrophages between 36 and 48 hours postinjury.[94,101] The absence of an early neutrophilic infiltration in the diffusely injured brain is thought to be a reflection of the less overt tissue disruption and only mild/moderate BBB compromise associated with this form of brain injury.

Experimental and clinical TBI investigations have implicated numerous factors in the inflammatory response to TBI. Notably, alterations in regional, intrathecal, and systemic concentrations of several inflammatory cytokines (interleukin-1, -1β, -6, -8, -10, -12, and tumor necrosis factor) have been observed in the acute (and some cases chronic) posttraumatic period following human and experimental TBI.[102–107] These cytokines (and related chemokines) mediate inflammation by promoting excitotoxicity, recruiting peripheral immune cells, increasing cerebrovascular permeability (leading to edema formation), and by further propagating the inflammatory response through the continued activation of immune cells. Although most cytokines have traditionally been associated with neuroinflammatory damage, more recent findings suggest that certain factors may also serve neuroprotective and neurotrophic roles in the injured brain.[104,108,109] Depending on their concentrations and the timing/conditions of their expression following TBI, such factors as interleukin-6 and tumor necrosis factor may also serve beneficial roles in the injured brain, possibly setting the stage for and promoting regenerative and reparative processes. The mechanisms underlying this dichotomy are poorly understood; however, a greater understanding of the duality of the inflammatory response is crucial to the development of therapeutic interventions aimed at reducing inflammation-mediated damage in the injured brain without sacrificing the potential beneficial aspects of the inflammatory response to recovery.

COMORBID FACTORS

Notwithstanding the previously detailed characterization of the pathophysiologic responses to TBI, these biologic responses occur in individuals who possess biologic differences that can modify their response to injury. Age is a major factor, with the elderly typically having a worse outcome than comparably injured young adults.[110] Genetic differences can also influence outcome. Although in its infancy, multiple sets of studies have implicated genetic variations as confounding factors, with APOE4, BDNF, and adenosine kinase genetic variation individually contributing to differences in patient outcomes.[111–114] Lastly, as reported by the TRACK-TBI study group, other factors, including, but not limited to, a previous history of a psychiatric disorder, socioeconomic status, and drug and substance abuse, can adversely impact outcome.[110]

REFERENCES

1. Teasdale G, Maas A, Lecky F, et al. The Glasgow Coma Scale at 40 years: standing the test of time. Lancet Neurol 2014;13(8):844–54.
2. Saatman KE, Duhaime AC, Bullock R, et al. Classification of traumatic brain injury for targeted therapies. J Neurotrauma 2008;25(7):719–38.
3. Povlishock JT, Katz DI. Update of neuropathology and neurological recovery after traumatic brain injury. J Head Trauma Rehabil 2005;20(1):76–94.
4. Fujisawa H, Maxwell WL, Graham DI, et al. Focal microvascular occlusion after acute subdural haematoma in the rat: a mechanism for ischaemic damage and brain swelling? Acta Neurochir Suppl (Wien) 1994;60:193–6.
5. Kurland D, Hong C, Aarabi B, et al. Hemorrhagic progression of a contusion after traumatic brain injury: a review. J Neurotrauma 2012;29(1):19–31.
6. Mondello S, Jeromin A, Buki A, et al. Glial neuronal ratio: a novel index for differentiating injury type in patients with severe traumatic brain injury. J Neurotrauma 2012;29(6):1096–104.
7. Papa L, Lewis LM, Falk JL, et al. Elevated levels of serum glial fibrillary acidic protein breakdown products in mild and moderate traumatic brain injury are associated with intracranial lesions and neurosurgical intervention. Ann Emerg Med 2012; 59(6):471–83.
8. Wang KK, Yang Z, Yue JK, et al. Plasma anti-glial fibrillary acidic protein autoantibody levels during the acute and chronic phases of traumatic brain injury: a transforming research and clinical knowledge in traumatic brain injury pilot study. J Neurotrauma 2016;33:1270–7.
9. Yuh EL, Cooper SR, Mukherjee P, et al. Diffusion tensor imaging for outcome prediction in mild traumatic brain injury: a TRACK-TBI study. J Neurotrauma 2014;31(17):1457–77.
10. Farkas O, Lifshitz J, Povlishock JT. Mechanoporation induced by diffuse traumatic brain injury: an irreversible or reversible response to injury? J Neurosci 2006;26(12):3130–40.
11. Farkas O, Povlishock JT. Cellular and subcellular change evoked by diffuse traumatic brain injury: a complex web of change extending far beyond focal damage. Prog Brain Res 2007;161:43–59.
12. Stoica BA, Faden AI. Cell death mechanisms and modulation in traumatic brain injury. Neurotherapeutics 2010;7(1):3–12.
13. Adams JH, Doyle D, Ford I, et al. Diffuse axonal injury in head injury: definition, diagnosis and grading. Histopathology 1989;15:49–59.
14. Blumbergs PC, Scott G, Manavis J, et al. Topography of axonal injury as defined by amyloid precursor protein and the sector scoring method in mild and severe closed head injury. J Neurotrauma 1995;12(4):565–72.
15. Adams JH, Graham DI, Murray LS, et al. Diffuse axonal injury due to nonmissile head injury in humans: an analysis of 45 cases. Ann Neurol 1982; 12(6):557–63.
16. Povlishock JT, Becker DP, Cheng CL, et al. Axonal change in minor head injury. J Neuropathol Exp Neurol 1983;42(3):225–42.
17. Povlishock JT, Kontos HA. The role of oxygen radicals in the pathobiology of traumatic brain injury. Hum Cell 1992;5(4):345–53.

18. Buki A, Povlishock JT. All roads lead to disconnection? Traumatic axonal injury revisited. Acta Neurochir (Wien) 2006;148(2):181–93 [discussion: 193–4].

19. Smith DH, Hicks R, Povlishock JT. Therapy development for diffuse axonal injury. J Neurotrauma 2013;30(5):307–23.

20. Buki A, Siman R, Trojanowski JQ, et al. The role of calpain-mediated spectrin proteolysis in traumatically induced axonal injury. J Neuropathol Exp Neurol 1999;58(4):365–75.

21. Povlishock JT, Erb DE, Astruc J. Axonal response to traumatic brain injury: reactive axonal change, deafferentation, and neuroplasticity. J Neurotrauma 1992;9(Suppl 1):S189–200.

22. Wang J, Fox MA, Povlishock JT. Diffuse traumatic axonal injury in the optic nerve does not elicit retinal ganglion cell loss. J Neuropathol Exp Neurol 2013; 72(8):768–81.

23. Niogi SN, Mukherjee P, Ghajar J, et al. Extent of microstructural white matter injury in postconcussive syndrome correlates with impaired cognitive reaction time: a 3T diffusion tensor imaging study of mild traumatic brain injury. AJNR Am J Neuroradiol 2008;29(5):967–73.

24. Spitz G, Maller JJ, Ng A, et al. Detecting lesions following traumatic brain injury using susceptibility weighted imaging: a comparison with FLAIR, and correlation with clinical outcome. J Neurotrauma 2013;30(24):2038–50.

25. Benson RR, Gattu R, Sewick B, et al. Detection of hemorrhagic and axonal pathology in mild traumatic brain injury using advanced MRI: implications for neurorehabilitation. NeuroRehabilitation 2012;31(3):261–79.

26. Marmarou CR, Walker SA, Davis CL, et al. Quantitative analysis of the relationship between intra-axonal neurofilament compaction and impaired axonal transport following diffuse traumatic brain injury. J Neurotrauma 2005;22(10): 1066–80.

27. Reeves TM, Phillips LL, Povlishock JT. Myelinated and unmyelinated axons of the corpus callosum differ in vulnerability and functional recovery following traumatic brain injury. Exp Neurol 2005; 196(1):126–37.

28. Nakamura T, Hillary FG, Biswal BB. Resting network plasticity following brain injury. PLoS One 2009;4(12):e8220.

29. Kasahara M, Menon DK, Salmond CH, et al. Altered functional connectivity in the motor network after traumatic brain injury. Neurology 2010;75(2): 168–76.

30. Kasahara M, Menon DK, Salmond CH, et al. Traumatic brain injury alters the functional brain network mediating working memory. Brain Inj 2011;25(12): 1170–87.

31. McDonald BC, Saykin AJ, McAllister TW. Functional MRI of mild traumatic brain injury (mTBI): progress and perspectives from the first decade of studies. Brain Imaging Behav 2012; 6(2):193–207.

32. Sharp DJ, Scott G, Leech R. Network dysfunction after traumatic brain injury. Nat Rev Neurol 2014; 10(3):156–66.

33. Bouma GJ, Muizelaar JP. Cerebral blood flow, cerebral blood volume, and cerebrovascular reactivity after severe head injury. J Neurotrauma 1992;9(Suppl 1):S333–48.

34. Overgaard J, Tweed WA. Cerebral circulation after head injury. 1. Cerebral blood flow and its regulation after closed head injury with emphasis on clinical correlations. J Neurosurg 1974;41(5):531–41.

35. Obrist WD, Langfitt TW, Jaggi JL, et al. Cerebral blood flow and metabolism in comatose patients with acute head injury. Relationship to intracranial hypertension. J Neurosurg 1984;61(2):241–53.

36. Bouma GJ, Muizelaar JP. Relationship between cardiac output and cerebral blood flow in patients with intact and with impaired autoregulation. J Neurosurg 1990;73(3):368–74.

37. DeWitt DS, Prough DS. Traumatic cerebral vascular injury: the effects of concussive brain injury on the cerebral vasculature. J Neurotrauma 2003;20(9): 795–825.

38. Armstead WM. Role of endothelin in pial artery vasoconstriction and altered responses to vasopressin after brain injury. J Neurosurg 1996;85(5): 901–7.

39. Kontos HA. Regulation of the cerebral circulation. Annu Rev Physiol 1981;43:397–407.

40. Kontos HA, Wei EP. Endothelium-dependent responses after experimental brain injury. J Neurotrauma 1992; 9(4):349–54.

41. Smith CJ, Xiong G, Elkind JA, et al. Brain injury impairs working memory and prefrontal circuit function. Front Neurol 2015;6:240.

42. Cohen AS, Pfister BJ, Schwarzbach E, et al. Injury-induced alterations in CNS electrophysiology. Prog Brain Res 2007;161:143–69.

43. Reeves TM, Lyeth BG, Phillips LL, et al. The effects of traumatic brain injury on inhibition in the hippocampus and dentate gyrus. Brain Res 1997; 757(1):119–32.

44. Reeves TM, Lyeth BG, Povlishock JT. Long-term potentiation deficits and excitability changes following traumatic brain injury. Exp Brain Res 1995;106(2):248–56.

45. Katayama Y, Becker DP, Tamura T, et al. Massive increases in extracellular potassium and the indiscriminate release of glutamate following concussive brain injury. J Neurosurg 1990;73(6):889–900.

46. Koura SS, Doppenberg EM, Marmarou A, et al. Relationship between excitatory amino acid

release and outcome after severe human head injury. Acta Neurochir Suppl 1998;71:244–6.

47. Bullock R, Zauner A, Myseros JS, et al. Evidence for prolonged release of excitatory amino acids in severe human head trauma. relationship to clinical events. Ann N Y Acad Sci 1995;765:290–7.

48. Chamoun R, Suki D, Gopinath SP, et al. Role of extracellular glutamate measured by cerebral microdialysis in severe traumatic brain injury. J Neurosurg 2010;113(3):564–70.

49. Faden AI, Demediuk P, Panter SS, et al. The role of excitatory amino acids and NMDA receptors in traumatic brain injury. Science 1989;244(4906): 798–800.

50. Palmer AM, Marion DW, Botscheller ML, et al. Traumatic brain injury-induced excitotoxicity assessed in a controlled cortical impact model. J Neurochem 1993;61(6):2015–24.

51. Bullock R, Zauner A, Woodward JJ, et al. Factors affecting excitatory amino acid release following severe human head injury. J Neurosurg 1998; 89(4):507–18.

52. Yi JH, Hazell AS. Excitotoxic mechanisms and the role of astrocytic glutamate transporters in traumatic brain injury. Neurochem Int 2006; 48(5):394–403.

53. Yi JH, Pow DV, Hazell AS. Early loss of the glutamate transporter splice-variant GLT-1v in rat cerebral cortex following lateral fluid-percussion injury. Glia 2005;49(1):121–33.

54. Rao VL, Baskaya MK, Dogan A, et al. Traumatic brain injury down-regulates glial glutamate transporter (GLT-1 and GLAST) proteins in rat brain. J Neurochem 1998;70(5):2020–7.

55. Rao VL, Dogan A, Bowen KK, et al. Antisense knockdown of the glial glutamate transporter GLT-1 exacerbates hippocampal neuronal damage following traumatic injury to rat brain. Eur J Neurosci 2001;13(1):119–28.

56. Nilsson P, Hillered L, Olsson Y, et al. Regional changes in interstitial K+ and Ca2+ levels following cortical compression contusion trauma in rats. J Cereb Blood Flow Metab 1993;13(2): 183–92.

57. Reinert M, Khaldi A, Zauner A, et al. High level of extracellular potassium and its correlates after severe head injury: relationship to high intracranial pressure. J Neurosurg 2000;93(5):800–7.

58. Saatman KE, Creed J, Raghupathi R. Calpain as a therapeutic target in traumatic brain injury. Neurotherapeutics 2010;7(1):31–42.

59. Cheng G, Kong RH, Zhang LM, et al. Mitochondria in traumatic brain injury and mitochondrial-targeted multipotential therapeutic strategies. Br J Pharmacol 2012;167(4):699–719.

60. Weber JT. Altered calcium signaling following traumatic brain injury. Front Pharmacol 2012;3:60.

61. Kawamata T, Katayama Y, Hovda DA, et al. Administration of excitatory amino acid antagonists via microdialysis attenuates the increase in glucose utilization seen following concussive brain injury. J Cereb Blood Flow Metab 1992; 12(1):12–24.

62. Kawamata T, Katayama Y, Hovda DA, et al. Lactate accumulation following concussive brain injury: the role of ionic fluxes induced by excitatory amino acids. Brain Res 1995;674(2):196–204.

63. Alessandri B, Doppenberg E, Bullock R, et al. Glucose and lactate metabolism after severe human head injury: influence of excitatory neurotransmitters and injury type. Acta Neurochir Suppl 1999; 75:21–4.

64. Hovda DA, Yoshino A, Kawamata T, et al. The increase in local cerebral glucose utilization following fluid percussion brain injury is prevented with kynurenic acid and is associated with an increase in calcium. Acta Neurochir Suppl (Wien) 1990;51: 331–3.

65. Bergsneider M, Hovda DA, Shalmon E, et al. Cerebral hyperglycolysis following severe traumatic brain injury in humans: a positron emission tomography study. J Neurosurg 1997;86(2):241–51.

66. Bergsneider M, Hovda DA, Lee SM, et al. Dissociation of cerebral glucose metabolism and level of consciousness during the period of metabolic depression following human traumatic brain injury. J Neurotrauma 2000;17(5):389–401.

67. Bergsneider M, Hovda DA, McArthur DL, et al. Metabolic recovery following human traumatic brain injury based on FDG-PET: time course and relationship to neurological disability. J Head Trauma Rehabil 2001;16(2):135–48.

68. Wu HM, Huang SC, Hattori N, et al. Subcortical white matter metabolic changes remote from focal hemorrhagic lesions suggest diffuse injury after human traumatic brain injury. Neurosurgery 2004; 55(6):1306–15.

69. Yoshino A, Hovda DA, Kawamata T, et al. Dynamic changes in local cerebral glucose utilization following cerebral conclusion in rats: evidence of a hyper- and subsequent hypometabolic state. Brain Res 1991;561(1):106–19.

70. Vespa P, McArthur DL, Alger J, et al. Regional heterogeneity of post-traumatic brain metabolism as studied by microdialysis, magnetic resonance spectroscopy and positron emission tomography. Brain Pathol 2004;14(2):210–4.

71. O'Connell MT, Seal A, Nortje J, et al. Glucose metabolism in traumatic brain injury: a combined microdialysis and [18F]-2-fluoro-2-deoxy-D-glucose-positron emission tomography (FDG-PET) study. Acta Neurochir Suppl 2005;95:165–8.

72. Wu HM, Huang SC, Hattori N, et al. Selective metabolic reduction in gray matter acutely following

human traumatic brain injury. J Neurotrauma 2004; 21(2):149–61.

73. Sanchez JJ, Bidot CJ, O'Phelan K, et al. Neuromonitoring with microdialysis in severe traumatic brain injury patients. Acta Neurochir Suppl 2013;118: 223–7.

74. Goodman JC, Valadka AB, Gopinath SP, et al. Extracellular lactate and glucose alterations in the brain after head injury measured by microdialysis. Crit Care Med 1999;27(9):1965–73.

75. Verweij BH, Amelink GJ, Muizelaar JP. Current concepts of cerebral oxygen transport and energy metabolism after severe traumatic brain injury. Prog Brain Res 2007;161:111–24.

76. Vespa PM, McArthur D, O'Phelan K, et al. Persistently low extracellular glucose correlates with poor outcome 6 months after human traumatic brain injury despite a lack of increased lactate: a microdialysis study. J Cereb Blood Flow Metab 2003;23(7):865–77.

77. Vespa P, Bergsneider M, Hattori N, et al. Metabolic crisis without brain ischemia is common after traumatic brain injury: a combined microdialysis and positron emission tomography study. J Cereb Blood Flow Metab 2005;25(6):763–74.

78. Vespa PM, O'Phelan K, McArthur D, et al. Pericontusional brain tissue exhibits persistent elevation of lactate/pyruvate ratio independent of cerebral perfusion pressure. Crit Care Med 2007;35(4): 1153–60.

79. Verweij BH, Muizelaar JP, Vinas FC, et al. Impaired cerebral mitochondrial function after traumatic brain injury in humans. J Neurosurg 2000;93(5): 815–20.

80. Hinzman JM, Wilson JA, Mazzeo AT, et al. Excitotoxicity and metabolic crisis are associated with spreading depolarizations in severe traumatic brain injury patients. J Neurotrauma 2016. [Epub ahead of print].

81. Feuerstein D, Manning A, Hashemi P, et al. Dynamic metabolic response to multiple spreading depolarizations in patients with acute brain injury: an online microdialysis study. J Cereb Blood Flow Metab 2010;30(7):1343–55.

82. Hartings JA, Watanabe T, Bullock MR, et al. Spreading depolarizations have prolonged direct current shifts and are associated with poor outcome in brain trauma. Brain 2011;134(Pt 5): 1529–40.

83. Hinzman JM, DiNapoli VA, Mahoney EJ, et al. Spreading depolarizations mediate excitotoxicity in the development of acute cortical lesions. Exp Neurol 2015;267:243–53.

84. Louveau A, Smirnov I, Keyes TJ, et al. Structural and functional features of central nervous system lymphatic vessels. Nature 2015;523(7560): 337–41.

85. Rock KL, Kono H. The inflammatory response to cell death. Annu Rev Pathol 2008;3:99–126.

86. Mathew P, Graham DI, Bullock R, et al. Focal brain injury: histological evidence of delayed inflammatory response in a new rodent model of focal cortical injury. Acta Neurochir Suppl (Wien) 1994; 60:428–30.

87. Kreutzberg GW. Microglia: a sensor for pathological events in the CNS. Trends Neurosci 1996; 19(8):312–8.

88. Nimmerjahn A, Kirchhoff F, Helmchen F. Resting microglial cells are highly dynamic surveillants of brain parenchyma in vivo. Science 2005; 308(5726):1314–8.

89. Streit WJ. Microglial response to brain injury: a brief synopsis. Toxicol Pathol 2000;28(1):28–30.

90. Nakajima K, Kohsaka S. Microglia: neuroprotective and neurotrophic cells in the central nervous system. Curr Drug Targets Cardiovasc Haematol Disord 2004;4(1):65–84.

91. Gehrmann J, Matsumoto Y, Kreutzberg GW. Microglia: intrinsic immuneffector cell of the brain. Brain Res Brain Res Rev 1995;20(3):269–87.

92. Benveniste EN. Cytokine actions in the central nervous system. Cytokine Growth Factor Rev 1998; 9(3–4):259–75.

93. Witcher KG, Eiferman DS, Godbout JP. Priming the inflammatory pump of the CNS after traumatic brain injury. Trends Neurosci 2015;38(10):609–20.

94. Holmin S, Soderlund J, Biberfeld P, et al. Intracerebral inflammation after human brain contusion. Neurosurgery 1998;42(2):291–8.

95. Royo NC, Wahl F, Stutzmann JM. Kinetics of polymorphonuclear neutrophil infiltration after a traumatic brain injury in rat. Neuroreport 1999;10(6): 1363–7.

96. Habgood MD, Bye N, Dziegielewska KM, et al. Changes in blood-brain barrier permeability to large and small molecules following traumatic brain injury in mice. Eur J Neurosci 2007;25(1):231–8.

97. Scholz M, Cinatl J, Schadel-Hopfner M, et al. Neutrophils and the blood-brain barrier dysfunction after trauma. Med Res Rev 2007;27(3):401–16.

98. Semple BD, Bye N, Ziebell JM, et al. Deficiency of the chemokine receptor CXCR2 attenuates neutrophil infiltration and cortical damage following closed head injury. Neurobiol Dis 2010;40(2):394–403.

99. Ransohoff RM, Tani M. Do chemokines mediate leukocyte recruitment in post-traumatic CNS inflammation? Trends Neurosci 1998;21(4):154–9.

100. Hausmann EH, Berman NE, Wang YY, et al. Selective chemokine mRNA expression following brain injury. Brain Res 1998;788(1–2):49–59.

101. Clark RS, Schiding JK, Kaczorowski SL, et al. Neutrophil accumulation after traumatic brain injury in rats: comparison of weight drop and controlled

cortical impact models. J Neurotrauma 1994;11(5): 499–506.

102. Kossmann T, Hans VH, Imhof HG, et al. Intrathecal and serum interleukin-6 and the acute-phase response in patients with severe traumatic brain injuries. Shock 1995;4(5):311–7.

103. Kossmann T, Stahel PF, Lenzlinger PM, et al. Interleukin-8 released into the cerebrospinal fluid after brain injury is associated with blood-brain barrier dysfunction and nerve growth factor production. J Cereb Blood Flow Metab 1997;17(3):280–9.

104. Morganti-Kossman MC, Lenzlinger PM, Hans V, et al. Production of cytokines following brain injury: beneficial and deleterious for the damaged tissue. Mol Psychiatry 1997;2(2):133–6.

105. Csuka E, Morganti-Kossmann MC, Lenzlinger PM, et al. IL-10 levels in cerebrospinal fluid and serum of patients with severe traumatic brain injury: relationship to IL-6, TNF-alpha, TGF-beta1 and blood-brain barrier function. J Neuroimmunol 1999; 101(2):211–21.

106. Fassbender K, Schneider S, Bertsch T, et al. Temporal profile of release of interleukin-1beta in neurotrauma. Neurosci Lett 2000;284(3):135–8.

107. Maier B, Schwerdtfeger K, Mautes A, et al. Differential release of interleukines 6, 8, and 10 in cerebrospinal fluid and plasma after traumatic brain injury. Shock 2001;15(6):421–6.

108. Lenzlinger PM, Morganti-Kossmann MC, Laurer HL, et al. The duality of the inflammatory response to traumatic brain injury. Mol Neurobiol 2001;24(1–3):169–81.

109. Morganti-Kossmann MC, Rancan M, Stahel PF, et al. Inflammatory response in acute traumatic brain injury: a double-edged sword. Curr Opin Crit Care 2002;8(2):101–5.

110. Lingsma HF, Yue JK, Maas AI, et al. TRACK-TBI Investigators. Outcome prediction after mild and complicated mild traumatic brain injury: external validation of existing models and identification of new predictors using the TRACK-TBI pilot study. J Neurotrauma 2015;32(2):83–94.

111. LoBue C, Denney D, Hynan LS, et al. Self-reported traumatic brain injury and mild cognitive impairment: increased risk and earlier age of diagnosis. J Alzheimers Dis 2016;51(3):727–36.

112. Failla MD, Kumar RG, Peitzman AB, et al. Variation in the BDNF gene interacts with age to predict mortality in a prospective, longitudinal cohort with severe TBI. Neurorehabil Neural Repair 2015;29(3): 234–46.

113. Diamond ML, Ritter AC, Jackson EK, et al. Genetic variation in the adenosine regulatory cycle is associated with posttraumatic epilepsy development. Epilepsia 2015;56(8):1198–206.

114. Yue JK, Pronger AM, Ferguson AR, et al. Association of a common genetic variant within ANKK1 with six-month cognitive performance after traumatic brain injury. Neurogenetics 2015;16(3):169–80.

Imaging Evaluation of Acute Traumatic Brain Injury

Christopher A. Mutch, MD, PhD[a], Jason F. Talbott, MD, PhD[b],*,
Alisa Gean, MD[b]

KEYWORDS

- Traumatic brain injury • TBI • Imaging • MRI • CT

KEY POINTS

- Multidetector CT remains the preferred first-line imaging study for moderate and severe traumatic brain injury because it can quickly identify patients who require urgent neurosurgical intervention.
- MRI is significantly more sensitive than CT for detection of pathoanatomic lesions in mild TBI.
- MRI is more sensitive than CT for many types of traumatic injuries and plays a complementary role. It is most indicated in the acute setting for mild TBI when a patient's symptoms and/or neurologic examination are not explained by CT findings.
- Emerging advanced neuroimaging techniques may improve the sensitivity for identifying mild TBI and offer prognostic information for all grades of injury.

INTRODUCTION

In the United States, traumatic brain injury (TBI) is estimated to affect 1.7 million people annually, leading to approximately 52,000 deaths and 275,000 hospitalizations. TBI plays a role in approximately one-third of all injury-related deaths.[1] Patients who survive the initial event can have debilitating long-term sequelae. TBI actually consists of multiple pathologic entities broadly defined by an "alteration in brain function, or other evidence of brain pathology, caused by an external force."[2] Imaging plays a crucial role in evaluation and diagnosis of TBI; particularly relevant is its role for triage in the acute setting for determination of which patients require emergent neurosurgical intervention. Thus, the treating practitioner and radiologist must be familiar with the various imaging manifestations of TBI pathology and their impact on clinical presentation, management, and prognosis.

The damage incurred by TBI is differentiated into primary and secondary mechanisms. Primary injury is typically defined as the direct mechanical damage caused by trauma. These injuries are usually apparent acutely and include fractures, intracranial hemorrhage, contusion, and traumatic axonal injury (TAI). This type of injury is best detected with conventional computed tomography (CT) and MRI structural imaging techniques. Secondary injury mechanisms are varied, and relate to disruption of the blood-brain barrier, production of reactive oxygen species and resultant oxidative stress, metabolic dysfunction, inflammation, and excitotoxicity.[3,4] These processes are mediated at the cellular level, which is currently below the resolution of conventional imaging;

J.F. Talbott is member of a data monitoring committee for StemCells, Inc. Phase II clinical trial for stem cells in spinal cord injury. C.A. Mutch and A. Gean have nothing to disclose.
[a] Department of Radiology, University of California, San Francisco, 505 Parnassus Avenue, M391, San Francisco, CA 94143, USA; [b] Department of Radiology, San Francisco General Hospital, University of California, San Francisco, 1001 Potrero Avenue, San Francisco, CA 94110, USA
* Corresponding author.
E-mail address: jason.talbott@ucsf.edu

however, they are believed to greatly contribute to the long-term morbidity and disability associated with TBI. When severe, macroscopic manifestations of secondary injuries may become apparent as diffuse cerebral hyperemia, cytotoxic and/or vasogenic edema, and tissue ischemia.

Clinical examination remains the cornerstone of acute TBI assessment. There are numerous clinical classification systems for TBI based on symptomology and severity, the most entrenched of which is the Glasgow Coma Scale (GCS).[5] The GCS is a clinical assessment tool with scores ranging from 3 to 15 based on three components of neurologic function: (1) eye opening to external stimuli, (2) motor response to stimuli, and (3) verbal response. TBI is commonly subdivided into mild ($\geq$13), moderate (9–12), and severe grade (3–8) using the GCS (**Table 1**). Although the GCS score has been shown to correlate with outcomes, it has limitations. Different varieties of pathoanatomic lesions can result in low GCS scores at admission.[6] For example, initial low GCS scores may be seen with subdural hematomas (SDHs), epidural hematomas (EDHs), cortical contusions, intracerebral hematomas (ICHs), and TAI, although these lesions may have different clinical courses

and long-term prognoses.[6,7] Evaluation is also limited by sedation, paralysis, and pre-existing injuries. Despite these limitations, the GCS has relatively high interrater reliability and does an adequate job of quickly and accurately stratifying patients broadly based on clinical severity of injury. GCS subscores should always be reported to convey a more granular description of neurologic impairment instead of simply reporting the composite score, which is less meaningful in isolation.

In conjunction with neurologic examination and clinical history, pathoanatomic characterization of TBI lesions with imaging is critical for triage and prognostication. To standardize definitions and imaging protocols for TBI classification and to promote research, the Interagency Common Data Elements Project was established in 2008.[8] Throughout the following descriptions of TBI injury classification and imaging protocols, we attempt to adhere to the common data element pathoanatomic terminologies and recommendations.[9,10] We begin with a brief summary of modality-specific indications for TBI. Technical considerations and neuroimaging protocols are also examined. Characteristic findings associated with the most frequently encountered extra-axial and intra-axial pathoanatomic lesions are then described. Finally, a brief review of advanced imaging techniques for TBI evaluation is reviewed. Throughout, we highlight how standardized imaging-based characterization of pathoanatomic lesions may complement clinical assessment for optimal triage and management of patients with TBI.

ROUTINE CLINICAL IMAGING

Routine clinical imaging for suspected TBI typically consists of noncontrast CT (NCCT) and MRI in select cases.[11,12] Cases of known and suspected primary vascular abnormality may require the addition of noninvasive angiography (CT angiography [CTA] or MR angiography [MRA]) or catheter angiography for diagnosis, and in some cases, treatment. In the past, skull radiographs were performed as a first-line study to evaluate for calvarial fractures in children (**Fig. 1**), although this has fallen out of favor because significant intracranial pathology can occur in absence of skull fracture.[13] In some cases of suspected pediatric nonaccidental trauma, skull radiographs are still performed as part of a skeletal survey in addition to CT; however, this does not supplant the need for CT when TBI is clinically suspected. Although radiographs may help differentiate accessory sutures from fractures, this too may

Table 1
Glasgow coma scale

Behavior	Response	Score
Eye opening response	Spontaneously	4
	To speech	3
	To pain	2
	No response	1
Best verbal response	Oriented to time, place, and person	5
	Confused	4
	Inappropriate words	3
	Incomprehensible sounds	2
	No response	1
Best motor response	Obeys commands	6
	Moves to localized pain	5
	Flexion withdrawal from pain	4
	Abnormal flexion (decorticate)	3
	Abnormal extension (decerebrate)	2
	No response	1
Total score	Best response	15
	Comatose patient	8 or less
	Totally unresponsive	3

Adapted from Teasdale G, Jennett B. Assessment of coma and impaired consciousness. A practical scale. Lancet 1974;2(7872):81–4.

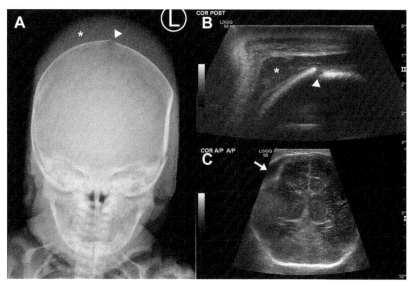

Fig. 1. Evaluation of neonatal traumatic brain injury with ultrasound and radiographs. Anteroposterior skull radiograph (*A*) and coronal ultrasound images (*B, C*) in a newborn reveal a traumatic injury suffered during a difficult forceps delivery. Skull radiograph (*A*) reveals a fracture of the parietal calvarium (*arrowhead*) and scalp soft tissue swelling compatible with a subgaleal hematoma (*asterisk*). (*B*) High-frequency (10 MHz) ultrasound of the scalp with a linear transducer shows the extracranial subgaleal hematoma in better detail (*asterisk*) and again demonstrates the fracture (*arrowhead*). (*C*) By positioning a lower frequency (6 MHz) vector transducer over a fontanel, images of the brain parenchyma and superior extra-axial spaces are obtained. These reveal a biconvex extra-axial collection (*arrow*) along the right parietal convexity, consistent with an epidural hematoma. Although ultrasound and radiographs generally do not play a role in the evaluation of TBI, they are useful for problem solving in limited pediatric imaging scenarios.

become obsolete as three-dimensional skull reformats are increasingly available in clinical practice.[14] In addition, the current CT "scout" view may often serve as a pseudoradiograph. Transfontanel ultrasound can detect some superficial lesions in neonates, such as extra-axial hemorrhage (see **Fig. 1**), and has some advocates,[15] but is limited by several blind spots including parenchymal, posterior fossa, and peripheral extra-axial lesions[16] and does not generally have a role in head trauma evaluation.[12]

Roles for Computed Tomography and MRI

Acute moderate and severe traumatic brain injury

Rapid imaging helps differentiate patients who require urgent/emergent neurosurgical intervention from those who can be safely monitored or sent home. Noncontrast multidetector CT (MDCT) has become the consensus choice[11,17] for the initial imaging study after acute moderate to severe TBI because it is fast; ubiquitous; very sensitive to calvarial injury and radiopaque foreign bodies (eg, gunshot fragments); and it is highly accurate for detecting injuries requiring emergent neurosurgical attention, such as namely hemorrhage, herniation, and hydrocephalus.

MDCT has also been shown to be useful for predicting clinical outcomes, and the NCCT findings have been incorporated into several outcome prediction rules.[18–21]

MRI is not typically indicated for the initial evaluation of TBI because it is less sensitive for fractures, takes longer to acquire, is generally less available, and is relatively expensive as a screening modality. MRI also requires additional safety screening for incompatible medical devices and metallic foreign bodies. However, MRI is exquisitely sensitive to pathologic changes related to even mild TBI (mTBI) and has demonstrated utility for assessing injury severity and prognostication (discussed later).

Acute mild traumatic brain injury

Mild TBI, as defined by a GCS greater than or equal to 13, is a misnomer in many cases because patients in this category often experience long-term debilitating symptoms that may interfere with normal daily activities.[22] Nor does this definition for mTBI imply an absence of structural abnormalities on imaging. In a recent prospective study evaluating imaging features in patients with mTBI, Yuh and colleagues[22] identified TBI–common data elements defined pathoanatomic features in 42% of patients when combining results from day-of-injury CT and semiacute MRI. Several guidelines, including the Canadian CT Head Rules,[20] New Orleans Criteria,[21] and National Emergency X-Ray Utilization Study (NEXUS)-II,[19] are routinely used to identify the cohort of patients who can safely bypass the initial noncontrast CT.[18] When imaging is clinically indicated, noncontrast CT is the primary initial modality of choice for evaluation of acute mTBI.[11,17] After clinical screening, most patients with mTBI for which imaging is indicated have normal noncontrast CTs (ie, "uncomplicated" mTBI).

Short-term follow-up imaging

Although MDCT is recommended in patients with neurologic deterioration following TBI, studies have shown little benefit for routine follow-up imaging.[23] Among patients with initial MDCT positive for intracranial traumatic injury, only certain attributes including subfrontal/temporal hemorrhagic contusion, use of anticoagulation, age older than 65 years, and volume of ICH greater than 10 mL have shown high risk for progression.[24] At many institutions it is commonplace to obtain routine follow-up MDCT in patients on anticoagulation, even when the initial MDCT is negative for acute intracranial pathology, although the clinical utility of this practice is not well established.[25] One recent prospective study evaluating patients with mild head trauma who were on anticoagulation found that repeat head CT imaging revealed hemorrhagic changes in only 1.4% of such patients after negative initial scan.[26]

MRI often plays a complementary role to CT and is most indicated in the acute setting for mTBI when a patient's symptoms and/or neurologic examination are not explained by CT findings. Compared with CT, MRI is far more sensitive for detection of acute traumatic pathology in mTBI, particularly for detection of nonhemorrhagic contusion and TAI.[27–33] For these reasons, MRI is also indicated within the first 2 weeks of any moderate or severe TBI for sensitive assessment of the degree of parenchymal injury.

Imaging subacute/chronic traumatic brain injury

Subacute and chronic TBI are best evaluated with MRI,[11,17,34] which outperforms CT in its ability to identify parenchymal atrophy, white matter injury, and microhemorrhage. Imaging is indicated in patients who experience new, persistent, or worsening symptoms. NCCT should be performed to evaluate subacute/chronic TBI if MRI is contraindicated or unavailable.

Vascular imaging

Intravenous contrast administration is not necessary or useful in the evaluation of TBI unless arterial or venous injury is suspected. NCCT findings can identify patients at increased risk for traumatic vascular injuries.[35] Patients with skull base fractures, particularly through the carotid canal, have much higher incidence of arterial injuries. Other findings that should raise suspicion for arterial injury include epistaxis, LeFort II and III facial fractures, high cervical spine fractures, GCS less than or equal to 8, or TAI.[36] Either CTA or MRA can be performed as an initial screening evaluation for arterial injury,[11,17] although CTA has gained popularity over the past decade with the proliferation of MDCT and the resultant high-quality, three-dimensional reformats (3D), rapid imaging of contrast bolus.[37] Conventional catheter angiography may be necessary for the diagnosis and treatment of certain lesions.

Venous injury should be suspected in patients with skull fractures extending across adjacent dural venous sinuses. A common injury involves an occipital fracture extending to the underlying transverse sinus (**Fig. 2**). Either CT venography or MRI venography are indicated to evaluate for dural venous sinus thrombosis in such cases.[11]

Pediatric imaging

Head trauma is a common imaging indication in children and recommended imaging studies largely mirror those recommended for adults for given indications.[12] Children are more susceptible to harmful effects of ionizing radiation than adults and every effort should be made to avoid unnecessary examinations, particularly CT. In balance, however, diagnostic head CT should not be avoided when clinically indicated because of an overemphasized concern for the relatively small radiation dose associated with modern scanners. When CT is performed, dedicated pediatric CT protocols should be used to keep the dose as low as possible (see http://www.imagegently.org for more information). MRI does not expose patients to ionizing radiation; however, it does present its own challenges in pediatric patients. Children may require general anesthesia to tolerate MRI examinations, which are much longer and more sensitive to motion than CT. "Rapid" MRI examinations with limited sequences and imaging time reduced to 3 to 4 minutes[38] may help with this in the future, but further studies are required to ensure diagnostic accuracy is on par with CT and standard MRI.

IMAGING PROTOCOLS FOR TRAUMATIC BRAIN INJURY

Optimal neuroimaging protocols for specific head injuries vary depending on individual patient and

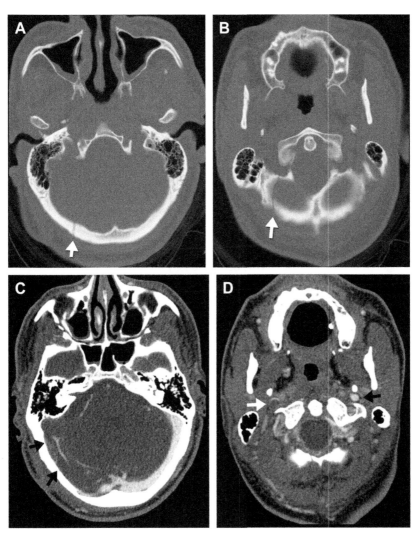

Fig. 2. Occipital fracture complicated by transverse sinus injury. A 42-year-old man presents after a fall with impact to the back of the head. Noncontrast head CT viewed at bone window technique (*A, B*) reveals a nondisplaced, linear right occipital fracture (*arrows*) adjacent to the expected location of the right transverse sinus. Therefore, a CT venogram was subsequently performed to evaluate for venous sinus injury. Note the thrombus, manifested as unopacified flow within the right transverse sinus (*C, arrows*) that extends into the right sigmoid sinus and the right jugular vein (*D, white arrow*.) The normal left jugular vein (*D, black arrow*) is shown for comparison.

environmental circumstances. This is particularly true for MRI, where there is a greater diversity in choice of available sequences and imaging parameters. It is important to always keep the patient's clinical condition in mind; at times, it is necessary to omit certain sequences in an abbreviated MRI examination or substitute CT to shorten the examination time.

Experts in TBI recently convened as part of the "Advanced Integrated Research on Psychological Health and Traumatic Brain Injury: Common Data Elements" joint workshop.[9] During this meeting, an expert panel proposed standardized CT and

MRI protocols for studying TBI. The panel defined different imaging protocols into a Tier 1 practical clinical imaging protocol and advanced research protocols (Tiers 2 through 4). In this section we describe the Tier 1 clinical imaging protocols. Description of some elements of the Tiers 2 to 4 protocols are discussed later in the advanced imaging subsections.

Routine Computed Tomography Protocol

CT imaging is typically acquired helically in the axial plane on an MDCT scanner. An axial slice thickness of 2.5 mm is commonly used for evaluating the brain parenchyma, although thinner reformats (0.625 mm) using a bone kernel is recommended for the detection of subtle fractures. Helical acquisition allows the generation of reformatted images in different planes (typically coronal and sagittal), and volume-rendered 3D reformats, which can aid in the detection of subtle intracranial hemorrhage and fractures.[39,40] Modern CT scanners also typically use dose reduction software, which reduces patient radiation exposure.

Routine MRI Protocol

The recommended clinical protocol (Tier 1) tailored for TBI evaluation (**Table 2**) incorporates multiplanar T1-weighted images (T1WI) (3D T1 if available), T2-weighted images (T2WI) (at 3 T, 3D T2 is recommended if available), T2 fluid-attenuated inversion recovery (FLAIR) weighted, and T2*-weighted gradient-recalled echo (GRE) or susceptibility-weighted (SWI) sequences, in addition to standard diffusion-weighted imaging (DWI). SWI sequences are rapidly being added to routine TBI imaging protocols and are preferred over GRE because of their increased sensitivity for blood products.[41] Detection, localization, and characterization of traumatic lesions benefit from the incorporation of multiple imaging planes, an advantage of 3D acquisitions.[9,27,29,30,32] Multiplanar imaging is particularly helpful in detecting small lesions (eg, traumatic brainstem injury [BSI]), which can be missed because of partial volume averaging effects or an interslice gap.[30]

Attributes of particular sequences for imaging specific pathologies is covered in detail later. Briefly, T1WI is commonly used to map brain anatomy, whereas T2WI is sensitive to pathology. Increased water content, as seen in cerebral edema, manifests as T2 prolongation and increased T2 signal intensity. 3D T1 sequences can be used for quantitative volumetric analysis of the brain (usually in research settings).[42]

FLAIR T2WI increases the conspicuity of lesions adjacent to, and within, the ventricles and subarachnoid spaces by suppressing cerebrospinal fluid (CSF) signal, which is normally bright on T2WI. GRE images and SWI sequences take advantage of artifacts associated with blood products to identify hematomas by their distinctive areas of magnetic susceptibility-induced hypointensity arising from paramagnetic iron.

DWI measures the freedom of molecular motion of water in tissue and is useful in identifying pathologic lesions including foci of axonal injury and infarction.[43,44] DWI is best used in conjunction with its associated apparent diffusion coefficient (ADC) map, which can distinguish between cytotoxic and vasogenic edema in the acute and subacute phases and is highly sensitive in the detection of secondary acute ischemic infarction associated with TBI.

Postcontrast T1WI is not recommended as part of routine TBI MRI protocol because it does not improve sensitivity for TBI lesions.[9] Postcontrast imaging is used as an optional sequence in certain situations, such as establishing chronicity of injury, subacute ischemia, or when nontraumatic intracranial pathologies are under consideration.[45]

Table 2
Recommended MRI protocol for TBI

Field Strength	1.5T			3T		
	Sequence	Orientation	Imaging Time (min)	Sequence	Orientation	Imaging Time (min)
Preferred sequences	3D T1W	Sagittal	8	3D T1W	Sagittal	4
	T2W FSE	Axial	3	3D T2W	Sagittal	4
	T2W FLAIR	Axial	3	T2W FLAIR	Axial	3
	DWI EPI	Axial	2	DWI EPI	Axial	2
	3D SWI	Axial	8	3D SWI	Axial	6
			Total: 24			Total: 19
Alternatives sequences	T1W SE[a]	Sagittal	3	T2W FSE[b]	Axial	3
	2D GRE[c]	Axial	3	2D GRE[c]	Axial	3

Abbreviations: DWI, diffusion-weighted imaging; EPI, echo-planar imaging; FLAIR, fluid-attenuated inversion recovery; FSE, fast spin echo; GRE, gradient-recalled echo; SE, spin echo; SWI, susceptibility-weighted images; T1W, T1 weighted; T2W, T2 weighted.
[a] Option if 3D T1W is not available.
[b] Option if 3D T2W is not available.
[c] Option if 3D SWI is not available.
Adapted from Haacke EM, Duhaime AC, Gean AD, et al. Common data elements in radiologic imaging of traumatic brain injury. J Magn Reson Imaging 2010;32(3):520–1.

IMAGING FINDINGS OF TRAUMATIC BRAIN INJURIES

Intracranial pathology is subdivided to anatomic location, the most basic distinction being whether it localizes to the brain parenchyma (intra-axial) or outside the brain tissue (extra-axial). Vascular injuries, although typically extra-axial, are addressed separately in this discussion to highlight differences in the imaging work-up.

Extra-Axial Lesions

Three intracranial, extra-axial spaces (epidural, subdural, and subarachnoid spaces) are potential sites for posttraumatic pathology, most often hemorrhage. NCCT is excellent at detecting acute hemorrhage, which appears hyperdense to the surrounding brain parenchyma typically measuring between 50 and 70 Hounsfield units. In general, the density of a hematoma decreases as it ages, which can create challenges for identifying subacute and chronic hemorrhages that may appear isodense to the surrounding brain parenchyma.

Although initially thought to be less sensitive than CT for acute hemorrhage, modern MRI now outperforms CT in identifying hemorrhage throughout all stages of its evolution, particularly small, subacute bleeds.[29,46] Additionally, because of biochemical changes in hemoglobin over time that alter T1 and T2 relaxation times in hematoma, the age of hemorrhage can be estimated with MRI (**Table 3**).[46]

Epidural hematoma

EDH form as blood collects in the potential spaces between the inner table of the skull and the dura.

EDHs are arterial or venous in origin, and may relate to direct bleeding from fractured bone into the epidural space. Arterial EDHs most commonly arise from laceration of meningeal arteries, typically the middle meningeal artery in the temporal or temporoparietal region.[47–52] In adults, an overlying skull fracture is present in most cases. Occasionally (9%), EDHs can occur from stretching and tearing of meningeal arteries in the absence of fracture. The latter occurs commonly in children because of transient deformation and depression of the calvarial vault.[47]

EDHs classically appear as a lenticular-shaped hematoma, which can cross dural attachment sites, but cannot cross cranial sutures (**Fig. 3**). On CT, acute EDHs generally appear hyperdense. Some hematomas can appear heterogeneous with intrinsic irregular areas of low density, termed the "swirl sign," an important imaging finding that corresponds to extravasation of hyperacute unclotted blood.[53] EDHs with this sign tend to rapidly expand and warrant urgent surgical consultation. Rarely, it may be difficult to differentiate a small EDH that does not have the classic shape from a SDH on CT. On MRI, the dura mater can often be visualized as a thin line of low signal intensity displaced away from the inner table of the skull, confirming the diagnosis of an EDH.[29,30]

Venous EDHs are less common than those of arterial origin.[47–52] They typically are caused by laceration of a dural sinus in conjunction with fracture of the overlying skull.[52,54] The posterior fossa (transverse or sigmoid sinus injury), middle cranial fossa (sphenoparietal sinus) (see **Fig. 3**G–I), and parasagittal region (superior sagittal sinus) are

Table 3
Appearance of aging blood on MRI sequences

	Time Frame	Molecular Species	Cellular Compartment	T1WI Signal[a]	T2WI Signal[a]
Hyperacute	<24 h	Oxyhemoglobin	Intracellular	Isointense	Isointense/hyperintense
Acute	1–3 d	Deoxyhemoglobin	Intracellular	Isointense/hypointense	Hypointense
Early subacute	3–7 d	Methemoglobin	Intracellular	Hyperintense	Hypointense
Late subacute	7–14 d	Methemoglobin	Extracellular	Hyperintense	Hyperintense
Chronic	>14 d				
Rim	—	Hemosiderin	Intracellular	Hypointense	Hypointense
Center	—	Hemichromes	Extracellular	Isointense	Hyperintense

[a] Compared with the signal intensity of normal brain parenchyma.
Adapted from Bradley WG Jr. MR appearance of hemorrhage in the brain. Radiology 1993;189(1):16.

416

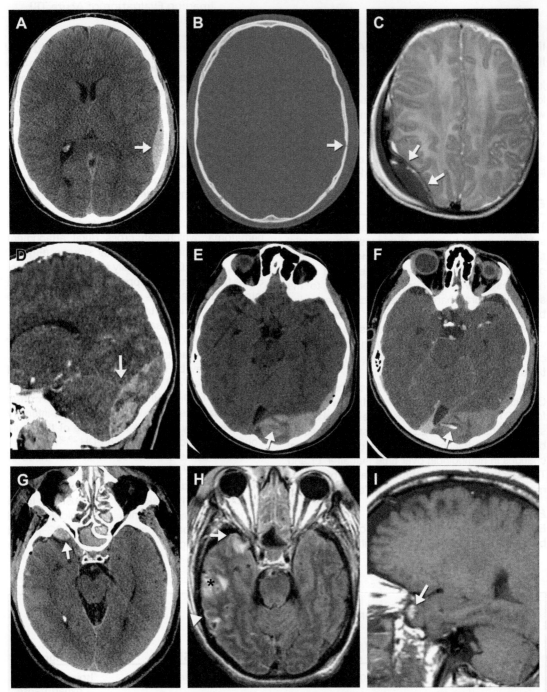

Fig. 3. CT and MRI appearance of epidural hematoma. Noncontrast CT (*A*, *B*) performed on a 26-year-old man who was "found down" with altered mental status. Note the classic biconvex hyperdense epidural hematoma with an overlying nondisplaced calvarial fracture (*arrows*). Axial T2WI (*C*) from a "rapid" MRI protocol in a different patient (3 month old accidentally dropped on her head) reveals a right parietal biconvex low-signal epidural collection. Note the position of the dura, seen as the *thin black line* deep to the collection (*arrows*); this allows confident determination that the collection is located in the epidural space. Sagittal (*D*) and axial (*E*) reformatted images from a noncontrast CT performed in a different patient (13-year-old boy after a skateboard accident) show a heterogeneous epidural hematoma in the occipital region. Areas of lower density within the hematoma likely represent hyperacute unclotted blood concerning for active bleeding and predictive of continued expansion of the hematoma. This is confirmed on the CTA of the head performed minutes later (*F*) where dense contrast material extravasates (*F, arrow*) into the area of low density on the earlier noncontrast study (*E, arrow*). The sagittal reformatted images (*D*) best demonstrate how the hematoma crosses the plane of the tentorium cerebelli (*arrow*) into the posterior fossa, characteristic

the most common locations for venous EHD.[54] Venous EDHs, unlike SDHs, are not bound by dural attachments and often extend above and below the tentorium. Posterior fossa EDHs occur less frequently (2%–29%), are more likely to be of venous origin (85%), and are associated with poorer outcomes than supratentorial lesions.[47,55,56] Differentiation of arterial and venous EDHs is usually possible with MRI and may have some therapeutic and prognostic significance because venous EDH typically do not progress as rapidly as arterial EDH.[52] Venous EDH may exhibit a more variable shape than those of arterial origin.[47,52] Invariably, venous EDH are found adjacent to a fracture transgressing a dural venous sinus.[47,55,56] These injuries have a high rate of associated dural sinus thrombosis or occlusion.[51] When in question, patency of the sinus can usually be established by CT venography or MRI venography. When evaluating for venous sinus injury, it is important to distinguish external sinus compression by epidural blood from traumatic venous sinus thrombosis. In the latter, the dural venous sinus is usually irregular with a central sinus filling defect correlating to the thrombus.

Subdural hematoma

Within the skull, the brain is relatively mobile and can move relative to the fixed dural sinuses. Injury to the bridging veins that traverse the subdural space connecting the brain to the dural sinuses results in the SDH.[57–59] Although SDHs are most often found along the supratentorial convexities, they can also occur in the posterior fossa, along the falx cerebri, and adjacent to the tentorium.[60,61] Interhemispheric and tentorial leaf SDH are common in children, including cases of abuse resulting from violent shaking (shaken-baby syndrome).[62–65] Although these hematomas are not specific for child abuse, their presence should lead to close consideration of the possibility.

Most SDHs manifest as a crescentic collection between the brain and the or inner table of the skull; interhemispheric and tentorial SDHs have a more linear morphology. All SDHs follow the typical appearance of evolving blood on CT and MRI (**Fig. 4**). Although large acute hyperdense SDHs are readily apparent on CT, small subacute SDHs are often isodense and difficult to identify (see **Fig. 4**C). MRI has been shown to be considerably more sensitive than CT for detection of SDH[29,30,66] and the MRI signal characteristics vary predictably with the age of the lesion (see **Table 3**). SDHs appear much more conspicuous on MRI because of high imaging contrast between the hematoma and signal void of the adjacent cortical bone (see **Fig. 4**E). Fortunately, SDHs not identified with CT almost always measure only 1 to 2 mm in diameter and are of doubtful clinical significance.[29] MRI also more clearly reveals the multicompartmental nature of subacute to chronic SDH, which can help establish the age of lesions and aid in planning for surgical drainage of these complex lesions.[27]

Subarachnoid and intraventricular hemorrhage

Subarachnoid hemorrhage (SAH) is a common finding in TBI. One large European series found evidence of SAH in 40% of patients with moderate-severe head injury.[67,68] Traumatic SAH is also the most common isolated finding in cases of mTBI and has been associated with poor outcome scores at 3 months after injury.[22] Acute traumatic SAH results from injury to small subarachnoid vessels or extension of intraparenchymal hemorrhage beyond the pial limiting membrane and into the subarachnoid space. Traumatic pseudoaneurysms typically do not occur in the acute setting.

Acute SAH appears as curvilinear hyperdensity within the cortical sulci, sylvian fissures, and basal cisterns on NCCT (**Fig. 5**F). Historically, SAH was considered far more difficult to detect with conventional MRI than with CT[69,70]; however, more recent technical improvements and additional sequences have shown MRI to be sensitive to SAH and hold some advantages over CT. FLAIR

---

of epidural hematomas (unlike subdural hematomas) because they are not constrained by dural boundaries. In contrast to arterial epidural hematomas, venous epidural hematomas bleed under lower pressure and are therefore less likely to increase in size. Noncontrast CT (*G*), axial FLAIR (*H*), and sagittal T1WI (*I*) performed on a 52-year-old victim of assault reveal a right sphenoparietal venous epidural hematoma (*arrows*). CT on the day of the injury (*G*) shows the characteristic well-defined, crescentic, high-density extra-axial collection (*arrow*) along the anterior margin of the middle cranial fossa. On MRI performed 2 days later (*H, I*), the same venous epidural hematoma (*arrow*) appears isointense to adjacent anterior temporal contusion on FLAIR (*H*) and hyperintense T1WI (*I*), consistent with intracellular methemoglobin blood products and it has not increased in size. In cases of trauma, multiple pathologic entities often are seen in the same examination. Notably, foci of subarachnoid hemorrhage (*arrowhead*) and temporal lobe contusions (*asterisk*) are much more visible on MRI (*H*) than CT.

418

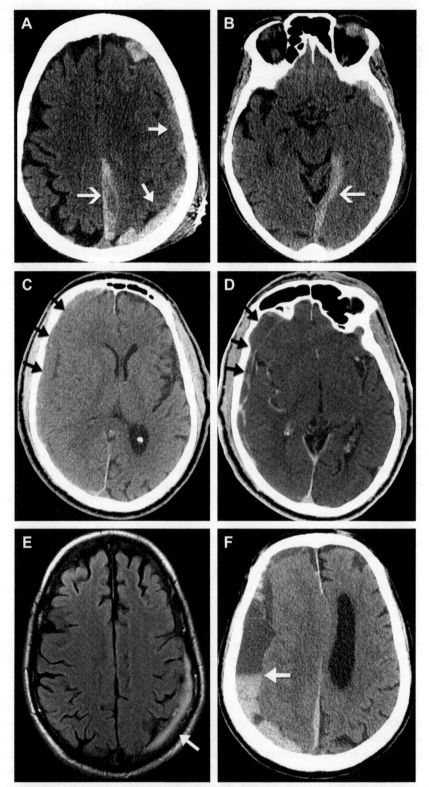

Fig. 4. CT and MRI appearance of subdural hematomas. Noncontrast CT (*A*, *B*) performed on a 90-year-old woman after a fall with left parietal scalp laceration reveals hyperdense blood along the left convexity (*A, closed arrows*), left posterior falx cerebri (*A, unfilled arrow*), and tentorium cerebelli (*B, unfilled arrow*). Note how the subdural hematomas do not cross the dural sinuses to the other side of the falx or tentorium. Noncontrast CT performed on an 82-year-old man after falling shows a right convexity subacute subdural hematoma that is isodense to the adjacent cortex (*C, arrows*). Postcontrast imaging is generally not required for

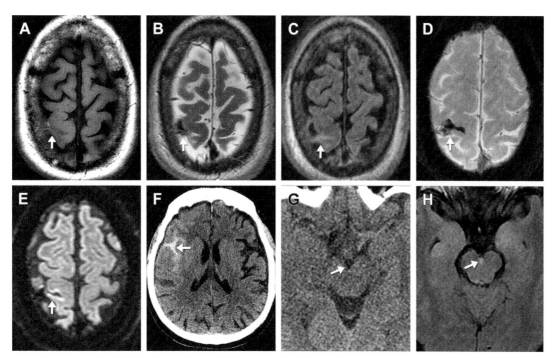

Fig. 5. CT and MRI appearance of subarachnoid hemorrhage. MRI (A–E) performed on a 58-year-old man who presented 3 days after a fall with altered mental status. Subacute subarachnoid hemorrhage appears hyperintense to brain on T1WI (A) and hypointense on T2WI (B). Subarachnoid hemorrhage does not suppress like normal CSF on FLAIR imaging (C) and it appears markedly hypointense on SWI (D). The linear area of reduced diffusion in the cortex adjacent to the subarachnoid hemorrhage likely represents adjacent cerebral contusion (E). This is a good example showing the appearance of early subacute subarachnoid blood products within the central sulcus on multiple pulse sequences (arrows). Noncontrast CT (F) from a 70-year-old man after syncope and fall with head injury shows the classic appearance of acute subarachnoid hemorrhage in the right sylvian fissure (arrow). Noncontrast CT (G) and FLAIR (H) images obtained the same day in a 33-year-old woman after a motor vehicle crash. The trace interpeduncular subarachnoid hemorrhage (arrow) is invisible on CT (G), but is readily apparent on MRI (H), highlighting the greater sensitivity of MRI to blood products.

sequences are highly sensitive to SAH (**Fig. 5**C) in acute and subacute periods,[71–73] whereas CT sensitivity falls sharply after the first few days.[74] CSF FLAIR signal hyperintensity is strongly suggestive of hemorrhage after trauma, although other processes that lead to increased CSF protein/cellularity, such as infection and leptomeningeal carcinomatosis, may have a similar appearance.[75] The combination of FLAIR and SWI sequences gives MRI (see **Fig. 5**) a better detection rate for SAH than NCCT.[76]

Intraventricular hemorrhage (IVH), considered a type of intra-axial injury by some authors, is addressed here because its pathophysiology and imaging findings largely overlap with SAH. IVH is also common in patients with head injury, occurring in from 3% to 35% of cases, depending on the severity of trauma.[27,28,30,60] Primary IVH may be caused by a variety of traumatic lesions including TAI, ICH, and contusions[27,28,30,60]; however, the most prevalent cause is thought to be the tearing of subependymal veins by rotational

evaluation of a subdural hematoma; however, it was obtained in this case. The postcontrast CT (D, arrows) images demonstrate peripheral enhancement of the collection without evidence of active extravasation, thus reinforcing a subacute injury. Axial FLAIR MRI (E) from a 69-year-old man after head trauma exemplifies the high-contrast difference on MRI between the FLAIR hyperintense subdural hematoma (arrow) and the adjacent hypointense calvarium. Axial noncontrast CT (F) from a different patient, a 73-year-old man with left-sided weakness, shows the appearance of a mixed-density, "acute-on-chronic" subdural hematoma along the right convexity and falx cerebri. Note the dependent layering of the acute, denser blood products within the chronic, hypodense collection; this is often referred to as the "hematocrit sign" (arrow).

strain.[31] Similar rotational forces are thought to cause callosal TAI and, indeed, one published series identified IVH in 60% of patients with TAI of the corpus callosum, but in only 12% of patients without callosal injury.[31] Interestingly, another study found that the presence of IVH on admission NCCT was the only CT imaging finding predictive of grade II or III TAI on subsequent MRI.[77] IVH appears similar to SAH with the blood products appearing hyperdense to CSF on CT and hyperintense to CSF on FLAIR and T1WI with MRI.[28] A CSF-blood fluid level is often seen layering within the posterior aspect of the occipital horns (remember that the images are acquired with the patient in the supine position). Because the subarachnoid and intraventricular CSF spaces communicate, delayed imaging may demonstrate IVH because of recirculation of SAH and vice versa.

Cerebrospinal fluid leak

CSF leak is a complication in approximately 1% to 3% of TBI cases[78] and is typically associated with a basilar skull fracture. These cases usually present with CSF rhinorrhea (~80%) or otorrhea (~20%) within the first 48 hours after traumatic injury, although cases can present months to years after the initial insult with meningitis or orthostatic headaches.[78,79] CSF rhinorrhea or otorrhea should prompt the search for a skull base fracture on thin-section maxillofacial or temporal bone CT.[11] Common fractures involve of anterior cranial fossa (especially the frontal sinus or cribriform plates), sella and sphenoid sinus, and temporal bone.[78]

CT cisternography is rarely used for initial evaluation, but is helpful for problem solving in patients with multiple skull defects, negative initial CT imaging, or to confirm a CSF fistula when the diagnosis is unclear. In this setting, intrathecal contrast media is injected to opacify the CSF spaces. A positive study shows abnormal increased attenuation within a paranasal sinus, nasal cavity, or middle ear secondary to contrast passage through the skull base defect (**Fig. 6**).[80]

Cisternography can also be performed as a nuclear medicine study, most commonly with In-111 DTPA. Positive studies show accumulation of tracer in the nasal cavity. Although radionucleotide cisternography lacks the anatomic specificity of CT, it is useful in certain difficult cases, particularly when combined with endoscopic placement of nasal pledgets. The pledgets are removed 24 hours after radionucleotide injection and activity associated with each pledget is counted to evaluate for occult CSF leak.[81]

MRI can be performed to assess for possible encephalocele or meningoencephalocele.[11] Some authors have advocated routinely obtaining MRI when CT shows complete or lobular, nondependent opacification of a sinus cavity adjacent to a bony defect because brain parenchymal herniation is challenging to differentiate from sinonasal secretions on CT.[78] MRI can also show secondary signs of intracranial hypotension resulting from a chronic CSF leak including diffuse pachymeningeal enhancement, subdural collections, "sagging" brainstem, and prominence of the dural sinuses and pituitary.[79]

Intra-Axial Injury

Intra-axial injuries refer to lesions within the brain parenchyma. Primary traumatic intra-axial lesions include the cortical contusion, ICH, TAI, and BSI. There are also secondary intra-axial injuries that can occur as a result of brain swelling and ischemia. Although CT and MRI are both sensitive for identification of extra-axial traumatic injury, MRI has a dominant role in evaluation of intra-axial pathology, because nonhemorrhagic and very small lesions can be occult on CT.

Parenchymal contusion

Parenchymal contusions (**Fig. 7**) occur when the brain forcibly impacts the irregular surface of the overlying skull, which typically occurs at (coup injury) or opposite (contrecoup) the site of blunt trauma. Contusions frequently are multifocal and bilateral, usually involving the superficial gray matter. They typically occur in the temporal (46%) and frontal (31%) lobes. These injuries tend to occur immediately adjacent to the petrous bone and posterior to the greater sphenoid wing in the temporal lobe and just superior to the cribriform plate, orbit roof, planum sphenoidale, and lesser sphenoid wing in the frontal lobe.[9,28,82] Contusions less often involve the parietal and occipital lobes (13%) and cerebellum (~10%).[28] Contusions frequently contain hemorrhagic foci ranging in size from punctate cortical surface petechiae to much larger confluent regions of hemorrhage occupying an entire lobe.

Intracerebral hematoma

ICH (**Fig. 8**)[83] results from injury to intraparenchymal arteries or veins secondary to rotational strain or penetrating trauma[27,84–86] and is usually located in the frontotemporal white matter[48] or basal ganglia.[84–86] Differentiation from hemorrhagic contusions or TAI is challenging[84–86]; ICHs collect between relatively intact parenchyma in contrast to hemorrhagic contusions wherein hemorrhage is within a larger area of injured edematous brain.[27] Prognosis of isolated ICH is generally good,[61] but worsens when the lesion coexists with marked

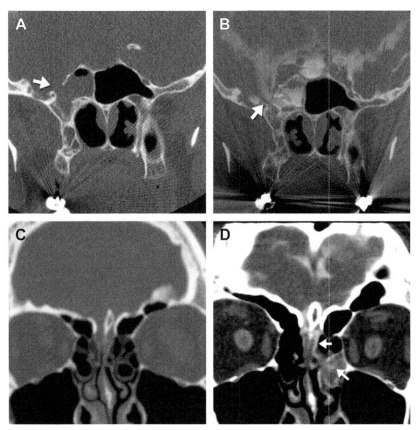

Fig. 6. Imaging evaluation of patients with CSF leaks. Coronal reformatted images from a noncontrast CT (*A, C*) and CT cisternograms (*B, D*) performed in two different patients with posttraumatic CSF leaks. The first patient (*A, B*) is a 55-year-old woman with a history of remote trauma and meningitis. Note the opacified right sphenoid sinus with a large bony defect between the lateral wall of the right sphenoid sinus and the middle cranial fossa (*A, arrow*). CT cisternography was performed (*B*), confirming abnormal leakage of CSF contrast from the middle cranial fossa into the sphenoid sinus (*arrow*). The second patient (*C, D*) is a 33-year-old woman with CSF rhinorrhea (confirmed with positive B_2-transferrin test) after facial trauma. Noncontrast CT (*C*) reveals subtle unilateral opacification of the left olfactory recess concerning for a possible cephalocele, but it did not show a definitive bony abnormality in that region. The patient returned 2 weeks later and a CT cisternogram was performed (*D*) revealing abnormal passage of CSF contrast (*arrows*) through the left cribiform plate through the left olfactory recess and into the nasal cavity.

mass effect, TAI, or multiple basal ganglia hemorrhages.[84,85] Temporal lobe hematomas are especially unpredictable, because even a relatively small lesion can lead to uncal herniation. When CTA is also performed, the "spot sign," or active extravasation of contrast into the hematoma, predicts future expansion of the hematoma and worsens clinical outcome.[87,88]

Traumatic axonal injury

TAI is one of the most common and important types of primary injury found in patients with all grades of head trauma. TAI typically results from rotational strain, and manifests as scattered, often bilateral, small white matter lesions with or without hemorrhagic components.[9] When there are

greater than three foci of radiographically evident TAI involving at least two separate lobes of the brain and the corpus callosum, the term diffuse axonal injury is used.

TAI tends to be multifocal. The severity of injury worsens as involvement of the deep anatomic structures become affected.[89–91] In the Adams Classification for TAI, grade 1 injuries involve the lobar white matter, particularly the gray-white junction frontal and temporal lobes (**Fig. 9**A–D). Grade 2 injuries extend to involve the corpus callosum, particularly the splenium (**Fig. 9**E–H). Grade 3 injuries (**Fig. 10**) involve the dorsolateral aspect of the upper brainstem.[89–91]

TAI lesions are usually ovoid with their long axis oriented in the direction of the involved axonal

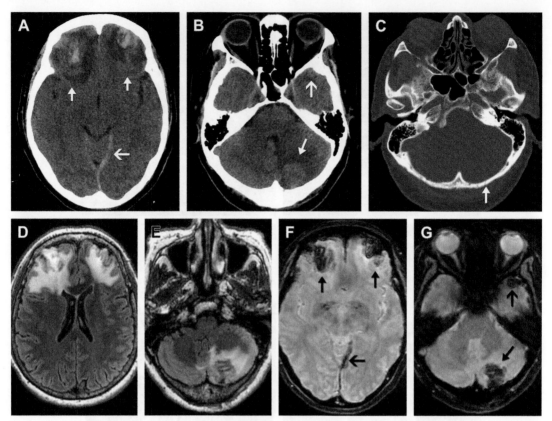

Fig. 7. CT and MRI appearance of cerebral and cerebellar contusion. Noncontrast CT (*A–C*) and FLAIR and susceptibility-weighted MRI (*D–G*) images obtained on a 59-year-old woman after a fall that occurred 5 days earlier. CT images show a nondisplaced left occipital fracture (*C, arrow*) with an underlying hemorrhagic contusion in the left cerebellar hemisphere (*B, closed arrow*) compatible with coup injury. There are also large, bifrontal, hemorrhagic contusions (*A, closed arrows*) and a small left anterior temporal hemorrhagic contusion (*B, open arrow*), compatible with contrecoup injuries. These lesions have a predictable appearance on MRI with low signal on SWI (*F, closed arrows; G, arrows*) and a large area of surrounding edema on FLAIR images (*D, E*). Also note the increased prominence of the left tentorial subdural hematoma (*unfilled arrow*) on MRI SWI (*F*) compared with CT (*A*).

tracts. They range in size from 2 to 15 mm, peripheral lesions tending to be smaller than more central ones. Overall, CT has poor sensitivity for TAI. Only about 10% of TAI display the classic CT findings of punctate hemorrhage (see **Fig. 9**) in the characteristic white matter loci.[92]

MRI has increased sensitivity for TAI compared with CT.[33,93,94] Hemorrhagic TAI appear as foci of increased magnetic susceptibility on GRE and SWI sequences in the characteristic white matter locations (see **Fig. 9**). FLAIR imaging may demonstrate foci of hyperintense signal for hemorrhagic and nonhemorrhagic TAI. Acute TAI lesions display reduced ADC values on DWI (see **Fig. 9**), a finding that is equal in sensitivity to FLAIR.[95] MRI may also be a useful prognostic tool. Several recent studies have shown a strong correlation between the burden of TAI lesions and worse clinical outcomes.[33,96,97]

Brainstem injury

BSI is divided into primary injuries that result directly from the initial impact and secondary injuries that develop subsequently.[30,98–100] Primary BSI is divided into four categories. The first type occurs when severe posterior displacement of the brain forces the dorsolateral upper brainstem to directly impact the tentorium producing laceration or contusion.[101] This mechanism is thought to be uncommon and, unlike brainstem TAI, it is not necessarily associated with more diffuse white matter injury.

The other types of BSI are indirect, the most common of which is brainstem TAI.[57,102] Brainstem TAI (**Fig. 11**) is invariably seen in the context of similar axonal lesions in the supratentorial white matter.[89–91] A third type of primary BSI is characterized by multifocal scattered petechial hemorrhages concentrated in the deep central white

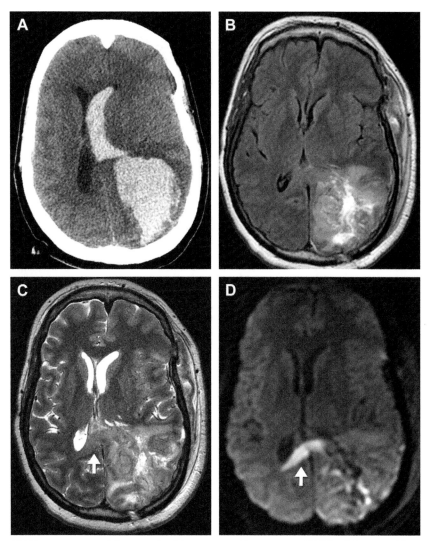

Fig. 8. CT and MRI appearance of intracerebral hematoma. Noncontrast CT (*A*) of 61-year-old man after head trauma reveals a large, hyperdense, acute left parietal hematoma with surrounding edema that has decompressed into the adjacent left lateral ventricle (intraventricular hemorrhage). MRI performed 11 days later (*B–D*) shows decreased edema with residual T2 hyperintense blood products (likely corresponding to "late subacute" extracellular methemoglobin). Increased T2 signal intensity (*C*) and reduced diffusion (*D*) in the splenium of the corpus callosum (*arrows*) is likely a result of wallerian degeneration of the axons leading away from the left parietal injury, and not traumatic axonal injury of the splenium.

matter, hypothalamus, thalamus, and periaqueductal rostral brainstem.[89–91,103] These lesions usually carry a grim prognosis.[89–91] Although both entities share a shear-strain cause, unlike brainstem TAI, this entity is not associated with lobar white matter, corpus callosum, or superior cerebellar peduncle lesions.[89–91] It is worth noting that distribution of these petechial hemorrhages differs from the secondary (Duret) hemorrhages described later. The final type of primary BSI is pontomedullary separation or rent, which is caused by a hyperextension-induced tear of the

ventral brainstem at the pontomedullary junction.[89–91,104,105] This injury may range from an incomplete tear to complete brainstem avulsion and is typically[105] but not invariably[104] fatal.

BSI is usually nonhemorrhagic making visualization with CT difficult.[28,30] The bulk of knowledge about these entities has been derived from autopsy studies; however, MRI has allowed evaluation of BSI in nonfatally injured patients.[30] MRI studies have shown that BSI is linked to poor clinical outcomes; dorsal hemorrhagic lesions and the bilateral BSI were particularly strongly associated

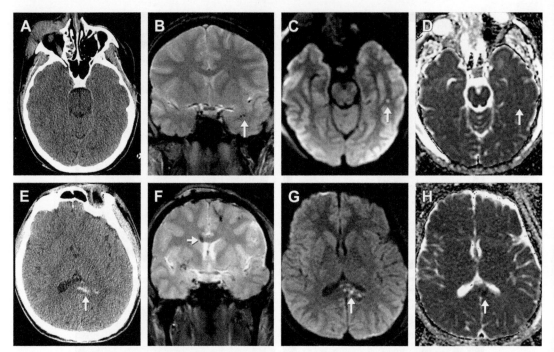

Fig. 9. CT and MRI appearance of traumatic axonal injury. Initial noncontrast CT (*A*) of a 24-year-old woman after a helmeted bicycle accident with brief loss of consciousness shows right periorbital soft tissue swelling, but is otherwise normal. MRI including T2*-weighted multiplanar gradient recall (MPGR) (*B*), DWI (*C*), and ADC map (*D*) obtained the following day shows scattered foci of reduced diffusion and increased susceptibility, compatible with traumatic axonal injuries. Example lesions include a focus of reduced diffusion (*C, arrow*) with low ADC value (*D, arrow*) and foci of increased susceptibility (*B, arrow*) in the left temporal stem subcortical white matter. A different patient presented after an assault (*E–H*). This patient's noncontrast CT shows multiple areas of hemorrhagic axonal shearing injury involving the splenium of the corpus callosum (*E, arrow*). This area shows reduced diffusion (*G, arrow*), low ADC value (*H, arrow*), and increased susceptibility on MPGR (*F, arrow*) on MRI performed the same day. The coronal MPGR image (*F*) also reveals numerous additional white matter shear injuries (low signal) compatible with diffuse axonal injury.

with poor outcomes.[106] Interestingly, BSI is not universally associated with poor outcomes, because nearly one-third of patients with MRI evidence for BSI actually had a good clinical outcome. Nonhemorrhagic lesions were the best predictor for benign clinical course.[106]

Secondary Injuries

Much of the morbidity and mortality associated with TBI relates to secondary injuries. Mass effect from hematoma or cerebral swelling in a fixed intracranial volume causes increased intracranial pressure and can lead to herniation. Herniation refers to the displacement of brain parenchyma into a different compartment. Subfalcine herniation (see **Fig. 11**A) occurs when the cingulate gyrus is displaced beneath the free edge of the falx cerebri. It can lead to further complications including distal anterior cerebral artery territory infarcts[107] (the callosomarginal branch runs along the cingulate sulcus) and contralateral hydrocephalus secondary

to obstruction of the foramen of Monro. Uncal herniation (**Fig. 12**) occurs when downward pressure forces the medial temporal lobes to descend below the tentorial incisura into the ambient cistern where they compress the brainstem or posterior cerebral artery.[108] Mass lesions or edema in the posterior fossa can result in upward herniation of the superior cerebellum through the incisura and compress the superior cerebellar arteries. Increased pressure from above can force the cerebellar tonsils inferiorly into the foramen magnum causing mass effect on the medulla and compression of the posterior inferior cerebellar arteries.

Downward transtentorial herniation can lead to BSI secondary to mechanical compression. Duret hemorrhages (see **Fig. 12**B, C) are typically centrally located collections of blood in the tegmentum of the rostral pons and midbrain associated with a grim prognosis.[30,89–91,103,109–111] These secondary brainstem hemorrhages are thought to result from stretching/tearing of upper

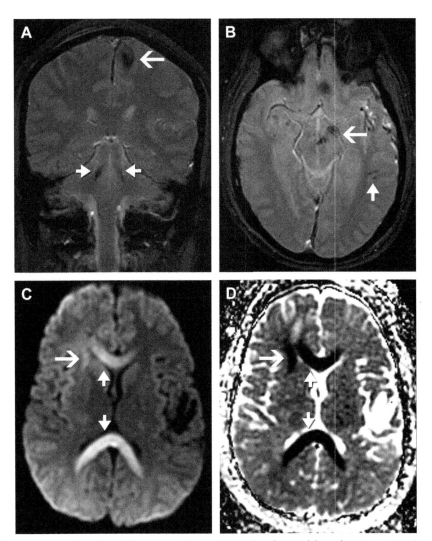

Fig. 10. MRI appearance of grade 3 diffuse axonal injury. MPGR (*A, B*), DWI (*C*), and ADC map MRI images of a 23-year-old man with head trauma after a motorcycle accident. MPGR images reveal foci of susceptibility in the subcortical white matter of the parietal (*A, unfilled arrow*) and temporal lobes (*B, closed arrow*) and infratentorial injury to the bilateral superior cerebellar peduncles (*A, closed arrows*) and midbrain and cerebral peduncle (*B, open arrow*) secondary to traumatic axonal injury. There are also extra-axial foci of susceptibility along the falx compatible with a subdural hematoma (*A, B*). DWI (*C*) and ADC map (*D*) from the same patient reveal marked reduced diffusion in the genu and splenium (*closed arrows*) of the corpus callosum also consistent with a combination of wallerian and axonal injury. Note how the entire right frontal lobe white matter shows abnormal reduced diffusion (*unfilled arrow* in *C, D*), with a more focal insult to the anterior subinsular region.

brainstem penetrating arteries during sudden downward transtentorial herniation.[30,103,110,111] Focal brainstem infarcts may also occur via the same mechanism.[30,103,112]

Both CT and MRI are excellent at evaluating for herniation and hydrocephalus, although MRI performs better in the posterior fossa where CT is limited by beam-hardening artifact.[82] Signs of herniation include midline shift, effacement of the basilar cisterns and cerebral sulci, and (often contralateral) ventricular entrapment.[113]

Hypoxic-ischemic brain injury typically results from a period of catastrophic cardiac or vascular compromise. On imaging it is associated with diffuse cerebral swelling and edema. Classic CT signs include the gray-white reversal sign[114] (ie, the white matter appears denser than the gray matter) and pseudo-SAH[115] (ie, the perimesencephalic and sylvian cisterns appear hyperdense to brain; the falx and tentorium also appear abnormally hyperdense). On MRI, the earliest imaging abnormality is reduced diffusion, particularly in

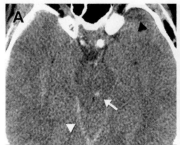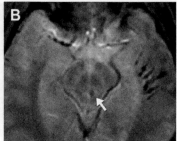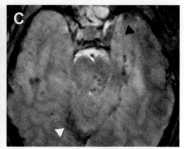

Fig. 11. CT and MRI appearance of brainstem injury with diffuse axonal injury. Axial noncontrast CT (*A*) and T2*-weighted MPGR MRI (*B, C*) images of 27-year-old man reveal posttraumatic brainstem injury. Hemorrhagic axonal injury in the midbrain tegmentum appears as rounded hyperdensity on CT (*A, arrow*) and as a focal area of susceptibility on MPGR sequence (*B, arrow*). Caudally, an axial MPGR image through the pons (*C*) reveals multiple additional foci of susceptibility in the dorsal pons that were not apparent on CT. Numerous additional foci of abnormal susceptibility (*B, C*) are present in the bilateral temporal supratentorial and infratentorial white matter consistent with diffuse axonal injury. Also note traumatic injuries including a right tentorial subdural hematoma (*white arrowheads*) and a left anterior temporal contusion (*black arrowheads*), which are better appreciated on MRI (*C*) than CT (*A*).

the cerebral cortex, cerebellar hemispheres, and basal ganglia.[116] Diffuse hypoxic-ischemic BSI usually occurs in conjunction with supratentorial ischemic injury. Brainstem involvement is usually a late event because the brainstem is usually spared until just before death.[30]

Vascular Injury

Traumatic arterial injury can result from several mechanisms including laceration by fracture fragments, blunt or penetrating trauma, vascular compression from brain herniation, and arterial strain.[27,117–119] Intracranial internal carotid artery (ICA) and vertebral segments are much less likely to suffer injury than the cervical segments.[120] Skull base fractures are among the most common causes of arterial injury; the presence of basilar fractures on NCCT should always prompt consideration of CTA or MRA for further evaluation.[117] Conventional angiography may be necessary in some cases, particularly when the lesion is subtle or endovascular therapy is the treatment of choice (eg, severe hemorrhage, epistaxis, or carotid-cavernous fistula [CCF]).

Arterial dissection

Dissection occurs when damage to the arterial intima allows blood products to accumulate within the vessel wall (intramural hematoma), which may narrow or occlude the lumen.[117] The intracranial ICAs are most vulnerable to fracture-related dissections and occlusions adjacent to the anterior clinoid process and clinocarotid canal.[35,117,118,121,122] Carotid injury in this region is associated with high incidence of concurrent traumatic optic nerve injury and vice versa, so injury to one of these structures should prompt increased

attention to the other.[27,35] Injuries of the vertebral arteries are also frequently encountered, producing a similar spectrum of injuries as seen with the carotid arteries.[117] These most commonly include traumatic dissection, laceration, and arteriovenous fistula (AVF).[117]

On CTA and MRA sequences, arterial dissection (**Fig. 13**) is identified by eccentric narrowing of the vascular lumen with an overall slight increase in the external diameter of the artery.[120] The addition of thin (<3 mm) T1WI with fat-saturation to highlight T1-shortening (beginning 48 hours after injury) within the subacute intramural hematoma is helpful to establish definitive vessel occlusion or dissection, which may obviate catheter angiography.[35] MRI with DWI is also excellent at identifying associated cerebral infarction related to distal emboli or decreased cerebral perfusion.

Traumatic pseudoaneurysm

Pseudoaneurysms occur when a tear in the inner wall of a vessel is covered by an intact outer adventitial layer.[35,117,118,121–123] These false aneurysms can develop gradually over a period of a few weeks to a few years. Symptoms, if any, are usually related to suprasellar mass effect causing vision changes and cranial neuropathies, epistaxis, or intermittent ischemic events caused by embolization of clot.[35,117,118,121,122] On NCCT, pseudoaneurysms appear as hyperdense round masses adjacent to vessels, but they may also have a somewhat irregular morphology (**Fig. 14**). Appearance of a nonacute pseudoaneurysm on MRI may vary, but generally it is identified by concentric laminated rings of hemorrhage in various stages of evolution.[35] A patent vessel lumen can usually be recognized by its associated

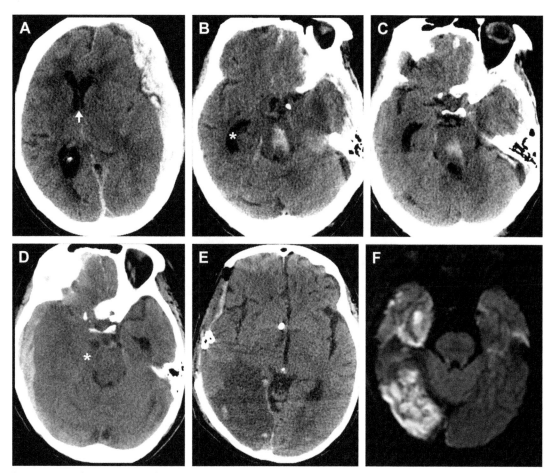

Fig. 12. Secondary traumatic brain injuries in patients with TBI. Axial noncontrast CT images (*A–C*) from an 80-year-old woman reveal left convexity holohemispheric and parafalcine subdural hematomas. Secondary complications resulting from mass effect from the hematomas include left to right midline shift (*arrow* shows position of the septum pelucidum) with subfalcine herniation (*A*), left uncal and downward transtentorial herniation (*B, C*), trapping of the temporal horn (*asterisk*) of the right lateral ventricle secondary to obstruction of the foramen of Monro (*B, C*), and a Duret hemorrhage in the midbrain (*B*) and pons (*C*). Images from a different patient show secondary complications in a 74-year-old woman after TBI. The preoperative noncontrast CT (*D*) images demonstrate mass effect from a right holohemispheric subdural hematoma resulting in right uncal herniation and trapping of the temporal horn of the left lateral ventricle. The right temporal horn is nearly midline in location (*asterisk*). The postoperative noncontrast CT obtained later that evening (*E*) reveals a decompressive craniectomy, ventricular drain placement, and a new large hypodensity involving the territory of the right posterior cerebral artery (PCA) vascular territory, consistent with infarction. Diffusion-weighted MRI (*F*) obtained 4 days after initial injury confirms the right PCA territory infarct, secondary to compression of the proximal PCA by the previously herniated right uncus.

flow void.[35] The tendency of these lesions to present long after trauma can lead to diagnostic confusion; familiarity with their imaging appearance is important to facilitate rapid intervention and prevent potentially catastrophic biopsy of these pseudotumors.

Carotid-cavernous fistula

The CCF is an AVF that results from a full-thickness arterial tear of the ICA located within the cavernous sinus. This allows high-pressure arterial blood direct access into the low-pressure cavernous sinus venous system.[35,117,119,124] The CCF is divided into direct and indirect types based on arterial supply. The direct CCF, as the name implies, features direct communication between the cavernous ICA and cavernous sinus. In the indirect CCF, connection between the carotid system and the cavernous sinus usually occurs via small branches of the external carotid artery or

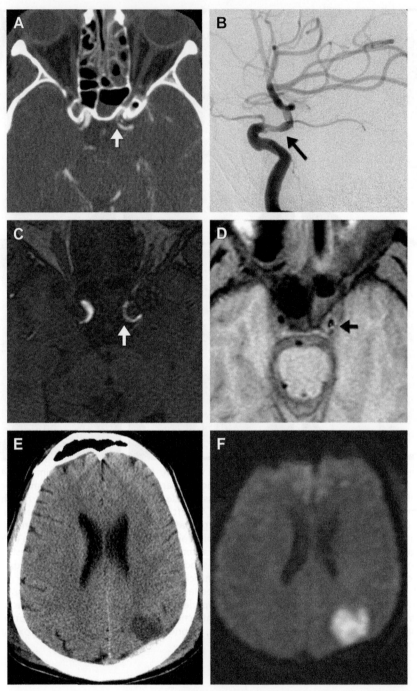

Fig. 13. Traumatic vascular dissection of the supraclinoid internal carotid artery. CTA (*A*) performed the day after injury shows asymmetric narrowing and luminal irregularity of the left ICA (*arrow*) just beyond the anterior clinoid process concerning for traumatic dissection. Note the air-hemorrhage level within the left sphenoid sinus (*A*), which should raise suspicion of anterior skull base fracture (not shown) and potential injury to the adjacent carotid artery. Dissection of the left supraclinoid ICA was confirmed the same day on digital subtraction angiography (*B*), which again revealed an irregular, narrowed lumen (*arrow*). Time of flight MRI angiogram (*C*) performed 3 days after injury shows a narrowed irregular lumen of the left supraclinoid ICA (*arrow*). T1WI (*D*) from the same examination reveals subtle T1-shortening (*arrow*) in the left ICA wall, consistent with early subacute methemoglobin blood products within a dissecting intramural hematoma. Noncontrast CT (*E*) and diffusion-weighted MRI (*F*) obtained 2 and 3 days after injury, respectively, show that the patient's dissection was complicated by an acute left middle cerebral artery territory embolic infarction.

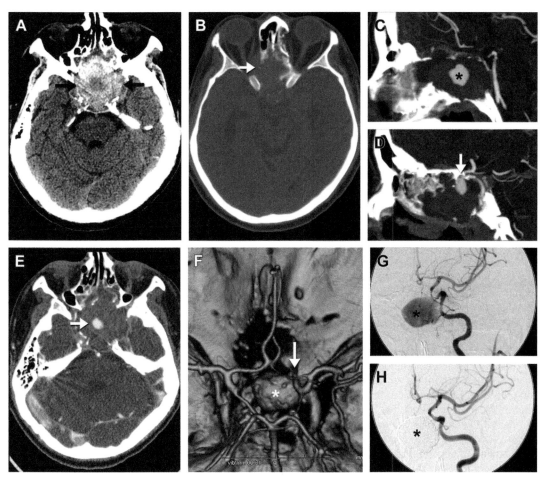

Fig. 14. Postraumatic pseudoaneurysm. This 43-year-old man presented with headache and visual symptoms 3 months after suffering facial fractures in a motor vehicle accident. Noncontrast CT reveals a large hyperdense mass (*arrows*) within the anterior skull base (*A*) eroding the sphenoid bone, sella, and the orbits (*arrow*) (*B*). Sagittal reformatted CT angiography images performed the same day show the central area of the mass enhancing (*asterisk*) to the same extent as the adjacent intracranial arteries (*C*). In addition, there is an apparent narrow-necked connection (*arrow*) between the enhancing portion and the left cavernous internal carotid artery (*D*), consistent with a pseudoaneurysm. Note that the central low density (*A*) within the higher density, thrombosed portion of the pseudoaneurysm correlates with the central nonthrombosed, enhancing area (*E, arrow*) on the postcontrast images. 3D reformatted images of the circle of Willis (*F*) highlight the relationship of the pseudoaneurysm (*asterisk*; note that only the nonthrombosed portion is visualized) to the left internal carotid artery (*arrow*). Catheter angiography images following injection of the left internal carotid artery show the appearance of the pseudoaneurysm (*asterisk*) before (*G*) and after (*H*) treatment with endovascular coil embolization.

extracavernous ICA. Nearly all direct CCFs occur secondary to trauma, whereas indirect CCF are much more likely to be nontraumatic.

The imaging appearance of the CCF depends the amount of flow shunted and the patient's venous collateral anatomy. High-flow lesions are suggested on CT and MRI imaging by enlargement of the ipsilateral cavernous sinus and surrounding venous structures, such as the superior ophthalmic vein and petrosal sinuses.[117] On a properly timed CTA, asymmetric early enhancement of the affected cavernous sinus and its draining veins may also be noted.[125] On MRI, abnormal flow voids connoting rapid flow may be seen within these enlarged draining veins,[119,122] and abnormal flow-related enhancement may be noted on MRA. Proptosis, extraocular muscle enlargement, stranding of the retro-orbital fat, and orbital preseptal soft tissue swelling may be identified because of elevated capillary and venous pressure. Bilateral enlargement of the superior ophthalmic veins is a classic finding indicating free communication of the fistula through the cavernous plexus of veins.[117] However, when the fistula drains predominately via the inferior petrosal sinus, the superior ophthalmic vein may not be abnormally enlarged. Less common "low flow" CCFs occur when the arterial source is a small-caliber intracavernous branch of the ICA rather than the cavernous ICA itself. Cross-sectional imaging findings may be much less obvious in these cases and conventional arteriography may be required for definitive diagnosis and potential endovascular treatment.

Dural arteriovenous fistula

Dural AVFs are rarely traumatic in etiology, although they can occur when an injured artery forms a connection with an adjacent draining vein or venous sinus. Most case reports in the literature involve a skull fracture that lacerates the middle meningeal artery and its associated venae comitantes.[126,127] These patients may not develop an EDH as would be expected with middle meningeal artery injury because the arterial extravasation evacuates through a dural (meningeal artery-to-meningeal vein) fistula. These injuries may remain asymptomatic or come to attention during work-up for tinnitus months later because of increased flow through the petrosal sinuses and internal jugular vein. Contrast-enhanced CT and conventional MRI findings in these cases are usually limited to venous distention.

Arterial spin labelling (ASL) is a promising, relatively new, advanced MRI technique used to measure cerebral perfusion. ASL electromagnetically tags arterial blood water proximal to the brain, which is used as a diffusible tracer to quantify blood flow. Typically, the labelling signal degrades before tagged water molecules can pass through the capillary bed into draining veins; however, in an AVF, the capillary bed is bypassed by the fistula connecting the artery directly to the vein. Therefore, the presence of ASL signal within venous structures should raise concern for an AVF. Indeed, one recent study found that inclusion of ASL sequences may improve sensitivity for small AVFs.[128]

Cerebral fat embolism syndrome

Comorbid long bone fractures are not infrequent with TBI polytrauma. The exact pathogenesis of cerebral fat emboli is controversial, but one favored hypothesis is traumatic introduction of bone marrow fat into the systemic and pulmonary circulations. Neurologic symptoms may include focal neurologic signs or generalized encephalopathy, which can range from drowsiness to coma.[129] The imaging manifestations are best appreciated on MRI as patchy or confluent regions of vasogenic edema involving deep white matter, basal ganglia, corpus callosum, and cerebellar hemispheres.[130–132] In addition, because of the embolic phenomenon, cytotoxic injury with reduced diffusion has been described.[133] As a manifestation of cerebral fat embolism syndrome (CFES), a diffuse pattern of multiple microsusceptibility lesions may be observed on GRE or SWI sequences related to microhemorrhage and/or secondary vascular stasis with increased intravascular deoxyhemoglobin content and microthrombi formation (**Fig. 15**). The MRI appearance may mimic that of TAI, which often coexists. Distinguishing between these two considerations may have management and prognostic implications.[133] Importantly, although TAI is present immediately after injury, CFES usually occurs in a slightly delayed fashion 48 to 72 hours after injury,[134] and is often associated with the characteristic pulmonary and cutaneous manifestations of CFES. On imaging, hemorrhagic TAI is usually irregular in size and distribution, with clustered foci of axonal injury in characteristic locations (juxtacortical, splenium, dorsal pons, and midbrain), whereas lesions related to CFES are more symmetric, uniform, and diffuse in appearance, consistent with a mechanism of cardioembolic showering. In addition, TAI is uncommon in the cerebellum, whereas it is a common location for CFES. The role of advanced imaging techniques, such as diffusion tensor imaging (DTI), for characterizing CFES is an area of active investigation.

ROLE OF ADVANCED IMAGING TECHNIQUES

Advanced imaging techniques are areas of active research and development and are currently targeted to two main areas: evaluating mTBI and obtaining prognostic information for all levels of TBI severity. Although promising, these techniques are limited for current clinical applications.[37] Presently, none of these advanced MRI techniques are recommended by the American College of Radiology appropriateness guidelines for routine evaluation of the patient with TBI.[11] Nevertheless, familiarity with these modalities and their application is worthwhile because they may benefit subsets of current patients and will likely be increasingly used in the future.

Diffusion Tensor Imaging

The discovery that diffusion of water molecules in cerebral white matter is directionally dependent (anisotropic), with the favored direction of diffusion parallel to the direction of axonal tracts in the brain, laid the foundation for DTI in the brain.[135]

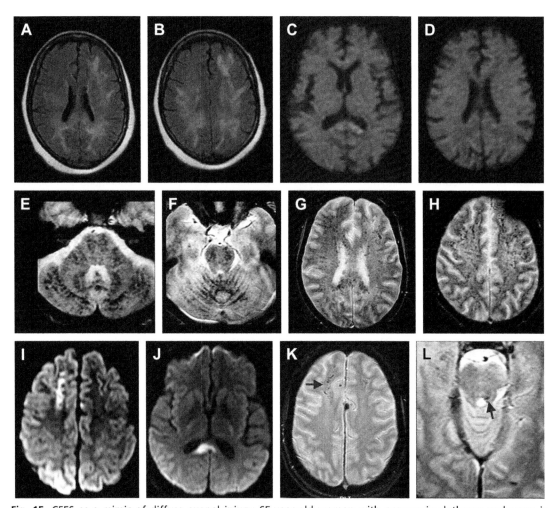

Fig. 15. CFES as a mimic of diffuse axonal injury: 65-year-old woman with progressive lethargy and coma in setting of multiple bone infarcts and cerebral fat embolism syndrome confirmed on autopsy. Axial FLAIR (*A, B*) and DWI (*C, D*) demonstrate confluent FLAIR hyperintense white matter signal abnormality with relatively little diffusion signal abnormality, which is isolated to the splenium of the corpus callosum. Axial susceptibility-weighted imaging (*E–H*) reveal innumerable foci of susceptibility artifact throughout the infratentorial and supratentorial brain consistent with a pattern of cardioembolic showering with resultant microhemorrhages. In comparison, axial DWI (*I, J*) from a brain MRI performed on a 42-year-old man 7 days after a motor vehicle collision shows clustered, confluent foci of reduced diffusion most prominent in the right juxtacortical frontal lobe and splenium of the corpus callosum related to diffuse axonal injury. T2*-weighted gradient echo sequences (*K, L*) reveal asymmetric clustered foci of susceptibility artifact in the right greater than left juxtacortical frontal lobe white matter (*K, arrow*) and dorsal pontomedullary junction near the left superior cerebellar peduncle (*L, arrow*). Compared with CFES, susceptibility artifact secondary to diffuse axonal injury tends to be more sparse, clustered, and irregular in distribution. In addition, CFES more commonly affects the cerebellum.

These properties have led to a great deal excitement for DTI as a potential biomarker for white matter pathology, including TBI.[136] DTI builds on conventional DWI by adding the ability to determine the 3D directionality and magnitude (tensor) of water motion. This is accomplished by acquiring at least six (but usually many more) noncollinear diffusion gradient directions. DTI can quantify diffusion using a variety of parameters, the most common of which are fractional anisotropy (FA), which quantifies the degree of anisotropy within a voxel, and mean diffusivity (MD), which quantifies the average magnitude of diffusivity over all sampled directions.

A complete review of the DTI literature related to TBI is beyond the scope of this article; for greater depth, there are several excellent reviews recently published on this topic.[136–138] To date, attempts to make generalizable conclusions about DTI in TBI in a single individual have been hindered by heterogeneity in study design with respect to patient populations, imaging parameters, analysis techniques, and imaging time points.[136] Although most studies of TBI have reported increases in MD and decreases in FA in areas of injury,[139–147] studies of acute/semiacute TBI can also be found in literature that report affected white matter FA values that are normal[148] and/or decreased[22,149] relative to normal controls. In part, these discrepancies likely reflect the intrinsic heterogeneity of TBI, although they also highlight the need for larger studies with standardized imaging and analysis protocols and consistent and proper outcome measures.[136]

Group analyses of patients with TBI have validated DTI as a robust measure of TAI at that level.[137] These studies have found abnormal MD and FA frontal and temporal lobe association areas that correlate with behavioral and cognitive outcome measures at follow-up.[22,142,150] A recent study of patients with mTBI by Yuh and colleagues[22] demonstrated that the prognostic utility of DTI parameters surpassed CT, clinical, demographic, and socioeconomic variables as predictors of 3- and 6-month outcome at group and individual patient levels. Such studies highlight the potential of DTI for diagnostic and prognostic purposes in individual patients and may soon lead to consensus guidelines for use of DTI parameters in TBI imaging.

Perfusion Imaging

TBI is associated with impaired cerebrovascular autoregulation, increased permeability of the blood-brain barrier, and vascular injuries, all of which can lead to altered cerebral blood flow, ischemia, and even infarction.[151] For these reasons, cerebral perfusion has long been a target for imaging interrogation. Numerous techniques have been used in the literature including single-photon emission CT (SPECT),[152–155] PET,[156] xenon-enhanced CT,[157] perfusion CT,[158] dynamic susceptibility contrast (DSC),[159] and ASL[160,161] perfusion MRI. Each of these techniques have relative advantages and disadvantages. SPECT and DSC perfusion studies only allow qualitative comparison between regions of the brain,[37] whereas $^{15}O_2$ PET, xenon-enhanced CT, perfusion CT, and ASL are quantitatively accurate. Xenon-enhanced CT and $^{15}O_2$ PET require specialized and expensive equipment that is not widely available, and in the case of $^{15}O_2$ the extremely short half-life of ^{15}O (2 minutes).

A large proportion of the current data relating to brain perfusion after TBI is derived from 99mTc-HMPAO SPECT,[152–155] xenon-enhanced CT, and perfusion CT imaging studies.[157,158] In these studies, regional hypoperfusion correlates with injury severity; favorable outcomes are seen in patients with TBI with hyperemia on baseline imaging, whereas oligemia portends a poor outcome.[157,158] Of these study types, perfusion CT is the most readily available; however, it requires repeated imaging over a narrow band of skull and does contribute to increased radiation dose.

Fewer studies have evaluated the utility of perfusion-weighted MRI techniques in TBI. The most common used MRI perfusion technique is DSC imaging. Using this technique, Garnett and colleagues[159] measured reduced cerebral blood volume in areas of contusion, and in a subset of patients with normal-appearing brain parenchyma. Although the sample size in this study was small, reduced cerebral blood volume was noted on DSC MRI, even in those patients with an otherwise normal MRI, and this correlated with worse clinical outcome.[159] ASL is an alternative MRI perfusion technique that does not require intravenous contrast (see technical description in the vascular injury section.) In patients with mTBI undergoing ASL imaging, decreased regional cerebral blood flow in the thalamus was found to be strongly correlated with neurocognitive impairment.[160,161] Although these studies were underpowered to evaluate prognostic capacity of ASL perfusion in patients with mTBI, the findings are enticing. As with other advanced imaging techniques, more prospective and longitudinal studies are needed to determine the role of perfusion imaging for TBI evaluation.

Magnetic Resonance Spectroscopy

Magnetic resonance spectroscopy (MRS) allows for quantification of certain tissue metabolites in vivo with standard clinical MRI hardware.[162,163] Most clinically relevant MRS applications use signal from the hydrogen proton (^1H) because of its natural abundance within biologic molecules of interest. This technique produces spectra with peaks corresponding to specific metabolites within a prescribed region of interest or voxel. The peaks for particular metabolites have characteristic locations along a spectrum (chemical shift) and their concentrations are measured as the area under their respective peak.

Spectroscopic analysis is performed on tissue within a single cubic volume of interest (single-voxel spectroscopy) or within a multivoxel grid placed over a larger region of interest (chemical shift imaging or MRS). Commonly measured metabolites in the brain include *N*-acetylaspartate

(NAA), a marker of neuronal viability; lactate, a marker of anaerobic glycolysis; choline (Cho), a marker of cellular membrane turnover; creatinine (Cr), a molecule involved in cellular energy use; myoinositol, a marker of membrane turnover and possibly reactive gliosis; and glutamate and glutamine (Glx), markers of excitatory neurotransmission. Cr, often used as a denominator to normalize the other peaks, should be interpreted with caution in MRS studies because its concentration can be altered after TBI.

Spectroscopic studies performed shortly after TBI show a consistent imaging pattern manifested by increased Cho and decreased NAA in regions of the adult brain known to be most susceptible to shear injury, such as the splenium of the corpus callosum and centrum semiovale.[164,165] These metabolic alterations are thought to reflect TAI, particularly when they occur in the absence of visible injury on conventional anatomic imaging.[166–169] Longitudinal studies in patients with mTBI have shown these changes to be transient with normalization of NAA, Cho, and Glx peaks.[165] Interestingly, Cho and myoinositol peaks remain elevated in the chronic stage, which has been attributed to proliferative astrogliosis.[170] For severe TBI, elevated Cho peaks in the parietal white matter, and elevated Glx peaks in the occipital gray matter, 7 days after injury have been shown to have prognostic value with respect to clinical outcome.[163,171] In children, the presence of abnormal lactate, Cho, and NAA is associated with poor long-term neuropsychological outcomes.[172,173] Evidence correlating MRS findings and mTBI outcomes is more limited. A recent prospective study found that centrum semiovale Cr levels positively correlated with decreased performance on neuropsychiatric metrics assessed 6 months after injury.[174] Clinical applications for MRS in TBI are also limited by significant overlap in spectral changes seen in several other brain disorders, lowering its specificity.

Positron Emission Tomography and Single-Photon Emission Computed Tomography

PET and SPECT are composed of tracer molecules tagged with radioisotopes and are typically used to image physiologic processes. Early studies using PET and SPECT in TBI primarily focused on perfusion imaging and metabolic imaging, primarily with fluorodeoxyglucose-PET.[175] Although the current clinical utility for these techniques in TBI is limited, they have a great deal of potential.[37] For example, recent studies have shown potential for PET radiotracers targeting tau and amyloid plaques,[176,177] which are known

to occur chronic traumatic encephalopathy, a form of chronic TBI. Like most areas of advanced imaging of TBI, these studies involve only small patient numbers and further validation is needed before they can clinically be used routinely.

DISCUSSION

Significant recent advances have been made in the imaging of TBI; still, there is much to improve. Advanced techniques, such as DTI, PET, and functional MRI hold a great deal of potential, and with more clinical validation and larger studies they will likely move from primarily research modalities to routine clinical use. Several specific injuries show particular promise for future innovations. Among these, mTBI and chronic traumatic encephalopathy are of interest because of their high prevalence and their lack of findings on conventional imaging. The ability to glean prognostic information from imaging studies is another promising area of active research. As new neurotherapeutic options for TBI are introduced, neuroimaging will likely guide which patients will benefit from these agents and also help follow their response to therapy.

REFERENCES

1. Faul MD, Xu L, Wald MM, et al. Traumatic brain injury in the United States: emergency department visits, hospitalizations and deaths 2002–2006. Atlanta (GA): Centers for Disease Control and Prevention; National Center for Injury Prevention and Control; 2010.
2. Menon DK, Schwab K, Wright DW, et al. Position statement: definition of traumatic brain injury. Arch Phys Med Rehabil 2010;91(11):1637–40.
3. Cornelius C, Crupi R, Calabrese V, et al. Traumatic brain injury: oxidative stress and neuroprotection. Antioxid Redox Signal 2013;19(8):836–53.
4. Readnower RD, Chavko M, Adeeb S, et al. Increase in blood–brain barrier permeability, oxidative stress, and activated microglia in a rat model of blast-induced traumatic brain injury. J Neurosci Res 2010;88(16):3530–9.
5. Hawryluk GWJ, Manley GT. Chapter 2-classification of traumatic brain injury: past, present, and future. In: Jordan G, Andres MS, editors. Handbook of clinical neurology, vol. 127. Elsevier; 2015. p. 15–21.
6. Lobato RD, Cordobes F, Rivas JJ, et al. Outcome from severe head injury related to the type of intracranial lesion. A computerized tomography study. J Neurosurg 1983;59(5):762–74.
7. Jennett B, Teasdale G, Braakman R, et al. Predicting outcome in individual patients after severe head injury. Lancet 1976;1(7968):1031–4.

8. Thurmond VA, Hicks R, Gleason T, et al. Advancing integrated research in psychological health and traumatic brain injury: common data elements. Arch Phys Med Rehabil 2010;91(11):1633–6.

9. Haacke EM, Duhaime AC, Gean AD, et al. Common data elements in radiologic imaging of traumatic brain injury. J Magn Reson Imaging 2010; 32(3):516–43.

10. Hicks R, Giacino J, Harrison-Felix C, et al. Progress in developing common data elements for traumatic brain injury research: version two–the end of the beginning. J Neurotrauma 2013;30(22):1852–61.

11. Vilaas S, Shetty M, Martin N, et al. ACR appropriateness criteria head trauma. American College of Radiology. Available at: https://acsearch.acr.org/docs/69481/Narrative/. Accessed November 18, 2015.

12. Maura E, Ryan M, Susan Palasis M, et al. ACR appropriateness criteria head trauma — child. American College of Radiology. Available at: https://acsearch.acr.org/docs/3083021/Narrative/. Accessed November 18, 2015.

13. Dunning J, Daly JP, Lomas J-P, et al. Derivation of the children's head injury algorithm for the prediction of important clinical events decision rule for head injury in children. Arch Dis Child 2006; 91(11):885–91.

14. Prabhu SP, Newton AW, Perez-Rossello JM, et al. Three-dimensional skull models as a problem-solving tool in suspected child abuse. Pediatr Radiol 2013;43(5):575–81.

15. Trenchs V, Curcoy AI, Castillo M, et al. Minor head trauma and linear skull fracture in infants: cranial ultrasound or computed tomography? Eur J Emerg Med 2009;16(3):150–2.

16. Ball WS Jr. Nonaccidental craniocerebral trauma (child abuse): MR imaging. Radiology 1989; 173(3):609–10.

17. Wintermark M, Sanelli PC, Anzai Y, et al. Imaging evidence and recommendations for traumatic brain injury: conventional neuroimaging techniques. J Am Coll Radiol 2015;12(2):e1–14.

18. Ro YS, Shin SD, Holmes JF, et al. Comparison of clinical performance of cranial computed tomography rules in patients with minor head injury: a multicenter prospective study. Acad Emerg Med 2011; 18(6):597–604.

19. Mower WR, Hoffman JR, Herbert M, et al. Developing a decision instrument to guide computed tomographic imaging of blunt head injury patients. J Trauma 2005;59(4):954–9.

20. Stiell IG, Wells GA, Vandemheen K, et al. The Canadian CT Head Rule for patients with minor head injury. Lancet 2001;357(9266):1391–6.

21. Haydel MJ, Preston CA, Mills TJ, et al. Indications for computed tomography in patients with minor head injury. N Engl J Med 2000;343(2):100–5.

22. Yuh EL, Cooper SR, Mukherjee P, et al. Diffusion tensor imaging for outcome prediction in mild traumatic brain injury: a TRACK-TBI study. J Neurotrauma 2014;31(17):1457–77.

23. Reljic T, Mahony H, Djulbegovic B, et al. Value of repeat head computed tomography after traumatic brain injury: systematic review and meta-analysis. J Neurotrauma 2014;31(1):78–98.

24. Washington CW, Grubb RL Jr. Are routine repeat imaging and intensive care unit admission necessary in mild traumatic brain injury? J Neurosurg 2012;116(3):549–57.

25. Menditto VG, Lucci M, Polonara S, et al. Management of minor head injury in patients receiving oral anticoagulant therapy: a prospective study of a 24-hour observation protocol. Ann Emerg Med 2012;59(6):451–5.

26. Kaen A, Jimenez-Roldan L, Arrese I, et al. The value of sequential computed tomography scanning in anticoagulated patients suffering from minor head injury. J Trauma 2010;68(4):895–8.

27. Gentry LR. Imaging of closed head injury. Radiology 1994;191(1):1–17.

28. Gentry LR, Godersky JC, Thompson B. MR imaging of head trauma: review of the distribution and radiopathologic features of traumatic lesions. AJR Am J Roentgenol 1988;150(3):663–72.

29. Gentry LR, Godersky JC, Thompson B, et al. Prospective comparative study of intermediate-field MR and CT in the evaluation of closed head trauma. AJR Am J Roentgenol 1988;150(3): 673–82.

30. Gentry LR, Godersky JC, Thompson BH. Traumatic brain stem injury: MR imaging. Radiology 1989; 171(1):177–87.

31. Gentry LR, Thompson B, Godersky JC. Trauma to the corpus callosum: MR features. AJNR Am J Neuroradiol 1988;9(6):1129–38.

32. Yuh EL, Hawryluk GW, Manley GT. Imaging concussion: a review. Neurosurgery 2014; 75(Suppl 4):S50–63.

33. Yuh EL, Mukherjee P, Lingsma HF, et al. Magnetic resonance imaging improves 3-month outcome prediction in mild traumatic brain injury. Ann Neurol 2013;73(2):224–35.

34. Le TH, Gean AD. Neuroimaging of traumatic brain injury. Mt Sinai J Med 2009;76(2):145–62.

35. Gentry LR. Facial trauma and associated brain damage. Radiol Clin North Am 1989;27(2): 435–46.

36. Bromberg WJ, Collier BC, Diebel LN, et al. Blunt cerebrovascular injury practice management guidelines: the eastern association for the surgery of trauma. J Trauma 2010;68(2):471–7.

37. Wintermark M, Sanelli PC, Anzai Y, et al. Imaging evidence and recommendations for traumatic brain injury: advanced neuro- and neurovascular

imaging techniques. AJNR Am J Neuroradiol 2015; 36(2):E1–11.

38. Cohen AR, Caruso P, Duhaime AC, et al. Feasibility of "rapid" magnetic resonance imaging in pediatric acute head injury. Am J Emerg Med 2015;33(7): 887–90.

39. Wei SC, Ulmer S, Lev MH, et al. Value of coronal reformations in the CT evaluation of acute head trauma. AJNR Am J Neuroradiol 2010; 31(2):334–9.

40. Zacharia TT, Nguyen DD. Subtle pathology detection with multidetector row coronal and sagittal CT reformations in acute head trauma. Emerg Radiol 2010;17(2):97–102.

41. Haacke EM, Mittal S, Wu Z, et al. Susceptibility-weighted imaging: technical aspects and clinical applications, Part 1. AJNR Am J Neuroradiol 2009;30(1):19–30.

42. Wang X, Xie H, Cotton AS, et al. Early cortical thickness changes after mild traumatic brain injury following motor vehicle collision. J Neurotrauma 2015;32(7):455–63.

43. Liu AY, Maldjian JA, Bagley LJ, et al. Traumatic brain injury: diffusion-weighted MR imaging findings. AJNR Am J Neuroradiol 1999;20(9): 1636–41.

44. Huisman TA. Diffusion-weighted imaging: basic concepts and application in cerebral stroke and head trauma. Eur Radiol 2003;13(10):2283–97.

45. Lang DA, Hadley DM, Teasdale GM, et al. Gadolinium DTPA enhanced magnetic resonance imaging in acute head injury. Acta Neurochir 1991; 109(1–2):5–11.

46. Gomori JM, Grossman RI, Goldberg HI, et al. Intracranial hematomas: imaging by high-field MR. Radiology 1985;157(1):87–93.

47. Zimmerman RA, Bilaniuk LT. Computed tomographic staging of traumatic epidural bleeding. Radiology 1982;144(4):809–12.

48. Baykaner K, Alp H, Ceviker N, et al. Observation of 95 patients with extradural hematoma and review of the literature. Surg Neurol 1988;30(5):339–41.

49. Lobato RD, Rivas JJ, Cordobes F, et al. Acute epidural hematoma: an analysis of factors influencing the outcome of patients undergoing surgery in coma. J Neurosurg 1988;68(1):48–57.

50. Bricolo AP, Pasut LM. Extradural hematoma: toward zero mortality. A prospective study. Neurosurgery 1984;14(1):8–12.

51. Servadei F, Faccani G, Roccella P, et al. Asymptomatic extradural haematomas. Results of a multicenter study of 158 cases in minor head injury. Acta Neurochir 1989;96(1–2):39–45.

52. Knuckey NW, Gelbard S, Epstein MH. The management of "asymptomatic" epidural hematomas. A prospective study. J Neurosurg 1989;70(3): 392–6.

53. Al-Nakshabandi NA. The swirl sign. Radiology 2001;218(2):433.

54. Gean AD, Fischbein NJ, Purcell DD, et al. Benign anterior temporal epidural hematoma: indolent lesion with a characteristic CT imaging appearance after blunt head trauma. Radiology 2010; 257(1):212–8.

55. Milo R, Razon N, Schiffer J. Delayed epidural hematoma. A review. Acta Neurochir 1987;84(1–2):13–23.

56. Pozzati E, Tognetti F, Cavallo M, et al. Extradural hematomas of the posterior cranial fossa. Observations on a series of 32 consecutive cases treated after the introduction of computed tomography scanning. Surg Neurol 1989;32(4):300–3.

57. Gennarelli TA, Spielman GM, Langfitt TW, et al. Influence of the type of intracranial lesion on outcome from severe head injury. J Neurosurg 1982;56(1): 26–32.

58. Holbourn AHS. Mechanics of head injuries. Lancet 1943;2:438–41.

59. Holbourn AHS. The mechanics of brain injuries. Br Med Bull 1945;3:147–9.

60. Cooper PR. Post-traumatic Intracranial Mass Lesions. In: Cooper PR, editor. Head injury. 2nd edition. Baltimore: Williams & Wilkins; 1987.

61. Seelig JM, Becker DP, Miller JD, et al. Traumatic acute subdural hematoma: major mortality reduction in comatose patients treated within four hours. N Engl J Med 1981;304(25):1511–8.

62. Sato Y, Yuh WT, Smith WL, et al. Head injury in child abuse: evaluation with MR imaging. Radiology 1989;173(3):653–7.

63. Bruce DA, Zimmerman RA. Shaken impact syndrome. Pediatr Ann 1989;18(8):482–4, 486-489, 492-484.

64. Zimmerman RA, Bilaniuk LT, Bruce D, et al. Computed tomography of craniocerebral injury in the abused child. Radiology 1979; 130(3):687–90.

65. Cohen RA, Kaufman RA, Myers PA, et al. Cranial computed tomography in the abused child with head injury. AJR Am J Roentgenol 1986;146(1): 97–102.

66. Zimmerman RA, Bilaniuk LT, Grossman RI, et al. Resistive NMR of intracranial hematomas. Neuroradiology 1985;27(1):16–20.

67. Murray GD, Teasdale GM, Braakman R, et al. The European Brain Injury consortium survey of head injuries. Acta Neurochir 1999;141(3):223–36.

68. Servadei F, Murray GD, Teasdale GM, et al. Traumatic subarachnoid hemorrhage: demographic and clinical study of 750 patients from the European brain injury consortium survey of head injuries. Neurosurgery 2002;50(2):261–7 [discussion: 267–9].

69. Chakeres DW, Bryan RN. Acute subarachnoid hemorrhage: in vitro comparison of magnetic

resonance and computed tomography. AJNR Am J Neuroradiol 1986;7(2):223–8.

70. Bradley WG Jr, Schmidt PG. Effect of methemoglobin formation on the MR appearance of subarachnoid hemorrhage. Radiology 1985;156(1):99–103.

71. Stuckey SL, Goh TD, Heffernan T, et al. Hyperintensity in the subarachnoid space on FLAIR MRI. AJR Am J Roentgenol 2007;189(4):913–21.

72. Maeda M, Yagishita A, Yamamoto T, et al. Abnormal hyperintensity within the subarachnoid space evaluated by fluid-attenuated inversion-recovery MR imaging: a spectrum of central nervous system diseases. Eur Radiol 2003;13(Suppl 4):L192–201.

73. Mitchell P, Wilkinson ID, Hoggard N, et al. Detection of subarachnoid haemorrhage with magnetic resonance imaging. J Neurol Neurosurg Psychiatry 2001;70(2):205–11.

74. van Gijn J, Kerr RS, Rinkel GJ. Subarachnoid haemorrhage. Lancet 2007;369(9558):306–18.

75. Tha KK, Terae S, Kudo K, et al. Differential diagnosis of hyperintense cerebrospinal fluid on fluid-attenuated inversion recovery images of the brain. Part II: non-pathological conditions. Br J Radiol 2009;82(979):610–4.

76. Verma RK, Kottke R, Andereggen L, et al. Detecting subarachnoid hemorrhage: comparison of combined FLAIR/SWI versus CT. Eur J Radiol 2013;82(9):1539–45.

77. Mata-Mbemba D, Mugikura S, Nakagawa A, et al. Intraventricular hemorrhage on initial computed tomography as marker of diffuse axonal injury after traumatic brain injury. J Neurotrauma 2015;32(5):359–65.

78. Lloyd KM, DelGaudio JM, Hudgins PA. Imaging of skull base cerebrospinal fluid leaks in adults. Radiology 2008;248(3):725–36.

79. Yuh EL, Dillon WP. Intracranial hypotension and intracranial hypertension. Neuroimaging Clin N Am 2010;20(4):597–617.

80. Stone JA, Castillo M, Neelon B, et al. Evaluation of CSF leaks: high-resolution CT compared with contrast-enhanced CT and radionuclide cisternography. AJNR Am J Neuroradiol 1999;20(4):706–12.

81. Glaubitt D, Haubrich J, Cordoni-Voutsas M. Detection and quantitation of intermittent CSF rhinorrhea during prolonged cisternography with 111In-DTPA. AJNR Am J Neuroradiol 1983;4(3):560–3.

82. Kim JJ, Gean AD. Imaging for the diagnosis and management of traumatic brain injury. Neurotherapeutics 2011;8(1):39–53.

83. Venkatasubramanian C, Kleinman JT, Fischbein NJ, et al. Natural history and prognostic value of corticospinal tract Wallerian degeneration in intracerebral hemorrhage. Journal of the American Heart Association 2013;2(4):e000090.

84. Jayakumar PN, Kolluri VR, Basavakumar DG, et al. Prognosis in traumatic basal ganglia haematoma. Acta Neurochir 1989;97(3–4):114–6.

85. Colquhoun IR, Rawlinson J. The significance of haematomas of the basal ganglia in closed head injury. Clin Radiol 1989;40(6):619–21.

86. Katz DI, Alexander MP, Seliger GM, et al. Traumatic basal ganglia hemorrhage: clinicopathologic features and outcome. Neurology 1989;39(7):897–904.

87. Wada R, Aviv RI, Fox AJ, et al. CT angiography "spot sign" predicts hematoma expansion in acute intracerebral hemorrhage. Stroke 2007;38(4):1257–62.

88. Park SY, Kong MH, Kim JH, et al. Role of 'spot sign' on CT angiography to predict hematoma expansion in spontaneous intracerebral hemorrhage. J Korean Neurosurg Soc 2010;48(5):399–405.

89. Adams H, Mitchell DE, Graham DI, et al. Diffuse brain damage of immediate impact type. Its relationship to 'primary brain-stem damage' in head injury. Brain 1977;100(3):489–502.

90. Adams JH, Graham DI, Murray LS, et al. Diffuse axonal injury due to nonmissile head injury in humans: an analysis of 45 cases. Ann Neurol 1982;12(6):557–63.

91. Adams JH, Graham DI, Scott G, et al. Brain damage in fatal non-missile head injury. J Clin Pathol 1980;33(12):1132–45.

92. Meythaler JM, Peduzzi JD, Eleftheriou E, et al. Current concepts: diffuse axonal injury–associated traumatic brain injury. Arch Phys Med Rehabil 2001;82(10):1461–71.

93. Mittl RL, Grossman RI, Hiehle JF, et al. Prevalence of MR evidence of diffuse axonal injury in patients with mild head injury and normal head CT findings. AJNR Am J Neuroradiol 1994;15(8):1583–9.

94. Orrison WW, Gentry LR, Stimac GK, et al. Blinded comparison of cranial CT and MR in closed head injury evaluation. AJNR Am J Neuroradiol 1994;15(2):351–6.

95. Kinoshita T, Moritani T, Hiwatashi A, et al. Conspicuity of diffuse axonal injury lesions on diffusion-weighted MR imaging. Eur J Radiol 2005;56(1):5–11.

96. Moen KG, Brezova V, Skandsen T, et al. Traumatic axonal injury: the prognostic value of lesion load in corpus callosum, brain stem, and thalamus in different magnetic resonance imaging sequences. J Neurotrauma 2014;31(17):1486–96.

97. Schaefer PW, Huisman TA, Sorensen AG, et al. Diffusion-weighted MR imaging in closed head injury: high correlation with initial Glasgow coma scale score and score on modified Rankin scale at discharge. Radiology 2004;233(1):58–66.

98. Cooper PR, Maravilla K, Kirkpatrick J, et al. Traumatically induced brain stem hemorrhage and the computerized tomographic scan: clinical, pathological, and experimental observations. Neurosurgery 1979;4(2):115–24.

99. Tsai FY, Teal JS, Quinn MF, et al. CT of brainstem injury. AJR Am J Roentgenol 1980;134(4):717–23.

100. Turazzi S, Alexandre A, Bricolo A. Incidence and significance of clinical signs of brainstem traumatic lesions. Study of 2600 head injured patients. J Neurosurg Sci 1975;19(4):215–22.

101. Saeki N, Ito C, Ishige N, et al. Traumatic brain stem contusion due to direct injury by tentorium cerebelli. Case report. Neurol Med Chir 1985;25(11):939–44 [in Japanese].

102. Gennarelli TA, Thibault LE, Adams JH, et al. Diffuse axonal injury and traumatic coma in the primate. Ann Neurol 1982;12(6):564–74.

103. Tomlinson BE. Brain-stem lesions after head injury. J Clin Pathol Suppl 1970;4:154–65.

104. Pilz P. Survival after ponto-medullary junction trauma. Acta Neurochir Suppl 1983;32:75–8.

105. Britt RH, Herrick MK, Mason RT, et al. Traumatic lesions of pontomedullary junction. Neurosurgery 1980;6(6):623–31.

106. Hilario A, Ramos A, Millan JM, et al. Severe traumatic head injury: prognostic value of brain stem injuries detected at MRI. AJNR Am J Neuroradiol 2012;33(10):1925–31.

107. Rothfus WE, Goldberg AL, Tabas JH, et al. Callosomarginal infarction secondary to transfalcial herniation. AJNR Am J Neuroradiol 1987;8(6):1073–6.

108. Wernick S, Wells RG. Sequelae of temporal lobe herniation: MR imaging. J Comput Assist Tomogr 1989;13(2):323–5.

109. Rosenblum WI, Greenberg RP, Seelig JM, et al. Midbrain lesions: frequent and significant prognostic feature in closed head injury. Neurosurgery 1981;9(6):613–20.

110. Friede RL, Roessmann U. The pathogenesis of secondary midbrain hemorrhages. Neurology 1966;16(12):1210–6.

111. Caplan LR, Zervas NT. Survival with permanent midbrain dysfunction after surgical treatment of traumatic subdural hematoma: the clinical picture of a Duret hemorrhage? Ann Neurol 1977;1(6):587–9.

112. Jellinger K, Seitelberger F. Protracted posttraumatic encephalopathy. Pathology, pathogenesis and clinical implications. J Neurol Sci 1970;10(1):51–94.

113. Johnson PL, Eckard DA, Chason DP, et al. Imaging of acquired cerebral herniations. Neuroimaging Clin N Am 2002;12(2):217–28.

114. Han BK, Towbin RB, De Courten-Myers G, et al. Reversal sign on CT: effect of anoxic/ischemic cerebral injury in children. AJR Am J Roentgenol 1990;154(2):361–8.

115. Given CA 2nd, Burdette JH, Elster AD, et al. Pseudo-subarachnoid hemorrhage: a potential imaging pitfall associated with diffuse cerebral edema. AJNR Am J Neuroradiol 2003;24(2):254–6.

116. Arbelaez A, Castillo M, Mukherji SK. Diffusion-weighted MR imaging of global cerebral anoxia. AJNR Am J Neuroradiol 1999;20(6):999–1007.

117. Davis JM, Zimmerman RA. Injury of the carotid and vertebral arteries. Neuroradiology 1983;25(2):55–69.

118. Goldberg HI, Grossman RI, Gomori JM, et al. Cervical internal carotid artery dissecting hemorrhage: diagnosis using MR. Radiology 1986;158(1):157–61.

119. Sklar EM, Quencer RM, Bowen BC, et al. Magnetic resonance applications in cerebral injury. Radiol Clin North Am 1992;30(2):353–66.

120. Rodallec MH, Marteau V, Gerber S, et al. Craniocervical arterial dissection: spectrum of imaging findings and differential diagnosis. Radiographics 2008;28(6):1711–28.

121. Barr HW, Blackwood W, Meadows SP. Intracavernous carotid aneurysms. A clinical-pathological report. Brain 1971;94(4):607–22.

122. Mokri B, Piepgras DG, Sundt TM Jr, et al. Extracranial internal carotid artery aneurysms. Mayo Clin Proc 1982;57(5):310–21.

123. Edwards JD, Sapienza P, Lefkowitz DM, et al. Posttraumatic innominate artery aneurysm with occlusion of the common carotid artery at its origin by an intimal flap. Ann Vasc Surg 1993;7(4):368–73.

124. Komiyama M, Hakuba A, Yasui T, et al. Magnetic resonance imaging of intracavernous pathology. Neurol Med Chir 1989;29(7):573–8.

125. Coskun O, Hamon M, Catroux G, et al. Carotid-cavernous fistulas: diagnosis with spiral CT angiography. AJNR Am J Neuroradiol 2000;21(4):712–6.

126. Feldman RA, Hieshima G, Giannotta SL, et al. Traumatic dural arteriovenous fistula supplied by scalp, meningeal, and cortical arteries: case report. Neurosurgery 1980;6(6):670–4.

127. Vassilyadi M, Mehrotra N, Shamji MF, et al. Pediatric traumatic dural arteriovenous fistula. Can J Neurol Sci 2009;36(6):751–6.

128. Le TT, Fischbein NJ, Andre JB, et al. Identification of venous signal on arterial spin labeling improves diagnosis of dural arteriovenous fistulas and small arteriovenous malformations. AJNR Am J Neuroradiol 2012;33(1):61–8.

129. Jacobson DM, Terrence CF, Reinmuth OM. The neurologic manifestations of fat embolism. Neurology 1986;36(6):847–51.

130. Citerio G, Bianchini E, Beretta L. Magnetic resonance imaging of cerebral fat embolism: a case report. Intensive Care Med 1995;21(8):679–81.

131. Stoeger A, Daniaux M, Felber S, et al. MRI findings in cerebral fat embolism. Eur Radiol 1998;8(9):1590–3.

132. Takahashi M, Suzuki R, Osakabe Y, et al. Magnetic resonance imaging findings in cerebral fat embolism: correlation with clinical manifestations. J Trauma 1999;46(2):324–7.

133. Bodanapally U, Shanmuganathan K, Saksobhavivat N, et al. MR imaging and differentiation of cerebral fat embolism syndrome from diffuse axonal injury: application of diffusion tensor imaging. Neuroradiology 2013;55(6):771–8.

134. Chen PC, Hsu CW, Liao WI, et al. Hyperacute cerebral fat embolism in a patient with femoral shaft fracture. Am J Emerg Med 2013;31(9):1420.e1-3.

135. Moseley ME, Cohen Y, Kucharczyk J, et al. Diffusion-weighted MR imaging of anisotropic water diffusion in cat central nervous system. Radiology 1990;176(2):439–45.

136. Hulkower MB, Poliak DB, Rosenbaum SB, et al. A decade of DTI in traumatic brain injury: 10 years and 100 articles later. AJNR Am J Neuroradiol 2013;34(11):2064–74.

137. Niogi SN, Mukherjee P. Diffusion tensor imaging of mild traumatic brain injury. J Head Trauma Rehabil 2010;25(4):241–55.

138. Shenton ME, Hamoda HM, Schneiderman JS, et al. A review of magnetic resonance imaging and diffusion tensor imaging findings in mild traumatic brain injury. Brain Imaging Behav 2012;6(2):137–92.

139. Arfanakis K, Haughton VM, Carew JD, et al. Diffusion tensor MR imaging in diffuse axonal injury. AJNR Am J Neuroradiol 2002;23(5):794–802.

140. Brandstack N, Kurki T, Tenovuo O. Quantitative diffusion-tensor tractography of long association tracts in patients with traumatic brain injury without associated findings at routine MR imaging. Radiology 2013;267(1):231–9.

141. Kumar R, Gupta RK, Husain M, et al. Comparative evaluation of corpus callosum DTI metrics in acute mild and moderate traumatic brain injury: its correlation with neuropsychometric tests. Brain Inj 2009;23(7):675–85.

142. Miles L, Grossman RI, Johnson G, et al. Short-term DTI predictors of cognitive dysfunction in mild traumatic brain injury. Brain Inj 2008;22(2):115–22.

143. Newcombe VF, Williams GB, Nortje J, et al. Analysis of acute traumatic axonal injury using diffusion tensor imaging. Br J Neurosurg 2007;21(4):340–8.

144. Wilde EA, Ramos MA, Yallampalli R, et al. Diffusion tensor imaging of the cingulum bundle in children after traumatic brain injury. Dev Neuropsychol 2010;35(3):333–51.

145. Wozniak JR, Krach L, Ward E, et al. Neurocognitive and neuroimaging correlates of pediatric traumatic brain injury: a diffusion tensor imaging (DTI) study. Arch Clin Neuropsychol 2007;22(5):555–68.

146. Henry LC, Tremblay J, Tremblay S, et al. Acute and chronic changes in diffusivity measures after sports concussion. J Neurotrauma 2011;28(10):2049–59.

147. Wilde EA, McCauley SR, Hunter JV, et al. Diffusion tensor imaging of acute mild traumatic brain injury in adolescents. Neurology 2008;70(12):948–55.

148. Perez AM, Adler J, Kulkarni N, et al. Longitudinal white matter changes after traumatic axonal injury. J Neurotrauma 2014;31(17):1478–85.

149. Toth A, Kovacs N, Perlaki G, et al. Multi-modal magnetic resonance imaging in the acute and sub-acute phase of mild traumatic brain injury: can we see the difference? J Neurotrauma 2013;30(1):2–10.

150. Lipton ML, Gulko E, Zimmerman ME, et al. Diffusion-tensor imaging implicates prefrontal axonal injury in executive function impairment following very mild traumatic brain injury. Radiology 2009;252(3):816–24.

151. Bigler ED, Maxwell WL. Neuropathology of mild traumatic brain injury: relationship to neuroimaging findings. Brain Imaging Behav 2012;6(2):108–36.

152. Abu-Judeh HH, Singh M, Masdeu JC, et al. Discordance between FDG uptake and technetium-99m-HMPAO brain perfusion in acute traumatic brain injury. J Nucl Med 1998;39(8):1357–9.

153. Hofman PA, Stapert SZ, van Kroonenburgh MJ, et al. MR imaging, single-photon emission CT, and neurocognitive performance after mild traumatic brain injury. AJNR Am J Neuroradiol 2001;22(3):441–9.

154. Jacobs A, Put E, Ingels M, et al. Prospective evaluation of technetium-99m-HMPAO SPECT in mild and moderate traumatic brain injury. J Nucl Med 1994;35(6):942–7.

155. Davalos DB, Bennett TL. A review of the use of single-photon emission computerized tomography as a diagnostic tool in mild traumatic brain injury. Appl Neuropsychol 2002;9(2):92–105.

156. Yamaki T, Imahori Y, Ohmori Y, et al. Cerebral hemodynamics and metabolism of severe diffuse brain injury measured by PET. J Nucl Med 1996;37(7):1166–70.

157. Rostami E, Engquist H, Enblad P. Imaging of cerebral blood flow in patients with severe traumatic brain injury in the neurointensive care. Front Neurol 2014;5:114.

158. Wintermark M, van Melle G, Schnyder P, et al. Admission perfusion CT: prognostic value in patients with severe head trauma. Radiology 2004;232(1):211–20.

159. Garnett MR, Blamire AM, Corkill RG, et al. Abnormal cerebral blood volume in regions of contused and normal appearing brain following traumatic brain injury using perfusion magnetic

resonance imaging. J Neurotrauma 2001;18(6):585–93.

160. Ge Y, Patel MB, Chen Q, et al. Assessment of thalamic perfusion in patients with mild traumatic brain injury by true FISP arterial spin labelling MR imaging at 3T. Brain Inj 2009;23(7):666–74.

161. Grossman EJ, Jensen JH, Babb JS, et al. Cognitive impairment in mild traumatic brain injury: a longitudinal diffusional kurtosis and perfusion imaging study. AJNR Am J Neuroradiol 2013;34(5):951–7. S951-953.

162. Lin AP, Liao HJ, Merugumala SK, et al. Metabolic imaging of mild traumatic brain injury. Brain Imaging Behav 2012;6(2):208–23.

163. Shutter L, Tong KA, Holshouser BA. Proton MRS in acute traumatic brain injury: role for glutamate/glutamine and choline for outcome prediction. J Neurotrauma 2004;21(12):1693–705.

164. Henry LC, Tremblay S, Leclerc S, et al. Metabolic changes in concussed American football players during the acute and chronic post-injury phases. BMC Neurol 2011;11:105.

165. Vagnozzi R, Signoretti S, Cristofori L, et al. Assessment of metabolic brain damage and recovery following mild traumatic brain injury: a multicentre, proton magnetic resonance spectroscopic study in concussed patients. Brain 2010;133(11):3232–42.

166. Signoretti S, Marmarou A, Fatouros P, et al. Application of chemical shift imaging for measurement of NAA in head injured patients. Acta Neurochir Suppl 2002;81:373–5.

167. Brooks WM, Stidley CA, Petropoulos H, et al. Metabolic and cognitive response to human traumatic brain injury: a quantitative proton magnetic resonance study. J Neurotrauma 2000;17(8):629–40.

168. Garnett MR, Corkill RG, Blamire AM, et al. Altered cellular metabolism following traumatic brain injury:

a magnetic resonance spectroscopy study. J Neurotrauma 2001;18(3):231–40.

169. Cecil KM, Hills EC, Sandel ME, et al. Proton magnetic resonance spectroscopy for detection of axonal injury in the splenium of the corpus callosum of brain-injured patients. J Neurosurg 1998;88(5):795–801.

170. Ashwal S, Holshouser B, Tong K, et al. Proton spectroscopy detected myoinositol in children with traumatic brain injury. Pediatr Res 2004;56(4):630–8.

171. Ross BD, Bluml S, Cowan R, et al. In vivo MR spectroscopy of human dementia. Neuroimaging Clin N Am 1998;8(4):809–22.

172. Babikian T, Freier MC, Ashwal S, et al. MR spectroscopy: predicting long-term neuropsychological outcome following pediatric TBI. J Magn Reson Imaging 2006;24(4):801–11.

173. Brenner T, Freier MC, Holshouser BA, et al. Predicting neuropsychologic outcome after traumatic brain injury in children. Pediatr Neurol 2003;28(2):104–14.

174. George EO, Roys S, Sours C, et al. Longitudinal and prognostic evaluation of mild traumatic brain injury: a 1H-magnetic resonance spectroscopy study. J Neurotrauma 2014;31(11):1018–28.

175. Byrnes KR, Wilson CM, Brabazon F, et al. FDG-PET imaging in mild traumatic brain injury: a critical review. Front Neuroenergetics 2013;5:13.

176. Hong YT, Veenith T, Dewar D, et al. Amyloid imaging with carbon 11-labeled Pittsburgh compound B for traumatic brain injury. JAMA Neurol 2014;71(1):23–31.

177. Small GW, Kepe V, Siddarth P, et al. PET scanning of brain tau in retired national football league players: preliminary findings. Am J Geriatr Psychiatry 2013;21(2):138–44.

Concussion—Mild Traumatic Brain Injury
Recoverable Injury with Potential for Serious Sequelae

Joshua Kamins, MD[a], Christopher C. Giza, MD[b],*

KEYWORDS

- Concussion • Mild TBI • Sequalae of concussion

KEY POINTS

- Concussion is a clinical syndrome induced by biomechanical force causing neurologic symptoms that recover in most individuals.
- A minority of patients with concussion go on to develop persistent symptoms that may be disabling.
- Proper management of concussion includes protecting the individual from repeated injury, assessment for risk factors or comorbidities that may prolong recovery, symptomatic care, reassurance, initial rest, and providing a planned gradual return to cognitive and physical demand.
- Remote deficits from mild traumatic brain injury include motor, cognitive, and endocrine dysfunction and potential neurodegeneration, for which the mechanisms are still being elucidated.

INTRODUCTION

Although the original contemplation of concussion originated in Ancient Greece (**Fig. 1**),[1] public and scientific awareness are finally gaining traction. The scientific establishment now recognizes that the consequences of mild traumatic brain injury (mTBI) might not always be so mild. With ongoing development of basic and clinical science, it becomes possible to provide better prevention, assessment, and treatment for concussions, particularly in higher-risk groups like military personnel, athletes, and pediatric patients.

DEFINITIONS

In order to proceed with a discussion of mTBI and concussion, one must establish working definitions, because mTBI and concussion are often used interchangeably. As seen in **Table 1**, mTBI is historically based on Glasgow Coma Score (GCS), whereas concussion is a clinical syndrome that may overlap with mild, moderate, and severe TBI.

EPIDEMIOLOGY

Whether from increased awareness or an increased risk, the rate of reported TBI in the United

Disclosure Statement: For full transparency, all funding sources are listed. Grants/Research Support: NIH, NCAA, DOD, NFL-GE, Today's and Tomorrow's Children Fund, UCLA BIRC, UCLA FGP, UCLA Steve Tisch BrainSPORT program; Consultant: NFL-NCP, NHLPA, Neural Analytics; Advisory Panel: LoveYourBrain, MLS, NBA, NCAA, Neural Analytics, USSF; Medicolegal: One or 2 cases annually; Speaker's Bureau: Medical Education Speakers Network; Stock Shareholder: None; Other Financial or Material Support: None; Other: Commissioner California State Athletic Commission (end 2/2015).
[a] Department of Neurology, University of California Los Angeles, 710 Westwood Plaza, Suite 1-240, Los Angeles, CA 90095-1769, USA; [b] Departments of Neurosurgery and Pediatrics, Mattel Children's Hospital-UCLA, University of California Los Angeles, Room 531 Wasserman, 300 Stein Plaza, Los Angeles, CA 90095, USA
* Corresponding author.
E-mail address: cgiza@mednet.ucla.edu

Neurosurg Clin N Am 27 (2016) 441–452
http://dx.doi.org/10.1016/j.nec.2016.05.005
1042-3680/16/$ – see front matter Published by Elsevier Inc.

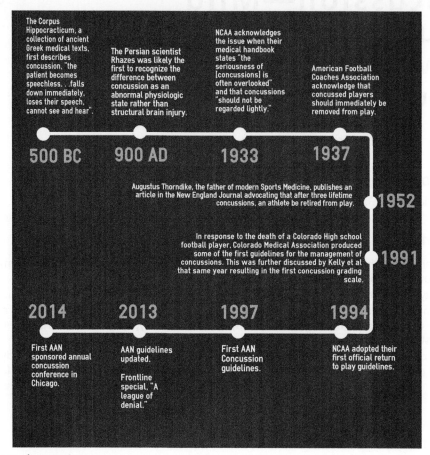

Fig. 1. History of concussions.

States has been increasing. From 2001 to 2009, the number of annual TBI-related emergency department (ED) visits related to sports and recreation activities increased from 153,375 to 248,418, with the highest rates among young men aged 10 to 19.[2] However, the ED is just the tip of the iceberg, because it is estimated that there are greater than 700,000 mTBIs per year in high school athletes alone, and more than 13% of these are in patients with recurrent concussions.[3]

Sports-related concussions have been on the increase, likely due to both increased recognition and increased power and strength in our athletes. In 2007, Hootman and colleagues[4] analyzed National Collegiate Athletic Association (NCAA) data from 1988 to 2004 regarding all injuries, including concussion. There was no significant change in overall rate of injury; however, concussions did increase significantly over this interval. Surprisingly, women's soccer had the highest risk of concussion per 1000 athlete exposures with a rate of 0.41, which was not only higher than men's soccer at 0.28, but on par with men's football's risk of 0.37.

This finding brought the idea to the forefront that women not only are at risk of concussion but may even be at a higher risk within the same activity compared with their male counterparts. Many theories have been proposed to explain this discrepancy, including hormonal differences, weaker neck muscles, and higher rate of symptom reporting among female athletes. Multiple investigators have confirmed that among comparable sports, in which rules of play are similar, women have a higher rate of concussions.[5,6]

PATHOPHYSIOLOGY

Concussion is a complicated syndrome of microstructural injury and functional impairment.[7,8] The initial event after impact is dominated by a massive flux of ions and excitatory neurotransmitters, resulting in a metabolic crisis. Rat models show that after fluid percussion injury (FPI), ionic flux of sodium, potassium, and calcium occurs, concomitant with a release of excitatory neurotransmitters, predominantly glutamate. Glutamate

Table 1
Traumatic brain injury and concussion definitions

	Definition
mTBI	Traumatic brain injury, GCS of 13–15 within 24 h of impact
Complicated mTBI	mTBI combined with intracranial imaging findings
Concussion	Clinical syndrome in which a biomechanical force, via acceleration-deceleration or rotational forces, transiently disturbs normal brain function, causing neurological-cognitive-behavioral signs and symptoms
Subconcussion	Proposed construct of biomechanical force causing subclinical injury in the absence of overt acute signs and symptoms

then generates further ionic imbalance transiently overwhelming the existing pumps on neurons and surrounding glial cells, whose purpose is to maintain a precise transmembrane ionic gradient.[9] NMDA receptor activation then leads to further calcium influx.

The ionic pumps being activated are ATP driven, and to keep up with ATP depletion, there is immediate hyperglycolysis. As TBI leads to decreased cerebral perfusion, this produces a neurovascular decoupling or metabolic mismatch, with high glucose demand and impaired delivery. This metabolic mismatch is exacerbated by mitochondrial dysfunction caused by secondary effects of calcium influx. Moreover, magnesium is depleted, which persists for days following TBI. This depletion of magnesium is important because in addition to its roles in glycolysis, oxidative generation of ATP, and providing stability to cellular membrane potential, magnesium is an NMDA antagonist. Thus, without magnesium, persistently open NMDA receptors lead to further calcium influx, intensifying the cycle described above.

In adult rats, the acute hypermetabolic state consisting of ion shifts, excitatory neurotransmitter activity, and hyperglycosis is followed by a hypometabolic state lasting 7 to 10 days. During this subacute period, there is upregulation of cytokines and inflammatory genes along with microglial activation. In addition to this inflammation and the metabolic dysfunction, there is microstructural

injury. Cytoskeletal damage can alter neurotransmission, and at the severe end, result in axonal disconnection triggered by dismantling of the axonal cytoskeleton via caspases and calpain.[10]

Although most of this neurometabolic cascade has only been demonstrated in humans after severe TBI, there is a cerebrovascular effect demonstrable after both severe and mTBI. It has been proposed that concussion symptoms acutely and subacutely are related to this metabolic mismatch,[11] which can be demonstrated in vivo with depressed cerebral blood flow (CBF), both acutely and persisting up to 30 days after injury.[12] Meier and colleagues[13] also demonstrated this depressed CBF at days 1 and 7 after injury with recovery in most subjects by 1 month. Those with persistent symptoms beyond 1 month were more likely to have persistently depressed CBF.

CLINICAL DIAGNOSIS OF THE ACUTE CONCUSSION

In order to accurately diagnose concussion, one must learn its common signs and symptoms and determine which tools are accurate and validated for assisting in this clinical diagnosis.

Of 544 high school sports concussions, the most common acute symptoms were headache in 93.4%, dizziness/unsteadiness in 74.6%, difficulty concentrating in 56.6%, vision changes including sensitivity to light in 37.5%, nausea in 28.9%, drowsiness in 26.5%, and amnesia in 24.3%. Loss of consciousness was only present in 4.6% of their patients.[5] In college athletes, the average number of symptoms and symptom resolution time do not differ by sex. However, a larger proportion of concussions in male athletes included amnesia and disorientation, whereas female athletes were more likely to report headache, excess drowsiness, and nausea/vomiting.[14]

There is no sign, symptom, or clinical tool that is 100% sensitive or specific for diagnosing a concussion. It remains a largely clinical diagnosis, and for this reason, the most important rule is "When in doubt, sit them out" to protect against the increased risk for a repeat concussion.

The provider should also be aware of available clinical tools to be used on the sideline or in clinic to aid in triage and diagnosis (**Table 2**). Tests are best used in combination. Most tests are intended for evaluation in a quieter location other than the sideline, although symptom checklists, Maddock's questions, and King-Devick have been used on the sideline or in locker rooms and clinics.

Table 2
Clinical tools for diagnosis

Test	Components	Pros	Cons
Standardized assessment of Concussion (SAC)	Orientation, immediate memory, concentration, and delayed recall	94% sensitivity and 76% specificity[10]	Requires trained practitioner
Sports Concussion Assessment Tool	Symptom checklist, cognitive assessment (SAC), balance examination (BESS), and coordination examination	Validated, thorough examination combining multiple systems	Requires trained practitioner
Maddocks Questions	Orientation and recent memory related to ongoing sporting event	Brief, easy to administer, and ideal for sideline	Low sensitivity in isolation
Balance Error Scoring System (BESS)[15]	Measurement of errors while balancing in 3 stances, on both firm ground and a foam pad	Practical test of vestibular networks, which are commonly affected in TBI	Poor interrater reliability
King-Devick[16]	Indicator of saccadic performance	Sensitive test and easy to administer	Practice effect
Dropstick test[17]	Measures clinical reaction time	Correlates with sport-related reactions	Requires extra hardware

Data from Refs.[5–17]

NEUROPSYCHOLOGICAL TESTING

A comprehensive examination of concussion patients would be incomplete without a thorough neuropsychological examination. The foundation of applying neuropsychological testing to concussed athletes began with Dr Jeffrey Barth in the 1980s. In 2008, Broglio and Puetz[18] published a meta-analysis of neuropsychological testing and showed that along with postural tests and symptom reporting, neurocognitive functioning was significantly depressed acutely and generally remained affected to a lesser degree for at least 14 days.

Computerized cognitive testing (CCT) is becoming widespread in a sports setting, with no particular brand showing a clear superiority. The main advantages of CCT are administration to large groups of athletes simultaneously, automated randomization of tests (alternate forms), accurate measurements of response and reaction time, and straightforward scoring and data storage,[19] whereas traditional pen and paper testing advantages are increased face-to-face time allowing customizable tests by the tester, the ability to judge fluency and verbal memory, the opportunity to take appropriate breaks, and extensive normative data for many demographic groups. As with any assessment tool, clinical context and judgment must be used when interpreting CCT, which is best done in consultation with a neuropsychologist. Studies have shown decreased CCT scores associated with orthopedic injury or even urge to void, rather than concussion.[20,21]

ACUTE IMAGING

Most mTBIs have no CT imaging findings. The Canadian Head CT Rule was directed to solve this dilemma.[22] Of 3121 adults with mTBI, 8% of patients had a clinically important brain injury (any acute finding on computed tomography [CT] requiring admission or neurologic follow-up); 1% required neurosurgical intervention, and 4% were found with clinically unimportant lesions (mostly small SAH or contusions not needing intervention, determined insignificant with no intervention needed and doing well at 14-day follow-up). The investigators found 5 high-risk features: failure to reach GCS of 15 within 2 hours of presentation, suspected open skull fracture, sign of basal skull fracture, vomiting greater than 2 episodes, or age greater than 65 years. In addition, there were 2 medium-risk factors: retrograde amnesia greater than 30 minutes and dangerous injury mechanism. Any single high-risk factor was 100% sensitive for the patient needing neurosurgical intervention, and medium-risk factors were 98.4% sensitive for a clinically important brain injury. In combination, the rule was found to be 92% sensitive for any injury on CT, including "clinically unimportant" lesions.

The New Orleans Criteria necessitates imaging for any patients with age greater than 60, vomiting, headache, intoxication, persistent anterograde amnesia, evidence of trauma above clavicle, or a seizure on presentation.[23] When compared with the New Orleans Criteria, the Canadian CT rule was found to have greater specificity for clinically important head trauma leading to less imaging and lower costs.

The Pediatric Emergency Care Applied Research Network (PECARN) resolved to differentiate low-risk pediatric mTBIs from those with clinically significant injury. This algorithm rules imaging out for patients with normal mental status, no loss of consciousness, no vomiting, a nonsevere injury mechanism, no signs of basilar skull fracture, and no severe headache. The negative predictive value was 99.5% with zero missed neurosurgical interventions.[24] Externally validated in 2014, the investigators found that "none of the children with a clinically important TBI were classified as very low risk by the PECARN TBI prediction rules."[25]

Acute MRI, while promising in several research studies comparing a cohort with clinical concussion with a control cohort, does not yet provide additional diagnostic or prognostic power in the evaluation of an individual patient. A study compared 75 mTBI patients to a control group with sprained ankles. CT and MRI were performed on all subjects, and MR sequences included not only fluid attenuated inversion recovery, T2 weighted imaging, susceptibility-weighted imaging, and diffusion-weighted imaging, but also diffusion tensor imaging (DTI). No significant differences were found between the 2 groups. Moreover, no differences were found in patients who turned out to have prolonged symptoms at 1 month, with the investigators suggesting there was no prognostic value of acute MRI with DTI.[26]

Conversely, the TRACK-TBI study enrolled 135 patients with mTBI who presented to a level I trauma center.[27] All patients enrolled received a CT scan and an "early MRI" (at 12 ± 3.9 days). Thirty-seven (27%) patients had abnormal head CT (31 intracranial, 6 isolated skull fractures). Of the 98 patients with negative head CTs, 28% had abnormal MRIs (23 hemorrhagic axonal injury, 3 contusions, 4 extra axial hematomas). Outside of socioeconomic and CT findings, the strongest predictor of poor outcome was MRI presence of one or more brain contusions or the presence of diffuse axonal injury.

REPEAT INJURY

The first step in management is always to remove the patient from any scenario where they risk further impact/contact to decrease risk of a second concussion, which has been associated with greater symptoms and prolonged recovery. In a prospective cohort study with 2905 NCAA football players, 184 had concussions, 12 had a second concussion in the same season, and 11 of 12 repeat concussions occurred within 10 days of the first injury.[28,29]

Moreover, following concussive brain injury in an animal model, there is a window of metabolic vulnerability.[30–32] A single mTBI resulted in significantly decreased cerebral metabolic rate of glucose (CMRglc), which returned to those of sham injuries by day 3. When a second mTBI was introduced within 24 hours of the first, CMRglc was further depressed, and recovery was prolonged. However, if the 2 impacts were introduced 120 hours apart, the CMRglc values recovered as if they were single impacts. In addition, the 24-hour repeat TBI (rTBI) rats had memory deficits beyond day 3, unlike the single mTBI or 120-hour rTBI animals. This study demonstrated increased physiologic risk during the metabolic window of vulnerability, with normal recovery if injuries were further apart.

In humans, magnetic resonance spectroscopy (MRS) was used to examine effects of concussion on brain metabolism.[33,34] Concussed athletes had significantly depressed metabolite ratios of N-acetylaspartate to creatinine or choline, lowest at day 3, and recovering to baseline by day 30. Athletes all reported symptom freedom between days 3 and 15 despite persistent metabolic changes on MRS. In a separate study, patients who had a second concussive injury before the 15-day mark did not recover NAA peaks until 45 days after injury. These data mirror that of Prins and colleagues[30–32] in that the compounded injury produced a more severe metabolic depression than the first, and required longer to recover.

SECOND IMPACT SYNDROME

Second Impact Syndrome (SIS) remains a controversial subject. It was first reported in 1984 by Saunders and Harbaugh, who described massive, fatal, cerebral edema after a second mTBI before recovery from a first mTBI.[35] In this initial case report, a 19-year-old football player, who allegedly suffered a concussion from a fight, returned to play 4 days later and suffered additional mTBI. This second concussion resulted in massive cerebral edema and death.

McCrory[36] argues that SIS is overreported, based on a recall bias of the first TBI, and that it shows a clear geographic bias, given no reports of this syndrome outside of the United States. If SIS were a risk in the general population, youth boxers should be at particular risk from this syndrome. Massive cerebral swelling after mTBI does occur rarely but may not always require repeated impacts. Multiple case reports have recounted disproportionate cerebral edema to a single mild head injury in patients with a personal or family history of hemiplegic migraine related to a familial or de novo mutation in one of the CACNA1A calcium channel subunit genes.[37–39] Based on current understanding of concussion pathophysiology, other types of ion channel dysfunction are plausible contributing mechanisms.

RECOVERING FROM INJURY: BALANCING REST AND EXERCISE

Regardless of the risk of SIS, the mainstay method for initial management of acute symptoms is cognitive and physical rest, given that symptoms may be worsened when the metabolic mismatch is challenged, followed by gradual return to cognitive and physical activity.

In an effort to answer the question of how much to rest their athletes, Majerske and colleagues[40] retrospectively assigned 95 adolescent student athletes with concussion to 1 of 5 groups based on after-injury activity levels.[40] All of the athletes' neurocognitive scores and symptom scores improved over time, but there was a significant relationship between those with the highest and lowest levels of activity and lower neurocognitive scores, particularly visual memory and reaction time. Those with moderate activity were associated with the best symptom scores and neurocognitive performance. Similarly, in a prospective cohort study, Brown and colleagues[41] concluded that those with the highest quartile of cognitive activity after injury had the longest duration of symptoms, while the subjects in the 3 lower quartiles all showed similar recovery rates. In a different study, patients with persistent symptoms showed benefit from a period of cognitive and physical rest, even months after concussion, although this study lacked a control group.[42]

In 2015, Thomas and colleagues[43] compared the result of 5 days of strict rest after injury versus "usual care" in which the patients had 1 to 2 days of rest and then returned in a stepwise manner. Patients in the strict rest group took significantly longer to recover compared with the usual care group. In addition, the strict rest subjects had a higher overall Post-Concussion Symptom Scale score and total number of symptoms in the 10-day follow-up, suggesting the possibility that strict rest may change symptom reporting patterns, too.

In summary, data demonstrate that it is likely beneficial for the patient to have some amount of cognitive and physical rest and then gradually transition back to full amount of activity.

It is well known that exercise has a beneficial role in a wide variety of psychiatric and neurologic diseases, varying from improving patient's negative response to stress, preserving cognitive function in aging and dementia,[44] recovering some of the observed depletion of important neurotransmitters in clinical major depression and anxiety, and functioning in a neuroprotective role in multiple sclerosis.[45–47] In the realm of concussion and TBI, there is uncertainty regarding how to advise our patients regarding exercise, given the fact that activity too early seems to hamper recovery, but the chronic symptoms may all benefit from exercise.

Preclinical studies showed that acute exercise after adult rat fluid percussion worsened performance on cognitive tasks. Given the fact that exercise normally upregulates brain growth factors (brain-derived neurotrophic factor, BDNF) and enhances expression of downstream plasticity markers, this was surprising. Interestingly, exercise within the first week after FPI appeared to interrupt the production of these intracellular signaling proteins, likely disrupting plasticity. In a follow-up study, delayed voluntary exercise was helpful in mitigating post-TBI spatial memory deficits. Moreover, when investigators used a BDNF inhibitor, this was found to block the effect of exercise.[48,49] In a small clinical study, human subjects with refractory and persistent after-concussive symptoms have been successfully and safely treated with 3 weeks of submaximal exercise.[50]

Current data suggest that, although very early cognitive and physical activity may delay recuperation and increase symptoms, exercise and activity can be beneficial for brain recovery and plasticity following concussion. Prolonged rest can have detrimental effects, as evidenced from other conditions such as low back pain.[51] It is important to avoid social isolation, worsening of the stress response, and depression and anxiety that can occur with prolonged restriction of normal activities, particularly in athletes.

COGNITIVE RESTRUCTURING

Cognitive restructuring is a therapeutic concept dating back to Bruner and Gage in the 1960s in which the patient is guided to challenge their own thoughts and misconceptions that can interfere with recovery.[52,53] In primary care, this is akin to the concept of anticipatory guidance, namely, providing the patient and family with information and expectations of what is likely to happen (used commonly for families with newborns going home, during normal development in children, and after vaccination). The goal with concussion is to facilitate recovery by teaching the patient to expect their symptoms will resolve.

As early as 1972, Relander and colleagues[54] published a series in *British Medical Journal* in which after-concussion symptoms were ameliorated by a combination of physiotherapy and daily meetings with a physician who emphasized a good prognosis. In 1996, Mittenberg and colleagues[55] contrasted 2 groups evaluated in the ED for mTBI. The control group received standard ED care, whereas the intervention group underwent a brief cognitive restructuring intervention. They reviewed the nature and incidence of expected symptoms, were taught techniques for reducing symptoms, and were given instructions for gradual resumption of activities. The patients in the intervention group reported significantly shorter average symptom duration and significantly fewer symptoms at follow-up. Furthermore, it has been shown in both children and adults that an intervention as simple as providing an information booklet at 1 week after injury that outlines common symptoms associated with mild head injury, their likely time course, and suggested coping strategies, results in improved outcome.[56,57]

POSTCONCUSSION SYNDROME

Despite the best efforts of clinicians, a significant minority of patients may develop chronic postconcussive symptoms and receive a diagnosis of postconcussion syndrome (PCS).[58] PCS is defined by ICD-10 (International Statistical Classification of Diseases and Related Health Problems, 10th revision) as organic and psychogenic disturbances observed after closed head injuries, including subjective physical complaints (ie, headache, dizziness), cognitive, emotional, and behavioral changes. Estimates of PCS incidence range widely from 10% to 40% of patients.[59] However, symptoms that would lead to a diagnosis of PCS[60] are not always specific, and even a portion of orthopedic injury control subjects reports moderate chronic symptoms. In addition, patients underreport premorbid symptoms that overlap with PCS. This underreporting suggests a role for maladaptive thoughts and misattribution of symptoms, and an even larger role for prevention of PCS with anticipatory guidance.

According to the American Academy of Neurology Guidelines, a history of prior concussion demonstrates the strongest evidence for more severe/longer duration of symptoms and cognitive deficits, while younger age, early posttraumatic headache, fatigue/fogginess, early amnesia, alteration in mental status, or disorientation demonstrated probable evidence for prolonged recovery.[29] Premorbid predictors of PCS also include personal or family history of migraine, mood disorders, or other psychiatric illness.[61]

Given that posttraumatic headaches are often the most refractory symptom, it is vital to recognize any patterns, whether it be a new primary headache syndrome or medication overuse headache (may contribute to up to 70% of chronic posttraumatic headaches).[62] Posttraumatic tension-type or migraine headaches should be managed similarly to nontraumatic headache syndromes with appropriate use of prophylactic and abortive agents.

Management of mood disorders, most commonly depression and anxiety,[63] is best done with a combination of continued cognitive restructuring and/or cognitive behavioral therapy, thorough evaluations by neuropsychologists, and consideration of referral for medical treatment by a psychiatrist.

As demonstrated above, exercise and cognitive therapy may play a large role in ameliorating persistent symptoms. Earlier this year, Gagnon and colleagues[64] organized a case series of 10 adolescents who were slow to recover from sport-related concussion, with symptoms lasting more than 4 weeks. The patients were provided with a structured exercise program, visualization and imagery techniques, and education for the patient and family. Significant and clinically relevant decrease in symptoms at 6-week follow-up was observed. Replicating these results in larger cohorts is important and may have strong implications for concussion rehabilitation.

POTENTIAL FOR LONG-TERM SEQUELAE

In addition to better identification and early management of concussion, there is growing concern of both the general public and the scientific community for the potential long-term consequences of repeated impacts and concussions. Professional athletes are reporting neurocognitive problems, culminating in class action lawsuits filed by former players in both football and hockey. Included in the nearly $1 billion settlement with the National Football League (NFL) are monetary awards for diagnoses of amyotrophic lateral sclerosis (ALS), Alzheimer disease (AD), Parkinson disease, dementia, and a postmortem diagnosis of chronic traumatic encephalopathy (CTE). Of note, there is no requirement to prove that the players' injuries were caused by playing football to receive compensation from the settlement.

It is important to distinguish between the multiple possible consequences of repeated brain impacts, because not every symptom or problem reported following concussion or contact sports exposure is a harbinger of a degenerative condition. A differential diagnosis for chronic neurocognitive problems in this scenario would include PCS, chronic headache disorders, chronic neurocognitive impairment (CNI), hormonal deficits, anxiety, depression, exacerbation of premorbid conditions, and neurodegenerative disorders (Parkinson, AD, ALS, CTE).

Mechanistically, persistent alterations of white matter signal are reported using DTI, suggesting axonal damage contributes to chronic problems. In a pediatric cohort, these changes are seen early after injury while the subjects were symptomatic, but persist at 4 months after injury, even after most symptoms resolve.[65] Moreover, "subconcussive injury" due to soccer heading has been associated with white matter microstructural and cognitive abnormalities in adults.[66] Other evidence of network dysfunction after remote sports concussion has been reported using detailed neuropsychological testing, event-related potential (ERP) testing, motor examination, and transcranial magnetic stimulation (TMS). Nineteen healthy former athletes who had sustained 1 to 5 concussions during their career, but all greater than 30 years prior, demonstrated subtle neuropsychological deficits in visual memory and executive function as well as corresponding differences on ERP. Moreover, they demonstrated decreased velocity of rapid alternating movements as well as altered activation patterns on TMS.[67]

In addition, preclinical studies suggest subacute and chronic endocrine impairment after TBI. Comparing a sham single injury to 4 repeat injuries with 24-hour intervals, investigators found that rTBI rats demonstrated a significant depression of circulating insulin-like growth factor-1 (IGF-1) acutely and reduced levels of growth hormone and IGF-1 at 1 month after injury.[31] Studies of human patients show endocrinopathies or pituitary damage after more severe TBI, with only a few case reports following concussive injury.

It is important to note that not all longitudinal studies have shown neurologic consequences from exposure to sports at risk of concussion. Investigators identified all male students who played high school football between 1946 and 1956 in their county. They found no significant difference in dementia, Parkinson, or ALS among the 438 football players compared with their non-football-playing counterparts. This absence of consequence for high school football likely demonstrates both a dose response to mTBI and a difference between amateur and professional athletes.

Many cognitive complaints are affected by anxiety, depression, and posttraumatic stress disorder. Recognition and treatment of any underlying psychiatric disease must be an important component of a comprehensive cognitive evaluation for remote effects of concussion.[68]

There has been mixed evidence with regards to risk for Parkinson disease. Overall, a history of TBI does seem to increase risk for PD; however, additional studies have shown no increase from mTBI. This evidence may suggest that the hazard originates from moderate to severe TBIs.[69,70]

With regards to chronic or remote neurocognitive consequences, there are distinctions described between CNI, which is diagnosed clinically in living patients, and CTE, which currently is a post-mortem pathologic diagnosis (**Table 3**).

Although multiple cohort studies describe a consistent pattern of neurocognitive impairment in athletes with exposure to contact and collision sports, due to an absence of longitudinal data leading to abnormality, the causal link between clinical and pathologic findings is yet to be fully established. The predominant theory is the presence of a unique neurodegenerative disorder, CTE, as opposed to the idea that multiple TBIs lead to diminished cerebral reserve and thus earlier clinical expression of age-related neurodegenerative diseases.

Proponents of the diminished cerebral reserve theory point to evidence that a history of moderate to severe TBI or stroke earlier in life may result in earlier expression of neurodegenerative diseases and that athletes often report lower force required

Table 3
Characteristics of chronic neurocognitive impairment and chronic traumatic encephalopathy

CNI	CTE
Decrement in function	Neurodegenerative disease
May be static	Presumed progressive
Detected in living patients	Detected post mortem
May be measured by neuropsychological testing or behavioral screening questionnaires	Characterized pathologically by tau accumulation
Causal link not yet established, but possible dose-dependent risk	Causal link not yet established, current data in case reports/series

with each subsequent concussion. This theory would predict an earlier expression of conventional age-related neurodegenerative diseases in patients with a history of head trauma compared with non-head-trauma controls.[71] Surveys of 513 retired NFL players implied cognitive impairment in 35.1%. A comparison of neurocognitive profiles in a subsample of this group to a clinical sample of patients with a diagnosis of mild cognitive impairment due to AD revealed a highly similar profile of impairments. The investigators contend this supports lowered cerebral reserve over a distinct diagnosis of CTE.

The science behind CTE has been advanced greatly in the last 2 decades by Drs Omalu and McKee, each with their own scores for CTE type and staging.[72] Dr McKee defines CTE clinically by symptoms of irritability, impulsivity, aggression, depression, short-term memory loss, and heightened suicidality that usually begin 8 to 10 years after experiencing repetitive mTBI. Pathologically, there is atrophy of the cerebral cortex, thinning of the corpus callosum, ventriculomegaly, cavum vergae, and fenestrated septum pellucidum. The 2015 NINDS/NIBIB (National Institute of Neurological Disorders and Stroke/National Institute of Biomedical Imaging and Bioengineering) consensus meeting gathered 25 blinded neuropathologists to attempt to differentiate a variety of abnormalities from CTE. The panel defined the pathognomonic lesion of CTE as an accumulation of abnormal hyperphosphorylated tau (p-tau) in neurons and astroglia distributed around small blood vessels at the depths of cortical sulci and in an irregular pattern.[73] Supporters propose this is a distinctive pattern that results from forces due to TBI, and detractors argue that these patterns overlap greatly with other known taopathies.[74,75] As mentioned, CTE currently remains a pathologic diagnosis, although efforts are underway to better characterize the clinical semiology associated with this syndrome. Recent advances in PET imaging, while not yet validated, show some promise to diagnose CTE in vivo, leading to earlier detection and better clinical characterization of the disease.[76]

SUMMARY

The moniker "mild TBI" was originally based on comparison using the GCS, which included severely injured patients rendered comatose by a traumatic injury. However, it is increasingly apparent that a subset of individuals with mTBI may develop persistent problems or, very rarely, a catastrophic outcome. It is critical to recognize that not every acute symptom is necessarily due to concussion pathophysiology, because many conditions may mimic concussion and are part of the differential diagnosis (migraine, attention deficit/hyperactivity disorder, anxiety, cervicogenic headaches, as well as rare but devastating cerebral edema with or without intracranial hemorrhage). Likewise, there is an extensive differential diagnosis for chronic symptoms after mTBI/concussion, including chronic headaches, exacerbation of premorbid conditions, anxiety, depression, misattribution of symptoms, PCS, CNI, CTE, and other neurodegenerative conditions. Careful consideration of all possibilities, with a focus on treatable conditions and symptomatic intervention, as well as cognitive restructuring and education, should be the mainstay for providing optimal clinical care for those experiencing concussion.

ACKNOWLEDGMENTS

The authors would like to thank Doug Polster, PhD and Talin Babikian, PhD for their assistance with the neuropsychology literature.

REFERENCES

1. McCrory PR, Berkovic SF. Concussion: the history of clinical and pathophysiological concepts and misconceptions. Neurology 2001;57:2283–9.
2. Gilchrist J, Thomas KE, Xu L, et al. Nonfatal TBI related to sports and recreation activities among persons aged ≤19 years. MMWR Morb Mortal Wkly Rep 2011;60(39):1337–42.
3. Castile L, Collins CL, McIlvain NM, et al. The epidemiology of new versus recurrent sports concussions among high school athletes, 2005-2010. Br J Sports Med 2012;46:603–10.
4. Hootman JM, Dick R, Agel J. Epidemiology of collegiate injuries for 15 sports: summary and recommendations for injury prevention initiatives. J Athl Train 2007;42(2):311–9.
5. Marar M, McIlvain NM, Fields SK, et al. Epidemiology of concussions among US High School Athletes. Am J Sports Med 2012;40(4):747–55.
6. Lincoln AE, Caswell SV, Almquist JL, et al. Trends in concussion incidence in high school sports: a prospective 11-year study. Am J Sports Med 2011;39(5):958–63.
7. Giza CC, Hovda DA. The neurometabolic cascade of concussion. J Athl Train 2001;36(3):228–35.
8. Giza CC, Hovda DA. The new neurometabolic cascade of concussion. Neurosurgery 2014;75(Suppl 4):S24–33.
9. Katayama Y, Becker DP, Tamura T, et al. Massive increases in extracellular potassium and the indiscriminate release of glutamate following concussive brain injury. J Neurosurg 1990;73(6):889–900.

10. Büki A, Povlishock JT. All roads lead to disconnection? Traumatic axonal injury revisited. Acta Neurochir (Wien) 2006;148(2):181–94.

11. Tan C, Meehan W III, Iverson G, et al. Cerebrovascular regulation, exercise, and mild traumatic brain injury. Neurology 2014;83:1665–72.

12. Maugans TA, Farley C, Altaye M, et al. Pediatric sports-related concussion produces cerebral blood flow alterations. Pediatrics 2012;129(1):28–37.

13. Meier TB, Bellgowan PSF, Singh R, et al. Recovery of cerebral blood flow following sports-related concussion. JAMA Neurol 2015;87106(5):530–8.

14. Wasserman EB, Kerr ZY, Zuckerman SL, et al. Epidemiology of sports-related concussions in National Collegiate Athletic Association athletes from 2009-2010 to 2013-2014: symptom prevalence, symptom resolution time, and return-to-play time. Am J Sports Med 2016;44(1):226–33.

15. Guskiewicz KM, Ross SE, Marshall SW. Postural stability and neuropsychological deficits after concussion in collegiate athletes. J Athl Train 2001;36(3): 263–73.

16. Galetta KM, Barrett J, Allen M, et al. The King-Devick test as a determinant of head trauma and concussion in boxers and MMA fighters. Neurology 2011; 76(17):1456–62.

17. Eckner JT, Lipps DB, Kim H, et al. Can a clinical test of reaction time predict a functional head-protective response? Med Sci Sports Exerc 2011;43(3):382–7.

18. Broglio SP, Puetz TW. The effect of sport concussion on neurocognitive function, self-report symptoms and postural control: a meta-analysis. Sports Med 2008;38(1):53–67.

19. Iverson GL, Schatz P. Advanced topics in neuropsychological assessment following sport-related concussion. Brain Inj 2015;29(2):263–75.

20. Hutchison M, Comper P, Mainwaring L, et al. The influence of musculoskeletal injury on cognition: implications for concussion research. Am J Sports Med 2011;39(11):2331–7.

21. Lewis M, Snyder PJ, Pietrzak RH, et al. The effect of acute increase in urge to void on cognitive function in healthy adults. Neurourol Urodyn 2011;30:183–7.

22. Stiell IG, Wells GA, Vandemheen K, et al. The Canadian CT Head Rule for patients with minor head injury. Lancet 2001;357(9266):1391–6.

23. Kavalci C, Aksel G, Salt O, et al. Comparison of the Canadian CT head rule and the New Orleans criteria in patients with minor head injury. World J Emerg Surg 2014;9(1):31.

24. Kuppermann N, Holmes JF, Dayan PS, et al. Identification of children at very low risk of clinically-important brain injuries after head trauma: a prospective cohort study. Lancet 2009;374(9696): 1160–70.

25. Schonfeld D, Bressan S, Da Dalt L, et al. Pediatric Emergency Care Applied Research Network head injury clinical prediction rules are reliable in practice. Arch Dis Child 2014;99(5):427–31.

26. Ilvesmäki T, Luoto TM, Hakulinen U, et al. Acute mild traumatic brain injury is not associated with white matter change on diffusion tensor imaging. Brain 2014;137(7):1876–82.

27. Yuh E, Mukherjee P, Lingsma HF, et al. Magnetic resonance imaging improves 3-month outcome prediction in mild traumatic brain injury. Ann Neurol 2013;73(2):224–35.

28. Guskiewicz KM, Mccrea M, Marshall SW, et al. Cumulative effects associated with recurrent concussion in collegiate football players: the NCAA Concussion Study. JAMA 2003;290(19):2549–55.

29. Giza CC, Kutcher JS, Ashwal S, et al. Summary of evidence-based guideline update: evaluation and management of concussion in sports. Neurology 2013;80(24):2250–7.

30. Prins ML, Alexander D, Giza CC, et al. Repeated mild traumatic brain injury: mechanisms of cerebral vulnerability. J Neurotrauma 2013;30(1):30–8.

31. Greco T, Hovda D, Prins M. The effects of repeat traumatic brain injury on the pituitary in adolescent rats. J Neurotrauma 2013;30(23):1983–90.

32. Prins ML, Hales A, Reger M, et al. Repeat traumatic brain injury in the juvenile rat is associated with increased axonal injury and cognitive impairments. Dev Neurosci 2011;32(5–6):510–8.

33. Vagnozzi R, Tavazzi B, Floris R, et al. Temporal Wendow of Metabolic Brain Vulnerability To Concussion : a Pilot 1 H-Magnetic Resonance Spectroscopic Study in Concussed Athletes - Part III. Neurosurgery 2008;62(6):1286–96.

34. Vagnozzi R, Signoretti S, Cristofori L, et al. Assessment of metabolic brain damage and recovery following mild traumatic brain injury: A multicentre, proton magnetic resonance spectroscopic study in concussed patients. Brain 2010;133(11):3232–42.

35. Bey T, Ostick B. Second impact syndrome. West J Emerg Med 2009;10(1):6–10.

36. McCrory P. Does second impact syndrome exist? Clin J Sport Med 2001;11(3):144–9.

37. Kors EE, Terwindt GM, Vermeulen FLMG, et al. Delayed cerebral edema and fatal coma after minor head trauma: role of the CACNA1A calcium channel subunit gene and relationship with familial hemiplegic migraine. Ann Neurol 2001;49(6):753–60.

38. Malpas TJ, Riant F, Tournier-Lasserve E, et al. Sporadic hemiplegic migraine and delayed cerebral oedema after minor head trauma: a novel de novo CACNA1A gene mutation. Dev Med Child Neurol 2010;52(1):103–4.

39. Curtain RP, Smith RL, Ovcaric M, et al. Minor head trauma–induced sporadic hemiplegic migraine coma. Pediatr Neurol 2006;34:329–32.

40. Majerske CW, Mihalik JP, Ren D, et al. Concussion in sports: postconcussive activity levels, symptoms,

and neurocognitive performance. J Athl Train 2008; 43(3):265–74.

41. Brown NJ, Mannix RC, O'Brien MJ, et al. Effect of cognitive activity level on duration of post-concussion symptoms. Pediatrics 2014;133(2): e299–304.

42. Moser RS, Glatts C, Schatz P. Efficacy of immediate and delayed cognitive and physical rest for treatment of sports-related concussion. J Pediatr 2012; 161(5):922–6.

43. Thomas DG, Apps JN, Hoffmann RG, et al. Benefits of strict rest after acute concussion: a randomized controlled trial. Pediatrics 2015;135(2):213–23.

44. Groot C, Hooghiemstra AM, Raijmakers PGHM, et al. The effect of physical activity on cognitive function in patients with dementia: a meta-analysis of randomized control trials. Ageing Res Rev 2016; 25:13–23.

45. Salmon P. Effects of physical exercise on anxiety, depression, and sensitivity to stress. Clin Psychol Rev 2001;21(1):33–61.

46. Giesser BS. Exercise in the management of persons with multiple sclerosis. Ther Adv Neurol Disord 2015;8(3):123–30.

47. Clark PJ, Amat J, McConnell SO, et al. Running reduces uncontrollable stress-evoked serotonin and potentiates stress-evoked dopamine concentrations in the rat dorsal striatum. PLoS One 2015;10(11): e0141898.

48. Griesbach GS, Gomez-Pinilla F, Hovda DA. The up-regulation of plasticity-related proteins following TBI is disrupted with acute voluntary exercise. Brain Res 2004;1016(2):154–62.

49. Griesbach GS, Hovda DA, Gomez-Pinilla F. Exercise-induced improvement in cognitive performance after traumatic brain injury in rats is dependent on BDNF activation. Brain Res 2009; 1288:105–15.

50. Leddy JJ, Kozlowski K, Donnelly JP, et al. A preliminary study of subsymptom threshold exercise training for refractory post-concussion syndrome. Clin J Sport Med 2010;20(1):21–7.

51. Malmivaara A, Aro T. The treatment of acute low back pain–bed rest, exercise therapy or ordinary activity? Duodecim 1995;111(22):2101–2.

52. Bruner JS. The process of education. Cambridge, Mass.: Harvard University Press; 1960.

53. Gage NL. Handbook of research on teaching. Chicago: Rand McNally; 1963.

54. Relander M, Troupp H, Af Björkesten G. Controlled Trial of Treatment for Cerebral Concussion. British Medical Journal 1972;4:777–9.

55. Mittenberg W, Tremont G, Zielinski RE, et al. Cognitive-behavioral prevention of postconcussion syndrome. Arch Clin Neuropsychol 1996;11(2):139–45.

56. Ponsford J, Willmott C, Rothwell A, et al. Impact of early intervention on outcome following mild head injury in adults. J Neurol Neurosurg Psychiatr 2002;73(3):330–2.

57. Ponsford J, Willmott C, Rothwell A, et al. Impact of early intervention on outcome after mild traumatic brain injury in children. Pediatrics 2001;108(6): 1297–303.

58. Mittenberg W, Strauman S. Diagnosis of mild head injury and the postconcussion syndrome. J Head Trauma Rehabil 2000;15(2):783–91.

59. Mittenberg W, Canyock EM, Condit D, et al. Treatment of post-concussion syndrome following mild head injury. J Clin Exp Neuropsychol 2001;23(6):829–36.

60. Dean PJA, O'Neill D, Sterr A. Post-concussion syndrome: prevalence after mild traumatic brain injury in comparison with a sample without head injury. Brain Inj 2012;26(1):14–26.

61. Morgan CD, Zuckerman SL, Lee YM, et al. Predictors of postconcussion syndrome after sports-related concussion in young athletes: a matched case-control study. J Neurosurg Pediatr 2015;15: 589–98.

62. Heyer GL, Idris SA. Does analgesic overuse contribute to chronic post-traumatic headaches in adolescent concussion patients? Pediatr Neurol 2014;50(5):464–8.

63. Fann JR, Katon WJ, Uomoto JM, et al. Psychiatric disorders and functional disability in outpatients with traumatic brain injuries. Am J Psychiatry 1995; 152:1493–9.

64. Gagnon I, Grilli L, Friedman D, et al. A pilot study of active rehabilitation for adolescents who are slow to recover from sport-related concussion. Scand J Med Sci Sports 2016;26(3):299–306.

65. Mayer AR, Ling JM, Yang Z, et al. Diffusion abnormalities in pediatric mild traumatic brain injury. J Neurosci 2012;32(50):17961–9.

66. Lipton M, Kim N, Zimmerman M, et al. Soccer heading is associated with white matter microstructural and cognitive abnormalities. Radiology 2013; 268(3):850–7.

67. De Beaumont L, Theoret H, Mongeon D, et al. Brain function decline in healthy retired athletes who sustained their last sports concussion in early adulthood. Brain 2009;132(3):695–708.

68. Ellis MJ, Ritchie LJ, Koltek M, et al. Psychiatric outcomes after pediatric sports-related concussion. J Neurosurg Pediatr 2015;709–18.

69. Gardner RC, Burke JF, Nettiksimmons J, et al. Traumatic brain injury in later life increases risk for Parkinson disease. Ann Neurol 2015;77(6): 987–95.

70. Marras C, Hincapié CA, Kristman VL, et al. Systematic review of the risk of Parkinson's disease after mild traumatic brain injury: results of the international collaboration on mild traumatic brain injury prognosis. Arch Phys Med Rehabil 2014;95(3): S238–44.

71. Randolph C, Karantzoulis S, Guskiewicz K. Prevalence and characterization of mild cognitive impairment in retired national football league players. J Int Neuropsychol Soc 2013; 19:873–80.

72. Jordan BD. The clinical spectrum of sport-related traumatic brain injury. Nat Rev Neurol 2013;9(4): 222–30.

73. McKee AC, Cairns NJ, Dickson DW, et al. The first NINDS/NIBIB consensus meeting to define neuropathological criteria for the diagnosis of chronic traumatic encephalopathy. Acta Neuropathol 2016; 131(1):75–86.

74. McKee AC, Stein TD, Nowinski CJ, et al. The spectrum of disease in chronic traumatic encephalopathy. Brain 2013;136(1):43–64.

75. Iverson GL, Gardner AJ, McCrory P, et al. A critical review of chronic traumatic encephalopathy. Neurosci Biobehav Rev 2015;56:276–93.

76. Barrio JR, Small GW, Wong K, et al. In vivo characterization of CTE using [F-18]FDDNP PET brain imaging. Proc Natl Acad Sci U S A 2015;112(22):E2981.

Cerebral Metabolism and the Role of Glucose Control in Acute Traumatic Brain Injury

Manuel M. Buitrago Blanco, MD, PhD*,
Giyarpuram N. Prashant, MD, Paul M. Vespa, MD

KEYWORDS

- Traumatic brain injury • Glucose control • Metabolism • Neurovascular unit • Metabolic crisis
- Outcome • Hyperglycolysis • Cerebral microdialysis

KEY POINTS

- Hyperglycemia is often observed in critical illness and severe TBIs, indicating systemic physiologic stress and severity of injury.
- Acute hyperglycemia has been found to be associated significantly with poor functional outcome and high mortality in severe TBI.
- Randomized clinical trials addressing hyperglycemia so far have failed to demonstrate improvement in neurologic outcomes after severe TBI, prompting further research to understand the disease process.
- Recent advancements in preclinical and clinical research shift the focus to the physiology of glucose use at the neurovascular unit level in the brain, where glucose metabolism is altered.
- Future research will shed light into the promise of alternative energy delivery methods.

INTRODUCTION

The human brain consumes about 25% of cardiac output, reflecting the high energetic demand that brain cells depend on to function at physiologic conditions. Energy demand and use are dramatically altered following severe traumatic brain injury (TBI) creating a biologic dilemma for neuronal survival and functional preservation.

Despite significant advances in the understanding of brain physiology and evidence demonstrating that blood flow regulation and oxygen delivery optimization improve the chances of survival after TBI, the most up-to-date Brain Trauma Foundation management guidelines do not include a formal recommendation in regards to systemic glucose control or brain glucose optimization.[1] Yet, mounting scientific experimental and clinical evidence demonstrate that systemic glucose derangements and deviation from a physiologic cerebral glucose metabolism further exert a negative impact in recovery from TBI, by exacerbating secondary tissue injury, hindering functional outcomes, and increasing the chance of mortality.

According to the Centers for Disease Control and Prevention, 2.2 million patients visit emergency rooms each year for TBI in the United States alone. Of those, about 250,000 are hospitalized and about 50,000 die as a result of their injury

Division of Neurocritical Care, Department of Neurosurgery, University of California Los Angeles, 757 Westwood Boulevard, Los Angeles, CA 90095, USA
* Corresponding author. Division of Neurocritical Care, Department of Neurosurgery, David Geffen School of Medicine, University of California Los Angeles, 757 Westwood Boulevard, Los Angeles, CA 90095.
E-mail address: mblanco@mednet.ucla.edu

Neurosurg Clin N Am 27 (2016) 453–463
http://dx.doi.org/10.1016/j.nec.2016.05.003
1042-3680/16/$ – see front matter © 2016 Elsevier Inc. All rights reserved.

(http://www.cdc.gov/traumaticbraininjury/data/). Improved protocols exist for management of intracranial pressure (ICP), cerebral perfusion pressure, and brain oxygenation. However, despite increased knowledge and understanding about glucose metabolism at the systemic level and in the brain, clinical trials aimed at controlling systemic hyperglycemia have failed to improve neurologic outcomes and survival after TBI. In a general critical care patient population, results have shown higher mortality with the intensive insulin therapy (IIT) strategy to control elevated serum glucose. In the neurologic population that suffers from severe TBI the results have been equally disappointing.

A thorough review of the pathophysiologic mechanisms behind cerebral metabolic failure supported by current scientific evidence and an outline toward future directions in management and research are discussed.

BRAIN GLUCOSE METABOLISM PRINCIPLES

Glycolysis is perhaps one the most preserved biologic processes from prokaryotes to mammals consisting of the biochemical steps that allow glucose use as a source of energy.[2–4] It occurs in the cytoplasm and results in production of pyruvate, lactate, and ATP. Pyruvate then diffuses across cellular compartments to reach the mitochondria where it is prepared to enter the citric acid cycle (Krebs cycle) in the form of acetyl-CoA. The end result is further generation of ATP, CO_2, and nicotinamide adenine dinucleotide. Nicotinamide adenine dinucleotide then enters the electron transport chain and through oxidative phosphorylation results in the production of large amounts of ATP. Oxygen is consumed as the electron acceptor allowing restoration of NAD^+ to maintain the cycle. This well-defined pathway constitutes aerobic respiration (**Fig. 1**).

The Krebs cycle is not only crucial for generation of chemical energy, but also to provide the cell with the necessary precursor materials to synthesize some amino acids, and in the case of neurons, neurotransmitters. Not all pyruvate generated by glycolysis enters the Krebs cycle; about 15% of pyruvate is converted to lactate, which in turn can be used to generate energy. Under anaerobic

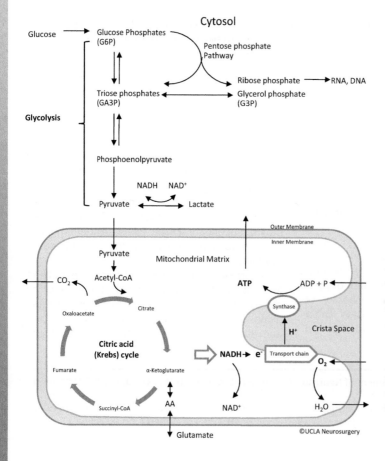

Fig. 1. Simplified diagram of glycolysis, citric acid cycle, and cellular respiration. All enzymes necessary for the glycolytic pathway are present in the cytosol allowing the metabolism of glucose into pyruvate and lactate. Pyruvate enters the mitochondrial matrix via a proton symporter where it is irreversibly oxidized to aceyl-CoA, the main substrate of the tricarboxylic (citric acid or Krebs) cycle. This cycle is important in the reduction of coenzymes necessary for the cellular respiration and other cellular processes. Cellular respiration occurs at the mitochondrial cristae with the end result of net production of 38-mol ATP (oxidative phosphorylation) for cellular energy use. Alternatively, lactate is the end product of glycolysis under anaerobic conditions leading to a net result of 2-mol ATP. AA, aminoacid; acetyl-CoA, acetyl coenzyme A; e$^-$, electron; G3P, glycerol 3-phosphate; G6P, glucose 6-phosphate; GA3P, glyceraldehyde 3-phosphate; NAD^+/NADH, nicotinamide adenine dinucleotide; P, phosphate. (*Courtesy of* Dr Manuel M. Buitrago Blanco, MD, PhD, Department of Neurosurgery, Neurological ICU, University of California, Los Angeles, 2016.)

conditions, the amount of pyruvate converted to lactate increases as a biologic mechanism to partially supply energy demand. Under the same conditions, glycerophosphate, an intermediate element of glycolysis, also dramatically accumulates.

Glucose is used at high rates by neurons and other brain cells. Strong evidence now shows that glycolysis in astrocytes and oxidative metabolism in neurons is increased as a function of neuronal activity.[5] The transport of glucose from the bloodstream across the blood-brain barrier is driven by a concentration gradient and mediated actively via the endothelial glucose transporter 1.[6] Because neurons are not able to synthesize glucose its transport mechanisms must be highly efficient to meet activity-driven demands. Shuttling from the extracellular space into astrocytes and neurons occurs through glucose transporter 1 and glucose transporter 3, respectively.[7] Efficient transport of fuel provides an essential element for generation of ATP and precursor molecules necessary for the synthesis of neurotransmitters essential for neuronal function.

GLUCOSE CONTROL IN CRITICAL ILLNESS

Energy demands and expenditure in critical illness differ significantly from normal physiologic states. States of organ dysfunction, trauma, infection, or a combination pose a challenge for the mechanisms responsible for glucose control. Hyperglycemia observed in acute illness may be caused by insulin insufficiency, insulin resistance, impaired glucose use, stress caused by hormonal dysregulation (eg, cortisol), and increased catecholamines.[8] Hyperglycemia is an independent predictor of adverse outcomes and increased mortality in survivors of myocardial infarction admitted to the intensive care unit (ICU) at 180 days,[9] 1 year,[10] and 2 years,[11] even in the absence of preexisting diabetes. Similar observations were confirmed in patients with critical illness of all causes, who had higher mortality rates at 180 days when hyperglycemia was observed in ICU.[12] Glucose elevation at any time throughout the ICU course has been shown to have a higher independent positive predictive value for mortality than the Acute Physiology and Chronic Health Evaluation II score.[13] The recognition of this relationship and the quest for glucose optimization in critical illness has been an area of intense investigation over the last decades, leading to large clinical trials aimed at testing whether glucose control could lead to improved survival and better outcomes. The first clinical trial in this area aimed at maintaining serum glucose levels in the range of 80 to 100 mg/dL using IIT. Mortality during intensive care was improved by about 50% (4.6% intensive therapy vs 8.0% standard therapy) highlighting the importance of stress-induced hyperglycemia and sparking further research interest in this area.[14] The indication for ICU stay in two-thirds of the patients included in this study was elective cardiac surgery. A large follow-up clinical trial by the same team failed to demonstrate a mortality benefit of using IIT in a medical ICU population with a more wide range of critical illness conditions.[15] Subsequent more inclusive clinical trials and a meta-analysis failed to support this observation in more heterogeneous groups of patients.[16,17] Adverse events were also more frequent in the patients with IIT.

An effort to address this important question was put forward with the NICE-SUGAR study, a large multicenter, international clinical trial in which 6104 patients were randomized to undergo tight glucose control (80–108 mg/dL) or standard therapy (goal 180 mg/dL).[18] This study found that intensive glucose control among adults in the ICU increased mortality at 90 days. Severe hypoglycemia (glucose <40 mg/dL) was significantly more frequent in the intensive control arm (6.8% vs 0.5%).

A salient aspect from these trials was the limited number of patients with a primary neurologic diagnosis or TBI, indicating that observations in the critically ill patient still remained widely inapplicable in neurologic patients. Recent evidence indicates that functional outcomes and mortality after TBIs are affected by systemic glucose derangements and that systemic glucose levels are not accurate indicators of brain glucose delivery or use. This has prompted active preclinical and clinical research to address these questions.

GLUCOSE METABOLISM IN TRAUMATIC BRAIN INJURY
Pathophysiology of Hyperglycemia in Traumatic Brain Injury

Similar to other critical illnesses, hyperglycemia in TBIs is a manifestation of severity of the disease and the mechanisms behind it have been under investigation for several decades. As a direct consequence of acute brain injury, an early surge in sympathetic activity leads to an increase in systemic circulating catecholamines. In experimental models of isolated brain injury, the degree of sympathoadrenal response seems to be graded in a linear relationship with severity of the brain injury.[19] The catecholamine surge occurs within minutes of the insult and may be transient, whereas the circulating glucose surge follows soon after in a sustained steady fashion.

In addition to the observation of spontaneous early hyperglycemia after TBI, now there is mounting evidence indicating this early anomaly may further worsen secondary injury.

Preclinical research in animal models of TBI has shown that induced hyperglycemia at the time of injury increased the accumulation of neutrophils in contusional areas potentially exacerbating inflammation and abnormalities in blood flow.[20] In this study, delayed hyperglycemia did not have the same effect, raising the question of an early time window of higher susceptibility to the negative effects from a glucose surge.

In experimental models of intracerebral hemorrhage hyperglycemia has been shown to worsen cerebral edema surrounding the hematoma and exacerbate neuronal death in these same brain regions.[21] In models of ischemic brain injury, early hyperglycemia resulted in a dramatic exacerbation of neocortical neuronal necrosis.[22] In humans with severe TBI hyperglycemia is associated with cerebral tissue acidosis; however, it is not clear whether there is a causal relationship.[23]

The observation that hyperglycemia exacerbates neuronal injury and death across several types of neurologic insults suggests a possible common underlying mechanism in secondary brain injury. One plausible mechanism that has been proposed for several decades now involves disruption of the blood-brain barrier leading to dysregulation in blood flow, glucose transport and use and excitotocity.[24,25] The modern concept of neurovascular unit dysfunction offers a more global and integrated physiologic explanation for the derangements observed in a wide range of neurologic insults including TBI.[26]

Association of Hyperglycemia and Brain Injury Outcomes

Systemic hyperglycemia has been associated with worse outcomes in a wide variety of acute neurologic insults, including intracranial hemorrhage, ischemic stroke, and aneurysmal subarachnoid hemorrhage.[26–30] In ischemic stroke this observation led to the design of pilot clinical trials aimed at testing safety of insulin infusions for targeted blood glucose control in the hours subsequent to the clinical event.[31,32] A more recent phase 2 trial has been completed demonstrating that tight glucose control is safe in acute ischemic stroke,[33] yet a definitive phase 3 trial is still ongoing.[34]

The association of spontaneous systemic hyperglycemia early after TBI and poor outcomes has been reported. In a study involving 59 subjects with moderate and severe brain injuries (Glasgow Coma Scale [GCS], 3–10) serum glucose levels greater than 200 mg/dL in the first 24 hours from hospital admission were associated with worse neurologic outcome at hospital discharge, 3 months, and 1 year.[35]

In a cohort of 169 patients with severe TBI (craniotomy for evacuation of mass occupying hematoma, ICP monitor placed), those with initial GCS less than 8 had significantly higher serum glucose than patients with GCS 12 to 15 on admission (192 vs 130 mg/dL). Furthermore, hyperglycemia was significantly worse in patients who died or remained in vegetative state when compared with those with good outcome or moderate disability (217 mg/dL vs 167 mg/dL).[36] These studies, however, were conducted at centers where administration of dextrose solutions and steroids were routine at the time, leaving open the possibility of a biologic effect of those interventions, despite statistical correction. Subsequent studies conducted rigorously avoided that issue. In a series of 267 patients with isolated moderate and severe TBI most of whom underwent craniotomy for evacuation of mass-occupying lesion, admission serum glucose was significantly higher in those with GCS less than or equal to 8 compared with moderate injury patients with GCS 9 to 12 (203 mg/dL vs 164 mg/dL). Furthermore, systemic glucose was significantly higher in patients with unfavorable outcome as measured by glasgow outcome scale (GOS) (GOS 3,2,1 = 204 mg/dL vs GOS 4, 5 = 179 mg/dL).[37] In a study involving 77 patients with severe TBI (admission GCS, $\leq$8), hyperglycemia within the first 5 ICU days, defined as two or more episodes of serum glucose greater than 170 mg/dL, was independently associated to increased hospital mortality at 21 days (survival rate 51% in patients with hyperglycemia vs 83% in patients without hyperglycemia).[38]

In a more recent study describing 380 patients admitted with TBI, peak glucose levels in the first 24 hours of hospital admission was an independent predictor of in-hospital mortality (cutoff glucose value for increased mortality, 160 mg/dL). Across brain injury severity groups, peak-glucose within 24 hours was significantly higher in nonsurvivors.[39] Similar observations have been made in the pediatric and adolescent population.[40]

Clinical Trials of Glucose Control in Traumatic Brain Injury

The observed association between hyperglycemia and worsened neurologic outcomes has led to clinical trials testing the neurologic effect of using of IIT in the neurologic ICU. In a clinical trial patients with TBIs were randomized to glucose goal less than 200 mg/dL or IIT (80–120 mg/dL). In this single center trial, the rate of hypoglycemic episodes per patient was nearly as twice as much on the IIT group; however, mortality rates were similar at hospital discharge and 6 months.[41] In a before/after study, designed to evaluate the effects of IIT implementation as part of routine practice (serum glucose goal, 80–120 mg/dL), 1957 patients in the "before" arm were compared with 1888 patients in the targeted "implementation arm." Use of the IIT protocol was associated to higher rates of hypoglycemia events and higher rate of mortality, specifically related to hypoglycemic events.[42]

In the first prospective clinical trial aimed at addressing the question of glucose control in a neurologically ill population, patients admitted to the neurologic ICU at a single center were randomized to IIT with serum glucose goal 80 to 110 mg/dL or conventional therapy with serum glucose goal less than 151 mg/dL. No benefit in mortality or functional outcome at 3 months was observed. Instead

a trend toward increased mortality in the IIT group was found.[43]

Cerebral Metabolic Energy Crisis: A Window Toward Goal-Targeted Therapies

The failure of clinical trials aimed at impacting outcomes by controlling hyperglycemia highlights the need to advance research efforts to elucidate the fate of glucose in the injured brain with focus on the neurovascular unit. Traditionally, the cornerstone in physiologic management of patients with severe TBI has been to focus on optimization of key physiologic brain variables: ICP, cerebral perfusion pressure, and brain oxygenation.[1] There is no evidence-based clinical guideline, at present, as to how glucose or other sources of energy should be delivered to the brain to sustain metabolic demands after TBI.

The neurovascular unit is the functional building block in the brain that ensures a proper match between energy supply and demand (**Fig. 2**).[26] The cascade of pathophysiologic changes that occur as the result of traumatic injury to the brain includes

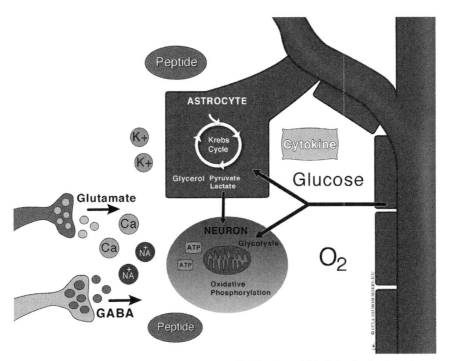

Fig. 2. The neurovascular unit. The neurovascular unit is the functional block in the brain. It is comprised of a capillary blood vessel, astrocytes (core of the blood-brain barrier), and neurons that are anatomically and physiologically coupled. Molecules present in the interstitium include electrolyte ions, oxygen, neurotransmitters, amino acids, peptides, immune system proteins, glucose, and cellular byproducts of glycolysis and oxidative metabolism. Information about physiologic states at tissue level can potentially be targeted and measured as surrogate measures of end organ function via noninvasive or minimally invasive techniques. (*Courtesy of* Dr Manuel M. Buitrago Blanco, MD, PhD and Josh Emerson, Department of Neurosurgery, Neurological ICU, University of California, Los Angeles, 2013.)

cytotoxic edema, macrovascular dysfunction, microvascular dysfunction, and cellular energetic failure.[44–46] These alterations, indicative of neurovascular unit dysfunction, are manifested at the organ level as increased ICP, cerebral vasospasm, cerebral blood flow autoregulatory failure, hypoxemia, cerebral tissue ischemia, and cerebral glucose metabolic dysfunction.[47] These physiologic derangements converge in a common pathway that leads to energetic failure, ultimately explained by either suboptimal delivery of oxygen and nutrients and/or cellular dissociation from normal glycolysis and oxidative metabolism.

The degree and type of metabolic disturbance after TBI may differ depending on proximity to areas of anatomic injury, the type of injury (focal vs diffuse), and timing from the initial insult. Abnormalities in brain glucose metabolism have been shown in experimental models of brain injury and in human subjects TBI.

In a rodent model of concussive brain injury, oxidative metabolism was transiently increased within minutes and subsequently decreased for several days mostly in neocortex and hippocampus ipsilateral to the impact.[48] The same group showed that glucose use follows a similar timecourse, with increased glucose use within 60 minutes, followed by a dramatic decrease that lasted several days.[49]

Bergsneider and colleagues,[50] at the University of California Los Angeles, were the first to report of hyperglycolysis after severe TBI in humans by using fluorodeoxyglucose (FDG)-PET. In that study, hyperglycolysis was defined as an abnormal state of increased glucose metabolism relative to the rate of oxygen use, thus representing a nonphysiologic decoupling between glycolytic and oxidative metabolism, as follows:

Metabolic Ratio (MR) = CMRO2/CMRG

Hyperglycolysis was defined as MR less than 0.35, where CMRO2 is the cerebral metabolic rate of oxygen and CMRG is the cerebral metabolic rate of glucose. Under that definition, about 50% of patients demonstrated hyperglycolysis within 1 week after the injury. Furthermore, hyperglycolysis was accentuated in areas adjacent to focal brain lesions. This finding was later confirmed by the Cambridge group in human severe brain injury using a combination of cerebral microdialysis and FDG-PET showing a likewise shift toward early increased glucose use.[51] This metabolic anomaly in glucose metabolism is now referred to as "cerebral metabolic energy crisis" and is thought to be a hallmark of profound cellular dysfunction after TBI.

Brain glucose levels measured with cerebral microdialysis reflect availability and glucose use. Vespa and colleagues[52] showed for the first time in humans that persistently low extracellular glucose levels in cerebral dialysate (<0.02 mmol/L at a perfusion rate of 2 µL/min) correlate with poor neurologic outcome at 6 months. In this study, however, low glucose levels were not correlated with increased cerebral lactate levels or brain ischemia, opening the question whether in a hyperglycolytic state (high glucose consumption) the injured human brain may be using the resulting lactate as a source of energy. Alternatively, it has also been shown that during metabolic crisis, glucose enters the pentose phosphate cycle potentially explaining the lack of lactate increase in tissue.[53] These observations represented a new departure from the standard brain hyperglycolysis hypothesis and have prompted the proposal that lactate may be considered as an alternative pathway of fuel to the injured brain.[54] Furthermore, the clinical severity of injury has been associated with lower cerebral microdialysis glucose levels in humans, and worsened outcome at hospital discharge.[55]

Another important pathophysiologic marker of stress is the cerebral tissue lactate/pyruvate ratio (LPR), which not only serves as an indicator of the metabolic state of cells but also predicts severity of injury and poor outcomes.[56] In a study involving a cohort of 223 patients (the largest to date) with severe TBI, LPR elevation had a significant association with death and unfavorable outcomes at 6 months.[57] In this study, a previously suggested physiologic threshold of LPR greater than or equal to 25[58] was used to discriminate outcomes, strongly predicting severe disability and death.

Early hyperglycolysis seems to be a transient phenomenon that within days is followed by a period of depression in cerebral glucose metabolism. Resembling the pattern seen in experimental models,[49] human data derived from FDG-PET suggest that glucose hypometabolism occurs several days after the insult and may last from weeks to months thereafter.[59]

Until recently, cerebral metabolic rate had not been investigated in relationship to neurophysiologic measures of cerebral activity. Vespa and colleagues,[60] have now found that periods of abnormally increased neuronal activity manifested as subclinical seizures are time-locked with the occurrence of cerebral metabolic crisis in human. This observation brings new fundamental understanding into the process of secondary injury and opens the opportunity for therapies aimed at controlling subclinical seizures, hence ameliorating secondary injury.

The existing scientific evidence derived from animal models and human data allows one to postulate a time-course for the anomalies observed in cerebral glucose metabolism (**Table 1**).

The dynamic nature of alterations in the physiology of glucose metabolism after brain injury and the nature of the tissue injury itself are factors that must be taken into consideration when designing studies to further understand this disease process and testing novel therapeutic interventions to improve functional outcomes in human. The use of multimodality monitoring in the neurologic ICU offers an insight into the evolution of brain injuries and will help better characteristic metabolic dysfunction in human TBI. The cerebral microdialysis technique has evolved since it was first described in the 1950s. A breakthrough in the field was made the 1970s when the tubular shaped membrane at the tip of the probe was first used by Ungerstedt and Pycock at the Karolinska Institute in Stockholm to monitor chemical events in brain tissue initially in animal models[61,62] and subsequently in humans.[63,64] The application in humans was reviewed during the joint American Association of Pharmaceutical Scientists–Food and Drug Administration workshop on microdialysis in 2005[65] and was more recently endorsed in the International Multidisciplinary Consensus Conference on Multimodality Monitoring in Neurocritical care.[66,67] The CMA/M Dialysis system (M Dialysis Inc, North Chelmsford, MA) is the only cerebral microdialysis system approved by the US Federal Drug Administration to monitor biochemical markers in the human brain and remains the gold standard in human clinical applications (**Fig. 3**).

Systemic Glucose Control and Cerebral Glucose Metabolism Optimization

Management of hyperglycemia and hypoglycemia is of high priority because cerebral metabolic state after brain injury can be significantly worsened by fluctuating arterial blood glucose levels.[68] Prior clinical evidence indicating adverse outcome associations with intensive glycemic control is now supported by biologic data from cerebral microdialysis demonstrating that cerebral metabolic crisis occurs as a result of tight glucose control in humans.[69,70] IIT after severe TBI has been shown to result in increased incidence of episodes of detrimental systemic hypoglycemia, and

Table 1
Triphasic hypothesis of glucose metabolism after TBI

Phase 1: Hypermetabolism	Phase 2: Hypometabolism	Phase 3: Normal Metabolism

• Hyperglycemia
• Abnormal brain metabolites
  ○ Low cerebral glucose
  ○ LPR increase
  ○ High glutamate
• Abnormal PET
  ○ High FDG uptake
	• Hyperglycemia/normoglycemia
	• Abnormal brain metabolites
	  ○ Normal/low cerebral glucose
	  ○ Normal/low LPR
	• Abnormal PET
	  ○ Low FDG uptake
		• Normoglycemia
		• Unknown brain metabolites
		• Improved PET
		  ○ Normalization of FDG update

Hours to days	Days to weeks	Weeks to months
• Control of systemic glucose • Control of ICP, oxygen, and temperature • Control of cerebral metabolic energy crisis • Control of seizures	• Optimization of systemic glucose • Control of ICP, oxygen, and temperature • Delivery of fuel and nutrition	• Rehabilitation and therapy

Glucose metabolism after TBI involves at least three distinct phases. A similar model was proposed earlier at University of California Los Angeles based on human data.[59] Broadly an early phase of hypermetabolism (phase 1) is supported by preclinical and clinical data suggesting early systemic derangement in glucose control (hyperglycemia), increased metabolic rate of glucose locally, and/or globally (CMRG) abnormal glucose metabolism in the brain characterized by low glucose and abnormal glycolysis metabolites (hyperglycolysis) and physiologic abnormalities manifested as subclinical seizures. The next stage is characterized by hypometabolism (phase 2) and consists of abnormal to normal glycemia, normalization of extracellular LPR or decrease, and decreased CMRG at the local and global level. Phase 3 or return to physiologic metabolism is less established and there are scarce data. At the bottom of the table, listed are potential strategies to address each specific stage.

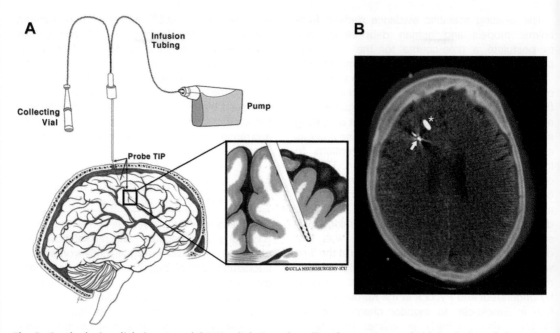

Fig. 3. Cerebral microdialysis system. (*A*) Microdialysis probes allow for continuous fluid circulation of electrolyte solutions through a two-way cannula adapted with a semipermeable tip, allowing for diffusion of solutes from the brain tissue across a semipermeable membrane. Brain tissue molecules present in the interstitial space diffuse across the membrane into the circulating fluid. Analysis of solutes present in the out-going fluid or "dialysate" is the cornerstone of cerebral microdialysis. Because the circulating dialysate flow is set at an arbitrary rate, solute concentrations are relative approximations to the actual tissue contents of the solute. A microdialysis system consists of the following components: microdialysis probe, precision pump, and tubing system. The microdialysis probes are designed to allow for circulation of fluid along a semipermeable membrane located at the tip of the probe. The membrane properties can vary according to the intended use. The size of the membrane pores can vary to allow molecules with sizes 6 kDa to about 100 kDa. Most recently, membranes with pore sizes up to 1 MDa have been made commercially available. The type of membrane chosen is an important factor in being able to retrieve specific molecules from the interstitial space. Most glycolysis metabolites and neurotransmitters freely diffuse across the 6-kDa pore size membranes. Such targets as peptides and proteins require larger pore membranes to be retrieved. (*B*) Example of microdialysis probe placement in the right frontal lobe. The probe has a radiopaque gold tip for easy visualization on CT (*arrow*) and it is ideally placed in gray-white matter junction, in this case adjacent to ventriculostomy catheter (*asterisk*). (*Courtesy of* Dr Manuel M. Buitrago Blanco, MD, PhD and Josh Emerson, Department of Neurosurgery, Neurological ICU, University of California, Los Angeles, 2013.)

not adding benefit in clinical outcomes.[41] In a microdialysis study arterial blood glucose levels between 108 mg/dL and 162 mg/dL correlated with optimal cerebral glucose levels and LPR suggesting a potential ideal range of glycemia for cerebral metabolism optimization in humans.[71] Furthermore, in a prospective randomized within-subject crossover trial using cerebral microdialysis and FDG-PET, tight glucose control resulted in metabolic crisis and hyperglycolytic state.[72]

Cerebral microdialysis has gained significant attention and offers an opportunity in the management of severe brain injury, including TBI, because it allows for detection of metabolic distress even with normal ICP or in the absence of cerebral ischemia.[73] In addition, patients with TBI often have increased cerebral metabolic demand and serum glucose levels that are considered to be normal be may relatively insufficient to meet increased requirements by the brain. It has also been suggested that rather than simply considering serum and brain interstitial glucose levels, the brain/serum glucose ratio may be a more sensitive measure of metabolic distress and is an independent predictor of mortality in TBI and patients with aneurysmal subarachnoid hemorrhages.[30,74] This ratio is presumably a reflection of brain glucose transport across the blood-brain barrier, but may be also be affected by hyperglycolysis or mitochondrial failure. Monitoring the brain/serum glucose ratio may provide a more specific therapeutic tool in the management of insulin therapy and glucose management.

A randomized clinical trial of systemic glucose optimization targeted to control cerebral metabolic energy crisis in TBI is yet to be carried out. The current guidelines for the management of TBI do not substantially address systemic glucose control or cerebral metabolic energy crisis.[1] The International Multidisciplinary Consensus Conference on Multimodal Monitoring in neurocritical care addresses systemic glucose control and the use of cerebral microdialysis for glucose metabolism optimization in TBI in two separate sections.[66,75] Extensive research gathered in this field has yielded new understanding into secondary injury, yet there is limited high level clinical evidence to support strong management recommendations. Although rigorous clinical trials still need to be designed to address key questions regarding brain metabolism after TBI, several conclusions are drawn from the existing literature. In doing so, we are also setting a path for further research:

1. Hyperglycemia greater than 200 mg/dL has been reported to worsen neurologic outcomes in TBI. A threshold for detrimental hyperglycemia needs to be defined and validated.
2. IIT for glucose control leads to a significantly higher number of hypoglycemic events (glucose <80 mg/dL) and offers no clinical benefit in long-term outcomes. Cerebral microdialysis may be of help to detect the optimum serum glucose below which metabolic crisis may ensue.
3. Cerebral metabolic energy crisis defined by low glucose levels and increased LPR greater than 25 in cerebral dialysate and hyperglycolysis observed in FDG-PET are associated with poor neurologic outcomes.
4. Subclinical seizures are associated with cerebral metabolic energy crisis and hence its nature and treatment must be investigated.
5. IIT is associated a higher rate of cerebral metabolic energy crisis and worsened outcomes and hence it is not recommended. Management protocols need to be validated and implemented

Future prospective clinical research is needed to define whether individualized goal-directed therapy aimed at decreasing the rate of cerebral metabolic energy crisis has an impact in neurologic outcomes. Furthermore, the use of alternative energy substrates and delivery methods is a field of future development and of high potential impact.

REFERENCES

1. Brain Trauma Foundation, American Association of Neurological Surgeons, Congress of Neurological Surgeons. Guidelines for the management of severe traumatic brain injury. J Neurotrauma 2007; 24(Suppl 1):S1.
2. Romano AH, Conway T. Evolution of carbohydrate metabolic pathways. Res Microbiol 1996;147:448.
3. Sparks S. The purpose of glycolysis. Science 1997; 277:459.
4. van Heerden JH, Wortel MT, Bruggeman FJ, et al. Lost in transition: start-up of glycolysis yields subpopulations of nongrowing cells. Science 2014; 343:1245114.
5. Kasischke KA, Vishwasrao HD, Fisher PJ, et al. Neural activity triggers neuronal oxidative metabolism followed by astrocytic glycolysis. Science 2004; 305:99.
6. McEwen BS, Reagan LP. Glucose transporter expression in the central nervous system: relationship to synaptic function. Eur J Pharmacol 2004;490:13.
7. Simpson IA, Carruthers A, Vannucci SJ. Supply and demand in cerebral energy metabolism: the role of nutrient transporters. J Cereb Blood Flow Metab 2007;27:1766.
8. Kavanagh BP, McCowen KC. Clinical practice. Glycemic control in the ICU. N Engl J Med 2010;363: 2540.
9. Ainla T, Baburin A, Teesalu R, et al. The association between hyperglycaemia on admission and 180-day mortality in acute myocardial infarction patients with and without diabetes. Diabet Med 2005;22:1321.
10. Bolk J, van der Ploeg T, Cornel JH, et al. Impaired glucose metabolism predicts mortality after a myocardial infarction. Int J Cardiol 2001;79:207.
11. Norhammar AM, Ryden L, Malmberg K. Admission plasma glucose. Independent risk factor for long-term prognosis after myocardial infarction even in nondiabetic patients. Diabetes Care 1999;22:1827.
12. Rady MY, Johnson DJ, Patel BM, et al. Influence of individual characteristics on outcome of glycemic control in intensive care unit patients with or without diabetes mellitus. Mayo Clin Proc 2005;80:1558.
13. Krinsley JS. Association between hyperglycemia and increased hospital mortality in a heterogeneous population of critically ill patients. Mayo Clin Proc 2003;78:1471.
14. Van den Berghe G, Wouters P, Weekers F, et al. Intensive insulin therapy in critically ill patients. N Engl J Med 2001;345:1359.
15. Van den Berghe G, Wilmer A, Hermans G, et al. Intensive insulin therapy in the medical ICU. N Engl J Med 2006;354:449.
16. Arabi YM, Dabbagh OC, Tamim HM, et al. Intensive versus conventional insulin therapy: a randomized controlled trial in medical and surgical critically ill patients. Crit Care Med 2008;36:3190.
17. Wiener RS, Wiener DC, Larson RJ. Benefits and risks of tight glucose control in critically ill adults: a meta-analysis. JAMA 2008;300:933.
18. Finfer S, Chittock DR, Su SY, et al. Intensive versus conventional glucose control in critically ill patients. N Engl J Med 2009;360:1283.

19. Rosner MJ, Newsome HH, Becker DP. Mechanical brain injury: the sympathoadrenal response. J Neurosurg 1984;61:76.

20. Kinoshita K, Kraydieh S, Alonso O, et al. Effect of posttraumatic hyperglycemia on contusion volume and neutrophil accumulation after moderate fluid-percussion brain injury in rats. J Neurotrauma 2002;19:681.

21. Song EC, Chu K, Jeong SW, et al. Hyperglycemia exacerbates brain edema and perihematomal cell death after intracerebral hemorrhage. Stroke 2003; 34:2215.

22. Pulsinelli WA, Waldman S, Rawlinson D, et al. Moderate hyperglycemia augments ischemic brain damage: a neuropathologic study in the rat. Neurology 1982;32:1239.

23. Zygun DA, Steiner LA, Johnston AJ, et al. Hyperglycemia and brain tissue pH after traumatic brain injury. Neurosurgery 2004;55:877.

24. Ginsberg MD, Welsh FA, Budd WW. Deleterious effect of glucose pretreatment on recovery from diffuse cerebral ischemia in the cat. I. Local cerebral blood flow and glucose utilization. Stroke 1980;11:347.

25. Welsh FA, Ginsberg MD, Rieder W, et al. Deleterious effect of glucose pretreatment on recovery from diffuse cerebral ischemia in the cat. II. Regional metabolite levels. Stroke 1980;11:355.

26. Attwell D, Buchan AM, Charpak S, et al. Glial and neuronal control of brain blood flow. Nature 2010; 468:232.

27. Bruno A, Levine SR, Frankel MR, et al. Admission glucose level and clinical outcomes in the NINDS rt-PA Stroke Trial. Neurology 2002;59:669.

28. Passero S, Ciacci G, Ulivelli M. The influence of diabetes and hyperglycemia on clinical course after intracerebral hemorrhage. Neurology 2003;61:1351.

29. Latorre JG, Chou SH, Nogueira RG, et al. Effective glycemic control with aggressive hyperglycemia management is associated with improved outcome in aneurysmal subarachnoid hemorrhage. Stroke 2009;40:1644.

30. Kurtz P, Claassen J, Helbok R, et al. Systemic glucose variability predicts cerebral metabolic distress and mortality after subarachnoid hemorrhage: a retrospective observational study. Crit Care 2014;18:R89.

31. Garg R, Chaudhuri A, Munschauer F, et al. Hyperglycemia, insulin, and acute ischemic stroke: a mechanistic justification for a trial of insulin infusion therapy. Stroke 2006;37:267.

32. Gray CS, Hildreth AJ, Sandercock PA, et al. Glucose-potassium-insulin infusions in the management of post-stroke hyperglycaemia: the UK Glucose Insulin in Stroke Trial (GIST-UK). Lancet Neurol 2007;6:397.

33. Johnston KC, Hall CE, Kissela BM, et al. Glucose Regulation in Acute Stroke Patients (GRASP) trial: a randomized pilot trial. Stroke 2009;40:3804.

34. Bruno A, Durkalski VL, Hall CE, et al. The Stroke Hyperglycemia Insulin Network Effort (SHINE) trial protocol: a randomized, blinded, efficacy trial of standard vs. intensive hyperglycemia management in acute stroke. Int J Stroke 2014;9:246.

35. Young B, Ott L, Dempsey R, et al. Relationship between admission hyperglycemia and neurologic outcome of severely brain-injured patients. Ann Surg 1989;210:466.

36. Lam AM, Winn HR, Cullen BF, et al. Hyperglycemia and neurological outcome in patients with head injury. J Neurosurg 1991;75:545.

37. Rovlias A, Kotsou S. The influence of hyperglycemia on neurological outcome in patients with severe head injury. Neurosurgery 2000;46:335.

38. Jeremitsky E, Omert LA, Dunham CM, et al. The impact of hyperglycemia on patients with severe brain injury. J Trauma 2005;58:47.

39. Liu-DeRyke X, Collingridge DS, Orme J, et al. Clinical impact of early hyperglycemia during acute phase of traumatic brain injury. Neurocrit Care 2009;11:151.

40. Seyed Saadat SM, Bidabadi E, Seyed Saadat SN, et al. Association of persistent hyperglycemia with outcome of severe traumatic brain injury in pediatric population. Childs Nerv Syst 2012;28:1773.

41. Bilotta F, Caramia R, Cernak I, et al. Intensive insulin therapy after severe traumatic brain injury: a randomized clinical trial. Neurocrit Care 2008;9:159.

42. Graffagnino C, Gurram AR, Kolls B, et al. Intensive insulin therapy in the neurocritical care setting is associated with poor clinical outcomes. Neurocrit Care 2010;13:307.

43. Green DM, O'Phelan KH, Bassin SL, et al. Intensive versus conventional insulin therapy in critically ill neurologic patients. Neurocrit Care 2010;13:299.

44. Pop V, Badaut J. A neurovascular perspective for long-term changes after brain trauma. Transl Stroke Res 2011;2:533.

45. Villapol S, Byrnes KR, Symes AJ. Temporal dynamics of cerebral blood flow, cortical damage, apoptosis, astrocyte-vasculature interaction and astrogliosis in the pericontusional region after traumatic brain injury. Front Neurol 2014;5:82.

46. Logsdon AF, Lucke-Wold BP, Turner RC, et al. Role of microvascular disruption in brain damage from traumatic brain injury. Compr Physiol 2015;5:1147.

47. Bouzat P, Sala N, Payen JF, et al. Beyond intracranial pressure: optimization of cerebral blood flow, oxygen, and substrate delivery after traumatic brain injury. Ann Intensive Care 2013;3:23.

48. Hovda DA, Yoshino A, Kawamata T, et al. Diffuse prolonged depression of cerebral oxidative metabolism following concussive brain injury in the rat: a cytochrome oxidase histochemistry study. Brain Res 1991;567:1.

49. Yoshino A, Hovda DA, Kawamata T, et al. Dynamic changes in local cerebral glucose utilization following

cerebral conclusion in rats: evidence of a hyper- and subsequent hypometabolic state. Brain Res 1991; 561:106.

50. Bergsneider M, Hovda DA, Shalmon E, et al. Cerebral hyperglycolysis following severe traumatic brain injury in humans: a positron emission tomography study. J Neurosurg 1997;86:241.

51. O'Connell MT, Seal A, Nortje J, et al. Glucose metabolism in traumatic brain injury: a combined microdialysis and [18F]-2-fluoro-2-deoxy-D-glucose-positron emission tomography (FDG-PET) study. Acta Neurochir Suppl 2005;95:165.

52. Vespa PM, McArthur D, O'Phelan K, et al. Persistently low extracellular glucose correlates with poor outcome 6 months after human traumatic brain injury despite a lack of increased lactate: a microdialysis study. J Cereb Blood Flow Metab 2003;23:865.

53. Dusick JR, Glenn TC, Lee WN, et al. Increased pentose phosphate pathway flux after clinical traumatic brain injury: a [1,2-13C2]glucose labeling study in humans. J Cereb Blood Flow Metab 2007; 27:1593.

54. Glenn TC, Kelly DF, Boscardin WJ, et al. Energy dysfunction as a predictor of outcome after moderate or severe head injury: indices of oxygen, glucose, and lactate metabolism. J Cereb Blood Flow Metab 2003;23:1239.

55. Sanchez JJ, Bidot CJ, O'Phelan K, et al. Neuromonitoring with microdialysis in severe traumatic brain injury patients. Acta Neurochir Suppl 2013;118:223.

56. Stein NR, McArthur DL, Etchepare M, et al. Early cerebral metabolic crisis after TBI influences outcome despite adequate hemodynamic resuscitation. Neurocrit Care 2012;17:49.

57. Timofeev I, Carpenter KL, Nortje J, et al. Cerebral extracellular chemistry and outcome following traumatic brain injury: a microdialysis study of 223 patients. Brain 2011;134:484.

58. Reinstrup P, Stahl N, Mellergard P, et al. Intracerebral microdialysis in clinical practice: baseline values for chemical markers during wakefulness, anesthesia, and neurosurgery. Neurosurgery 2000;47:701.

59. Bergsneider M, Hovda DA, McArthur DL, et al. Metabolic recovery following human traumatic brain injury based on FDG-PET: time course and relationship to neurological disability. J Head Trauma Rehabil 2001;16:135.

60. Vespa P, Tubi M, Claassen J, et al. Metabolic crisis occurs with seizures and periodic discharges after brain trauma. Ann Neurol 2016;79(4):579–90.

61. Ungerstedt U, Pycock C. Functional correlates of dopamine neurotransmission. Bull Schweiz Akad Med Wiss 1974;30:44.

62. Ungerstedt U. Microdialysis: principles and applications for studies in animals and man. J Intern Med 1991;230:365.

63. Hillered L, Persson L, Ponten U, et al. Neurometabolic monitoring of the ischaemic human brain using microdialysis. Acta Neurochir (Wien) 1990;102:91.

64. Meyerson BA, Linderoth B, Karlsson H, et al. Microdialysis in the human brain: extracellular measurements in the thalamus of parkinsonian patients. Life Sci 1990;46:301.

65. Chaurasia CS, Muller M, Bashaw ED, et al. AAPS-FDA Workshop White Paper: microdialysis principles, application, and regulatory perspectives. J Clin Pharmacol 2007;47:589.

66. Hutchinson P, O'Phelan K. International multidisciplinary consensus conference on multimodality monitoring: cerebral metabolism. Neurocrit Care 2014;21(Suppl 2):S148.

67. Le Roux P, Menon DK, Citerio G, et al. Consensus summary statement of the International Multidisciplinary Consensus Conference on Multimodality Monitoring in Neurocritical Care: a statement for healthcare professionals from the Neurocritical Care Society and the European Society of Intens. Neurocrit Care 2014;21(Suppl 2):S1.

68. Holbein M, Bechir M, Ludwig S, et al. Differential influence of arterial blood glucose on cerebral metabolism following severe traumatic brain injury. Crit Care 2009;13:R13.

69. Vespa P, Boonyaputthikul R, McArthur DL, et al. Intensive insulin therapy reduces microdialysis glucose values without altering glucose utilization or improving the lactate/pyruvate ratio after traumatic brain injury. Crit Care Med 2006;34:850.

70. Oddo M, Schmidt JM, Carrera E, et al. Impact of tight glycemic control on cerebral glucose metabolism after severe brain injury: a microdialysis study. Crit Care Med 2008;36:3233.

71. Meierhans R, Bechir M, Ludwig S, et al. Brain metabolism is significantly impaired at blood glucose below 6 mM and brain glucose below 1 mM in patients with severe traumatic brain injury. Crit Care 2010;14:R13.

72. Vespa P, McArthur DL, Stein N, et al. Tight glycemic control increases metabolic distress in traumatic brain injury: a randomized controlled within-subjects trial. Crit Care Med 2012;40:1923.

73. Vespa P, Bergsneider M, Hattori N, et al. Metabolic crisis without brain ischemia is common after traumatic brain injury: a combined microdialysis and positron emission tomography study. J Cereb Blood Flow Metab 2005;25:763.

74. Kurtz P, Claassen J, Schmidt JM, et al. Reduced brain/serum glucose ratios predict cerebral metabolic distress and mortality after severe brain injury. Neurocrit Care 2013;19:311.

75. Badjatia N, Vespa P. Monitoring nutrition and glucose in acute brain injury. Neurocrit Care 2014; 21(Suppl 2):S159.

Role of Metabolomics in Traumatic Brain Injury Research

Stephanie M. Wolahan, PhD[a,b], Daniel Hirt, MD[a,b],
Daniel Braas, PhD[c,d], Thomas C. Glenn, PhD[a,b],*

KEYWORDS

- Small molecules • Spectroscopy • Metabolism • Principal component analysis • Biomarkers

KEY POINTS

- Metabolomics is the study of the small molecules, which are reactants, intermediaries, and end products of biological processes. Metabolomics can define healthy and disease states. The genome and proteome, along with environmental factors, contribute to the metabolome. Metabolomic studies can be untargeted or targeted.
- Metabolomic analytical techniques include nuclear magnetic resonance spectroscopy and mass spectroscopy, including gas chromatography or liquid chromatography.
- The following 3 major components are required for conducting metabolomics studies: good specimens collected in an accepted manner; a strong analytical facility; and knowledgeable statisticians.
- Common data elements, biobanks, and collaborations/multidisciplinary teams will be necessary to produce meaningful results.
- Heterogeneity of disease and progressive nature mean that applying metabolomics to predicting secondary events and/or long-term risks could be highly impactful.

INTRODUCTION

The explosion of "omics" in various fields of biology has led to new and exciting areas of research. In addition to genomics and proteomics, metabolism, or the biology of small molecules, was an early adapter to the "omics" mania. The overarching aims of "omics" studies are to characterize large collections of molecules and describe their role(s) in biological systems during normal health and disease. The number of molecules quantified in each sample can easily outnumber the subjects, and sophisticated analytical and statistical techniques must be used to exploit the rich information found in the biological specimens. The goal of this article is to briefly describe the current state-of-the-art regarding metabolomics and frame it in the context of traumatic brain injury (TBI).

Metabolomics is concerned with a diverse set of endogenous, low-molecular-weight biochemicals that serve as substrates and intermediates of

The authors have nothing to disclose.
[a] UCLA Brain Injury Research Center, David Geffen School of Medicine at UCLA, 10833 Le Conte Ave, Los Angeles, CA 90095, USA; [b] Department of Neurosurgery, David Geffen School of Medicine at UCLA, 300 Stein Plaza, Los Angeles, CA 90095-6901, USA; [c] Department of Molecular and Medical Pharmacology, David Geffen School of Medicine at UCLA, 570 Westwood Plaza, Los Angeles, CA 90095-1735, USA; [d] UCLA Metabolomics and Proteomics Center, 570 Westwood Plaza, University of California, Los Angeles, Los Angeles, CA 90095, USA
* Corresponding author. Department of Neurosurgery, David Geffen School of Medicine at UCLA, PO Box 956901, 300 Stein Plaza, Room 533, Los Angeles, CA 90095-6901.
E-mail address: TGlenn@mednet.ucla.edu

Neurosurg Clin N Am 27 (2016) 465–472
http://dx.doi.org/10.1016/j.nec.2016.05.006
1042-3680/16/$ – see front matter © 2016 Elsevier Inc. All rights reserved.

biochemical pathways and/or as signaling molecules. Within the systems biology approach, metabolomics is at the top of the biological continuum and represents a snapshot of the systemic environment created by the genome, transcriptome, and proteome.[1] Following TBI, particularly in the acute setting, biochemical homeostasis is disrupted and reflected in the metabolome.

There are 2 general designs in metabolomics studies[2]:

- Untargeted, or exploratory, metabolomics studies seek to identify a global metabolite fingerprint by quantifying as many metabolites as possible in the same biological sample.
- Targeted metabolomics studies limit the number of metabolites included in analysis to improve data interpretation and answer well-defined clinical questions.

Untargeted studies are used to test whether 2 groups (eg, healthy subject vs TBI patient) can be discriminated from one another on the basis of biofluid metabolites by including as many metabolites as possible no matter the biochemical pathway involved, independent of molecular identity, and assuming bias-free metabolite quantification. Targeted studies will focus on a set of endogenous metabolites and/or may include exogenous isotopically labeled metabolites to track biochemical pathway activity.

Study of the small molecules that enter biochemical pathways has a long history in TBI research, although application of modern metabolomics techniques to these research questions is sparse. For example, glucose and lactate dynamics in the acute period have been studied with respect to outcome, to disease progression, and to mechanisms.

In the first week after injury, hyperglycolysis was reported to occur in 56% of patients.[3] The hyperglycolytic transient response increases cerebral glucose utilization but, despite adequate oxygenation, is not matched by an increase in the metabolic rate of oxygen. The high energy demands are caused by TBI-induced ionic and neurochemical imbalances,[4–6] and increased nonoxidative metabolism of glucose produces excess lactate. High-lactate cerebral spinal fluid (CSF) concentrations have been associated with cerebral lactic acidosis and, when prolonged, with poor outcomes.[7–9]

Global and regional hyperglycolysis are followed by global cerebral metabolic depression, independent of level of consciousness, that can persist for a month following injury.[10–12] Cerebral uptake of both oxygen and glucose is depressed compared with healthy adults, and glucose is relatively more depressed.

Throughout the acute after-injury period, TBI causes metabolic crisis that is long lasting and unresolved by standard clinical resuscitation and control of intracranial pressure (ICP).[13,14] Cerebral metabolic crisis is the coincidence of low cerebral glucose concentration and high lactate:pyruvate ratio (LPR). Nonischemic metabolic crisis results from mitochondrial dysfunction and is exacerbated by and/or increases risk for secondary insults, and prolonged acute metabolic crisis is linked to increased brain atrophy 6 months following injury.[15–18]

In a later publication on blood glucose, lactate, and oxygen, most TBI patients showed cerebral lactate uptake (arteriovenous difference >0) at least once, and the patients with favorable outcome were associated with cerebral lactate uptake at moderately elevated arterial lactate concentrations.[19] The ability of the injured brain to oxidize lactate, and the potential benefits associated with lactate as a cerebral fuel, was recently investigated using the dual isotope tracer technique.[20,21]

Based on the prior interest in small molecules in TBI research, metabolomics is well suited to expand the current understanding of dysfunctional cerebral metabolism.

DISCUSSION
Biospecimen Sources in Traumatic Brain Injury

Table 1 summarizes possible biospecimens for use in metabolomics studies in TBI research. Targeted metabolomics analysis of cerebral tissue has been applied to TBI research on animal models.[22–28]

The range of biofluids typically used for metabolomic analysis includes blood (plasma or serum), urine, saliva, CSF, and microdialysate. Standard operating procedures for collecting and storing biofluids should be followed.[29,30]

Cerebral microdialysate studies based on the hourly metabolite measurements could be considered a type of metabolomics study.[31,32] Metabolic crisis is defined as low microdialysis glucose (less than 0.8 mM considered abnormal) coincident with a high LPR (greater than 40 critical; greater than 25 abnormal) and has been associated with poor recovery.[13–18] Glutamate, glycerol, and urea are also available with the ICSUSflex Microdialysis Analyzer (M Dialysis AB, Stockholm, Sweden), and microdialysis is considered a valuable tool in the neurologic intensive care unit (ICU).[33] The Cambridge group has published research using pooled cerebral microdialysate (generally over a period of 24 hours) and has introduced tracer

Table 1
Biospecimen sources for application of metabolomics in traumatic brain injury research

Biospecimen	Pros	Cons
Tissue	The most direct relevance to the injury, can compare injured hemisphere to uninjured hemisphere	Not applicable to clinical research; rarely would tissue be available and unclear how a metabolomics study could be designed
Blood	Easily obtained	Systemic vs brain
Arteriovenous differences	Systemic minus cerebral metabolites	Jugular catheter is invasive
Cerebrospinal fluid	Drained as a treatment for high ICP, would otherwise be discarded	Commonly available with severe injuries; invasive to obtain otherwise
Urine	Easily obtained	Concentration of metabolites a function of systemic dilution; within sample normalization is common
Cerebral microdialysate	From the cerebral tissue, as close to the source as possible	Low volumes obtained leading to pooling biofluid over a large period of time; perfusate and not directly sampling extracellular fluid

metabolites to the tissue through the microdialysis catheter itself.[34]

Biospecimen banks may contain multiple biospecimens from the same individual, allowing longitudinal metabolomics studies and/or comparison of metabolite profiles between biofluids.[35] **Figs. 1** and **2** present spectra of biofluids collected simultaneously, including arterial blood plasma, jugular venous blood plasma, CSF, and urine (see **Fig. 1**). The cerebral microdialysate spectrum is the result of pooling 12 hours of fluid, from midnight to noon, and the corresponding plasma was drawn at 9:30 AM (see **Fig. 2**).

Integration of metabolomics datasets from different biofluids and integration of metabolomics datasets collected on different platforms are an exciting avenue for TBI researchers, particularly for understanding dysfunction in biochemical pathways and for working toward a systems-level understanding of the cerebral and systemic responses to neurotrauma.

Technologies Used in Metabolomics

Mass spectrometry (MS) and nuclear magnetic resonance (NMR) are the most common

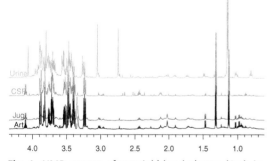

Fig. 1. NMR spectra of arterial blood plasma (Art), jugular venous blood plasma (Jug), cerebrospinal fluid (CSF), and urine. Biospecimens were obtained from a TBI patient within a 5-minute period. The UCLA Brain Injury Research Center research nurse and a research assistant visit the bedside together and, following biofluid draws by the research nurse, samples are immediately placed on ice and processed by the research assistant. Urine and CSF are transferred to Falcon tubes, centrifuged, frozen on dry ice, and transferred to a −80°C freezer as soon as possible. Blood is transferred to lithium heparin coated tubes and centrifuged, and plasma is retained for the freezer.

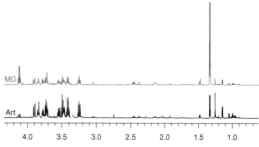

Fig. 2. NMR spectra of arterial blood plasma (Art) and cerebral microdialysate (MD) pooled over a period of 12 hours. Cerebral microdialysis vials are immediately analyzed by the ICSUS flex microdialysis analyzer for glucose, lactate, and pyruvate as routine clinical practice and frozen on dry ice and transferred to a −80°C freezer as soon as possible after that.

technologies used in metabolomics. Applying these technologies to metabolomics studies requires careful consideration of study goals and the expertise available, and detailed reviews are available.[36,37]

Table 2 compares MS-based methods and NMR. MS-based methods identify metabolites by the mass-to-charge ratio (*m/z*) and, when using a chromatography step, the retention time is also required. The intensity of the MS peak at a particular retention time and *m/z* are proportional to the concentration.

NMR methods identify metabolites by the spectral peak pattern; all chemicals present in the biofluid containing hydrogen are present in the NMR spectrum. Metabolites with similar chemical structures overlap one another (for example, L-lactate and L-threonine overlap at 1.3 ppm). The integrated area of the spectral peak is proportional to concentration.

Because of the complexity and specialization required for MS-based metabolomics methods, there are companies, such as Metabolon Inc (Durham, NC, USA), that analyze samples and return high-quality data, statistical analysis, and chemical identification to their customers. Companies offering fee-for-service analysis generally provide reduced pricing to academic institutions. In addition, there are National Institutes of Health–funded facilities such as the West Coast Metabolomics Center at UC Davis that can also conduct analysis as a fee for service.

Statistical Data Analysis

With the aim to better understand disease pathology, both implementing and interpreting advanced statistical modeling techniques are required. The large size of the raw data makes all stages of data processing nontrivial.

Table 2
Comparison between mass spectrometry and nuclear magnetic resonance as it applies to metabolomics research

	MS	NMR
Sensitivity	$\geq$ picoMole concentrations	$\geq$ microMole concentrations
Sample preparation	Minimal to extensive: deproteinization, derivatization possibly required for targeted studies	Minimal: addition of a buffered deuterium oxide solution, deproteinization optional
Sample volume	On the order of 10 μL	On the order of 100 μL or more
Quantification	Relative concentrations are most common, absolute quantification requires internal chemical standard at known concentration for each metabolite	Absolute concentrations are standard; internal chemical standard at known concentration routinely added during sample preparation[44]
Chromatography?	Yes, either liquid or gas chromatography used before injection into the instrument	Not common
Sample recovered?	No: principle relies on fragmentation of molecules and physical interaction with the instrument	Yes: principle relies on nuclear spin, a fundamental property of certain nuclei, and excitation/emission of photons is nondestructive
Quality control	Interbatch and intrabatch variability requires periodically testing a set of standards and correcting for changes in sensitivity over time after data collection	Not required
Global	Yes, but requires quality control and instrument expertise	Yes
Targeted: endogenous	Highly sensitive and specific	Depends on the location of the resonance peaks in the spectrum
Targeted: exogenous	Yes	Depends, and NMR-active isotopes (^{13}C or ^{15}N) at low natural abundance are helpful

Before statistical exploration of the data, extensive spectral processing is required.[38] These steps ensure that (a) high-quality datasets with minimal biases are used, (b) spectral features are assigned to metabolites correctly, and (c) all spectra are aligned before metabolite concentration extraction.

Univariate comparisons are helpful in data exploration and may be helpful in discussing an interpretation of the data, but the increasing number of metabolites that modern analytical techniques allow makes univariate analyses laborious. Multiple testing corrections, including the Bonferroni correction and the q value,[39] should be used in order to minimize spurious results in these cases.[40]

Multivariate regression methods are more likely to discern statistically significant changes and minimize false positives. Multivariate regression methods include principal components analysis (PCA), partial least squares, and orthogonal projections to latent structures, and although these methods are widely available in statistical computing packages, using the method properly is not trivial and perhaps more important than which method is used.[41]

Unsupervised methods, such as PCA, seek out patterns in the variance of the data without any other prior knowledge about the data. PCA in particular parses out the variance from largest to smallest. Supervised methods identify patterns in the variance associated with a certain trait or variable of interest while down weighting other (perhaps larger) sources of variance.

For metabolomics to meaningfully impact TBI research, results must be reported numerically, not only as a principal components (PC) scores plot, and statistical significance must be reported. Without an attempt at interpreting metabolite loadings within the biological context, metabolomics studies lose scientific impact.

In order for metabolomics techniques to enter the clinic, the discrimination must be superior to the current gold standard. In the case that a metabolomics test does not significantly improve diagnosis accuracy, further research in the area could clarify which biochemical pathways are associated with a disease.

Role of Metabolomics in Clinical Research

Metabolomics has been applied to the diagnosis of several diseases, including diabetes and cardiovascular disease.[41] Diagnosis of mild TBI or concussions is an area of active research where metabolomics could be applied.[42]

This powerful modern research technique, metabolomics, could serve many roles in contemporary TBI clinical research (**Box 1**). The TBI patient population is heterogeneous for several reasons, both because of the injury itself and because the disease progresses over time differently between individuals. Furthermore, the metabolome is reflective of active biochemical pathways and is also influenced by a subject's environment, which means large patient cohorts will be required to detect small effects.

It is important for real clinical applications to convert the numerical "significance" to whether this could actually improve things for patients, not only improve sensitivity/specificity, but also whether it could improve on current gold standard.

Example of Metabolomics Applied to Traumatic Brain Injury Research

The authors conducted an observational feasibility study aimed at identifying differences in the metabolite profile of TBI patients and healthy control individuals. Six TBI patients (mean age 31; mean Glasgow Coma Score (GCS): 3.8) and 2 healthy controls were consented for arterial and jugular venous blood sampling. The University of California, Los Angeles (UCLA) institutional review board (IRB) for human research approved this study. TBI subjects were identified and consented by proxy, and enrolled. Eligible patients were mechanically ventilated, head injured adults (aged 18 and older) with GCS less than or equal 8. Normal volunteers were recruited under UCLA IRB approval.

A total of 90 metabolites were identified by liquid chromatography–MS,[43] analyzed with an UltiMate 3000RSLC (Thermo Scientific) coupled to a Q

Box 1
Possible applications of metabolomics in traumatic brain injury research

Acute injury setting (in the neurologic ICU):

- Monitoring acute pathophysiology
- Predicting onset of secondary injuries, such as high ICP, edema, vasospasm
- Monitoring treatments: identifying candidate treatments and treatment success
- Prognosis, long-term outcomes

Chronic injuries:

- Monitoring evolving pathophysiology
- Rehabilitation suitability
- Association between TBI and later-in-life health issues

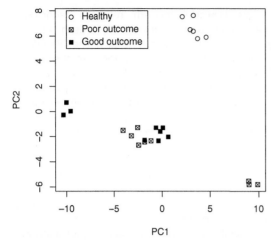

Fig. 3. Principal components score plot. Eight arterial plasma samples (2 healthy controls) were run in triplicate.

Exactive mass spectrometer (Thermo Scientific). The Q Exactive was run with polarity switching (+4.00 kV/−4.00 kV) in full-scan mode with an m/z range of 70–1050. Separation was achieved using (a) 5 mM NH_4AcO (pH 9.9) and (b) acetonitrile. The gradient started with 15% (a) going to 90% (b) over 18 minutes, followed by an isocratic step for 9 minutes and reversal to the initial 15% (a) for 7 minutes. Metabolites were quantified with TraceFinder 3.1 using accurate mass measurements (≤ 3 ppm) and retention times

established by running pure standards. PCA was performed using the statistical language R.

PCA revealed significant separation of the metabolite contributions of TBI versus normal patients in principal component 2 (PC2) ($P<.0001$, **Fig. 3**). Principal component 1 (PC1) discriminated between individuals included in the analysis (explaining 26% of the total variance, PC2 explaining 15%). The authors were unable to discriminate between subjects with 6-month Glasgow Outcome Scale extended scores between 2 and 4 (poor outcome) and those between 5 and 8 (good outcome).

Investigation of the metabolite loadings revealed that metabolites of glycolysis and the TCA cycle, such as fumarate, lactate, and 2-oxoadipate, were the most negative metabolite loadings (**Fig. 4**), and thus, make large contributions to the PC scores of brain-injured patients, ranging from approximately −6 to 1 (scores are unitless). In contrast, citrate and aconitate, metabolites in these same pathways, had the largest metabolite loadings and thus, were decreased in TBI patients compared with normal individuals. Other differences that were identified between these 2 groups included changes in numerous amino acids (phenylalanine, tyrosine, cysteine), metabolites involved in glycerophospholipid metabolism (phosphoenthanolamine and choline phosphate), and metabolites involved in pyrimidine metabolism (cytosine and orotidine), as presented in **Fig. 4**.

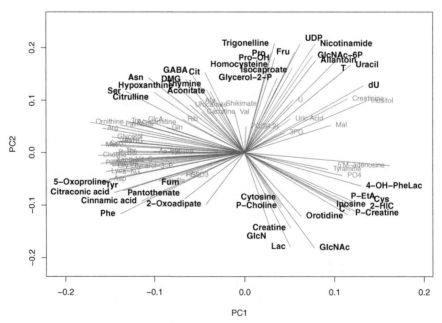

Fig. 4. Principal components loadings plot. Loadings in the top PC2 quartile and bottom PC2 quartile are highlighted.

SUMMARY

There are 3 major components required for conducting metabolomics studies:

- Good specimens collected in an accepted manner
- A strong analytical facility
- Knowledgeable statisticians

Understanding the metabolomic profile of TBI is an important quest. From the moment of physical insult to rehabilitation and recovery, metabolomics can yield useful information about the pathophysiology of this disease. Metabolomics is an underlying component of precision medicine that allows the clinician scientist the ability to tailor medical care and treatment. Many more metabolomic studies need to be conducted across the entire spectrum of TBI in order to better understand and treat TBI.

REFERENCES

1. Serkova NJ, Standiford TJ, Stringer KA. The emerging field of quantitative blood metabolomics for biomarker discovery in critical illness. Am J Respir Crit Care Med 2011;184:647–55.
2. Bowling FG, Thomas M. Analyzing the metabolome. Chapter 3. In: Trent R, editor. Clinical bioinformatics. 2nd edition. New York: Humana Press; 2014. p. 31–45.
3. Bergsneider M, Hovda DA, Shalmon E, et al. Cerebral hyperglycolysis following severe traumatic brain injury in humans: a positron emission tomography study. J Neurosurg 1997;86:241–51.
4. Katayama Y, Becker DP, Tamura T, et al. Massive increases in extracellular potassium and the indiscriminate release of glutamate following concussive brain injury. J Neurosurg 1990;73:889–900.
5. Kawamata T, Katayama Y, Hovda DA, et al. Lactate accumulation following concussive brain injury: the role of ionic fluxes induced by excitatory amino acids. Brain Res 1995;20:196–204.
6. Sunami K, Nakamura T, Ozawa Y, et al. Hypermetabolic state following experimental head injury. Neurosurg Rev 1989;12(Suppl 1):400–15.
7. De Salles AA, Kontos HA, Becker DP, et al. Prognostic significance of ventricular CSF lactic acidosis in severe head injury. J Neurosurg 1986;65:615–24.
8. De Salles AA, Muizelaar JP, Young HF. Hyperglycemia, cerebrospinal fluid lactic acidosis, and cerebral blood flow in severely head-injured patients. Neurosurgery 1987;21:45–50.
9. Inao S, Marmarou A, Clarke GD, et al. Production and clearance of lactate from brain tissue, cerebrospinal fluid, and serum following experimental brain injury. J Neurosurg 1988;69:736–44.
10. Bergsneider M, Hovda D, McArthur D, et al. Metabolic recovery following human traumatic brain injury based on FDG-PET: time course and relationship to neurological disability. J Head Trauma Rehabil 2001;16:135–48.
11. Bergsneider M, Hovda DA, Lee SM, et al. Dissociation of cerebral glucose metabolism and level of consciousness during the period of metabolic depression following human traumatic brain injury. J Neurotrauma 2000;17:389–401.
12. Yoshino A, Hovda DA, Kawamata T, et al. Dynamic changes in local cerebral glucose utilization following cerebral concussion in rats: evidence of a hyper- and subsequent hypometabolic state. Brain Res 1991; 561:106–19.
13. Stein NR, McArthur DL, Etchepare M, et al. Early cerebral metabolic crisis after TBI influences outcome despite adequate hemodynamic resuscitation. Neurocrit Care 2012;17:49–57.
14. Vespa PM, Bergsneider M, Hattori N, et al. Metabolic crisis without brain ischemia is common after traumatic brain injury: a combined microdialysis and positron emission tomography study. J Cereb Blood Flow Metab 2005;25:763–74.
15. Marcoux J, McArthur DA, Miller C, et al. Persistent metabolic crisis as measured by elevated cerebral microdialysis lactate-pyruvate ratio predicts chronic frontal lobe brain atrophy after traumatic brain injury. Crit Care Med 2008;36:2871–7.
16. Vespa PM, McArthur DL, O'Phelan K, et al. Persistently low extracellular glucose correlates with poor outcome 6 months after human traumatic brain injury despite a lack of increased lactate: a microdialysis study. J Cereb Blood Flow Metab 2003;23:865–77.
17. Vespa PM, Miller C, McArthur D, et al. Nonconvulsive electrographic seizures after traumatic brain injury result in a delayed, prolonged increase in intracranial pressure and metabolic crisis. Crit Care Med 2007;35:2830–6.
18. Xu Y, McArthur DL, Alger JR, et al. Early nonischemic oxidative metabolic dysfunction leads to chronic brain atrophy in traumatic brain injury. J Cereb Blood Flow Metab 2010;30:883–94.
19. Glenn TC, Kelly DF, Boscardin WJ, et al. Energy dysfunction as a predictor of outcome after moderate or severe head injury: indices of oxygen, glucose, and lactate metabolism. J Cereb Blood Flow Metab 2003;23:1239–50.
20. Glenn TC, Martin NA, Horning MA, et al. Lactate: brain fuel in human traumatic brain injury. A comparison to normal healthy control subjects. J Neurotrauma 2015; 32(11):820–32.
21. Glenn TC, Martin NA, McArthur DL, et al. Endogenous nutritive support following traumatic brain injury: peripheral lactate production for glucose supply via gluconeogenesis. J Neurotrauma 2015;32(11):811–9.
22. Bartnik BL, Hovda DA, Lee PW. Glucose metabolism after traumatic brain injury: estimation of pyruvate carboxylase and pyruvate dehydrogenase flux by

mass isotopomer analysis. J Neurotrauma 2007;24: 181–94.

23. Bartnik BL, Lee SM, Hovda DA, et al. The fate of glucose during the period of decreased metabolism after fluid percussion injury: a ^{13}C NMR study. J Neurotrauma 2007;24:1079–92.

24. Bartnik BL, Sutton RL, Fukushima M, et al. Upregulation of pentose phosphate pathway and preservation of tricarboxylic acid cycle flux after experimental brain injury. J Neurotrauma 2005;22:1052–65.

25. Bentzer P, Davidsson H, Grande P. Microdialysis-based long-term measurement of energy-related metabolites in the rat brain following a fluid percussion trauma. J Neurotrauma 2000;17:441–7.

26. Clausen F, Hillered L, Gustafsson J. Cerebral glucose metabolism after traumatic brain injury in the rat studied by 13C-glucose and microdialysis. Acta Neurochir 2011;153:653–8.

27. Tavazzi B, Signoretti S, Lazzarino G, et al. Cerebral oxidative stress and depression of energy metabolism correlate with severity of diffuse brain injury in rats. Neurosurgery 2005;56:582–9.

28. Viant MR, Lyeth BG, Miller MG, et al. An NMR metabolomic investigation of early metabolic disturbances following TBI in a mammalian model. NMR Biomed 2005;18:507–16.

29. Manley GT, Diaz-Arrastia R, Brophy M, et al. Common data elements for traumatic brain injury: recommendations from the biospecimens and biomarkers working group. Arch Phys Med Rehabil 2010;91:1667–72.

30. Yue JK, Vassar MJ, Lingsma HF, et al. Transforming research and clinical knowledge in traumatic brain injury pilot: multicenter implementation of the common data elements for traumatic brain injury. J Neurotrauma 2013;30:1831–44.

31. Jalloh I, Helmy A, Shannon RJ, et al. Lactate uptake by the injured human brain: evidence from an arteriovenous gradient and cerebral microdialysis study. J Neurotrauma 2013;30:2031–7.

32. Timofeev I, Carpenter K, Nortje J, et al. Cerebral extracellular chemistry and outcome following traumatic brain injury: a microdialysis study of 233 patients. Brain 2011;134:484–94.

33. Hutchinson P, O'Phelan K, Participants of the International Multi-disciplinary Consensus Conference on Multimodality Monitoring. International

multidisciplinary consensus conference on multimodality monitoring: cerebral metabolism. Neurocrit Care 2014;21:S148–58.

34. Gallagher CN, Carpenter KL, Grice P, et al. The human brain utilizes lactate via the tricarboxylic acid cycle: a ^{13}C-labelled microdialysis and high-resolution nuclear magnetic resonance study. Brain 2009;132:2839–49.

35. Robinette SL, Lindon JC, Nicholson JK. Statistical spectroscopic tools for biomarker discovery and systems medicine. Anal Chem 2013;85:5297–303.

36. Dettmer K, Aronov PA, Hammock BD. Mass spectrometry-based metabolomics. Mass Spectrom Rev 2007;26:51–78.

37. Zhang S, Gowda GAN, Ye T, et al. Advances in NMR-based biofluid analysis and metabolite profiling. Analyst 2010;135:1490–8.

38. Alonso A, Marsal S, Julia A. Analytical methods in untargeted metabolomics: state of the art in 2015. Front Bioeng Biotechnol 2015;3:23.

39. Storey J, Tibshirani R. Statistical significance for genomewide studies. Proc Nat Acad Sci 2003;100: 9440–5.

40. Broadhurst DI, Kell DB. Statistical strategies for avoiding false discoveries in metabolomics and related experiments. Metabolomics 2006;2:171–96.

41. Madsen R, Lundstedt T, Trygg J. Chemometrics in metabolomics—a review in human disease diagnosis. Anal Chim Acta 2010;659:23–33.

42. Jeter CB, Hergenroeder GW, Ward NH, et al. Human mild traumatic brain injury decreases circulating branched-chain amino acid and their metabolite levels. J Neurotrauma 2013;30:671–9.

43. Thai M, Graham NA, Braas D, et al. Adenovirus E4ORF1-induced MYC activation promotes host cell anabolic glucose metabolism and virus replication. Cell Metab 2014;19:694–701.

44. Wolahan SM, Hirt D, Glenn TC. Translational metabolomics of head injury: exploring dysfunctional cerebral metabolism with ex vivo NMR spectroscopy-based metabolite quantification. In: Kobeissy FH, editor. Brain neurotrauma: molecular, neuropsychological, and rehabilitation aspects. Boca Raton (FL): CRC Press; Taylor & Francis; 2015. p. 25.

Cerebral Edema in Traumatic Brain Injury
Pathophysiology and Prospective Therapeutic Targets

Ethan A. Winkler, MD, PhD[a,b], Daniel Minter, BS[b],
John K. Yue, BA[a,b], Geoffrey T. Manley, MD, PhD[a,b],*

KEYWORDS

- Cerebral edema • Traumatic brain injury • Pathophysiology • Therapeutic targets
- Blood-brain barrier

KEY POINTS

- The development of cerebral edema following TBI is an important factor which contributes to evolution of brain injury following initial trauma.
- Post-traumatic cerebral edema arises from disruption of the blood-brain barrier or dysfunction of cellular ionic pumps and may be classified as vasogenic or cytotoxic edema, respectively.
- Vasogenic and cytotoxic edema arise from unique molecular pathways which which may be targeted therapeutically in pre-clinical models.
- Future studies are needed to determine which therapies targeting cerebral edema may have clinical efficacy in human TBI.

INTRODUCTION

Traumatic brain injury (TBI) is a complex and heterogeneous disorder with a tremendous public health burden. It is grossly defined as an alteration in brain function or other evidence of brain pathology caused by an external force which may occur in a multitude of settings – including the highway, at home, at work, during sports activities, and on the battlefield.[1,2] Despite extensive measures taken to prevent these injuries, TBI continues to have an unacceptably high morbidity and mortality. As of 2010, the Centers for Disease Control and Prevention estimated that 2.5 million emergency department visits, hospitalizations, or deaths were associated with TBI, either alone or in combination with other injuries. TBI was a diagnosis in more than 280,000 admissions. A total of 1.7 million people each year sustain a TBI in the United States. Of those, 275,000 are hospitalized and 52,000 die. It is thought that TBI is a contributing factor in nearly a third of all injury-related deaths in the United States.[3] Furthermore, many of those individuals who survive their initial injury will have clinically evident disability later in life; it has been estimated that up to 5.3 million people are currently living with TBI-related disability in the United States alone.[4]

The deleterious effects of a TBI are not confined to the initial traumatic event. Initial brain trauma initiates a complex cascade of pathophysiologic pathways that lead to evolution

[a] Brain and Spinal Injury Center, San Francisco General Hospital, 1001 Potrero Avenue, Building 1, Room 101, San Francisco, CA 94110, USA; [b] Department of Neurological Surgery, University of California, San Francisco, 505 Parnassus Avenue, M779, San Francisco, CA 94143, USA
* Corresponding author. Department of Neurological Surgery, University of California, San Francisco, 1001 Potrero Avenue, Building 1, Room 101, San Francisco, CA 94110.
E-mail address: manleyg@neurosurg.ucsf.edu

Neurosurg Clin N Am 27 (2016) 473–488
http://dx.doi.org/10.1016/j.nec.2016.05.008

of brain injury.[5] These effects have led to the adoption of the crude temporal categories of injury known as primary and secondary injury. Primary injuries are brain injuries that occur at the time of the initial trauma, including cerebral contusions, diffuse axonal injury, penetrating or tissue crushing wounds, extra-axial hematomas, and damage to the cerebral vasculature.[5,6] Short of preventive measures to mitigate and/or avoid initial injury, in the absence of regenerative therapy very few, if any, therapeutic options are available to reverse injury. Secondary injuries are those that occur in the hours to days following the initial insult and are composed of a diverse array of pathophysiologic phenomena, including hypoperfusion, mitochondrial dysfunction, oxidative injury, as well as disruptions to the blood-brain barrier (BBB).[5–8]

One process central to the pathogenesis of secondary injury is the development of cerebral edema.[9] In accordance with the Monro-Kellie Doctrine,[10] an increase in brain volume as a result of cerebral edema rapidly leads to an increase in intracranial pressure (ICP). As brain volume begins to increase, cerebrospinal fluid (CSF) is displaced into the spinal thecal sac and blood is compressed from the distensible cerebral veins with little increase in ICP. Once these compensatory mechanisms are exceeded, ICP increases exponentially—a common deleterious cascade observed in severe TBI—and has been shown to correlate with increased mortality and poor functional outcomes.[11] Increases in ICP, in turn, lead to the compression of brain vasculature and decrease the cerebral perfusion pressure, defined as mean arterial blood pressure subtracted by ICP. Mechanical compression of the vasculature and/or reductions in cerebral perfusion pressure may give rise to either focal or global ischemia, which may lead to further edema and ultimately irreversible brain injury.[12]

Evolving brain edema also leads to the genesis of pressure gradients across different intracranial compartments and mechanical displacement of brain structures across compartments, a phenomenon known as *herniation*. This herniation leads to further neurologic injury through axonal stretch, vascular disruption or compression, and/or a combination thereof and often represents a penultimate event to significant neurologic injury, coma, or death. Despite its importance in neurologic decline, treatment of traumatic intracranial hypertension predominately consists of hyperosmolar therapy, for example, hypertonic saline and mannitol, which lead to the efflux of water from the brain into the systemic circulation and/or surgical decompression. Efforts to expand the treatment armamentarium

for intracranial hypertension, including hypothermia and barbiturate induced coma, have largely been unsuccessful. In the present article, the authors focus on the cellular and molecular mechanisms underlying cerebral edema following TBI derived from review of both clinical and preclinical animal models. Special attention is devoted to the cellular and molecular mechanisms underlying its pathogenesis as well as future therapeutic targets.

PATHOGENESIS OF CEREBRAL EDEMA

Cerebral edema is broadly categorized as being either vasogenic or cytotoxic.[13,14] Vasogenic edema results from disruption to the BBB formed by cerebrovascular endothelial cells (ECs) and leads to an influx of protein-rich fluid from circulating blood into the brain interstitial fluid.[15] Cytotoxic edema, on the other hand, is a product of failure of homeostatic ion channels and pumps resulting in failure of ionic gradients and an intracellular osmotic shift resulting in cellular swelling, a process more prominent in astrocytes and glial cells.[16,17]

TBI is a complex and multifaceted injury that leads to dysfunction and/or disruption of multiple cell types.[5] Although TBI-associated brain edema was initially thought to arise predominantly from vasogenic mechanisms, more recent clinical and preclinical studies have demonstrated that cytotoxic edema plays a significant role.[18–20] For example, MRI studies of patients with closed-head injury revealed a mixed picture of both cytotoxic and vasogenic edema by imaging criteria.[21] However, in the absence of vasogenic edema, a process that depends exclusively on cytotoxic edema would be self-limiting.[22] Similarly, it is likely that the contributions of vasogenic and cytotoxic processes make differential relative contributions through different phases of evolution of edema following brain trauma. In TBI, brain edema is thought to follow a bimodal time course, with one study showing that half of patients had their highest mean ICP recorded during the first 3 days after injury, whereas 25% of patients showed their highest mean ICP after postinjury day 5.[23] In the ensuing subsections, the authors describe in detail the molecular and cellular mechanisms underlying the pathogenesis of posttraumatic vasogenic and cytotoxic edema.

The Blood-Brain Barrier and Neurovascular Unit

The BBB is formed by a continuous lining of brain ECs with specialized properties.[24,25] Tight junctional complexes composed of transmembrane occludin and claudin proteins are linked to the actin cytoskeleton through adapter proteins, such as zonula occludens-1. Adjacent cells are further connected through adherens junctions composed of cell adhesion molecules, for example, vascular endothelial cadherin molecules. Tight and adherens junctions limit unregulated paracellular flow of circulating proteins and cells from blood into brain.[26] Unlike peripheral vascular beds, brain ECs do not possess fenestrae and display low rates of pinocytosis and nonspecific vesicular transport, so-called bulk flow transcytosis.[24,25] As a result, molecules that are not sufficiently lipophilic and greater than 40 kDa are excluded from the brain in the absence of highly specialized and regulated transmembrane transport systems in brain ECs.[25]

EC function, however, is further influenced by adjacent cells. Brain endothelium is surrounded by vascular basement membrane, pericytes, and astrocyte end feet.[24,27,28] Recent research has demonstrated that pericytes are necessary for establishment and maintenance of endothelial barrier properties.[24,26,27,29] Astrocytes also contribute to barrier functionality and polarity of endothelial transport systems.[30] Their end feet also have a high concentration of aquaporin (AQP) channels that facilitate movement for brain free water in and out of the vascular compartment as well as through the para-vascular compartment.[31,32] This growing knowledge of the multicellular structure of the cerebrovasculature has led to the coining of the term *neurovascular unit*, which represents the interconnected relationship of ECs, mural cells (pericytes and vascular smooth muscle cells), glial cells, and neurons.[24,25,28] Coordinated bidirectional signaling between cell types is necessary for preservation of vascular structure and function, and injury and/or dysfunction of one cell type influences the structure and function of cells. For example, several signaling molecules, such as cytokines, matrix metalloproteinases (MMPs), and various secondary messengers, may lead to disruption of endothelial barrier properties.[24,28]

Vasogenic Edema

Vasogenic edema results from disruption of the BBB with extravasation of plasma-derived factors and circulating erythrocytes and immune cells that are normally excluded from the brain parenchyma.[13,14] Accumulation of protein-rich fluids increases oncotic pressure of the extracellular space and increases total brain volume. The mechanism of vasogenic edema involves (1) mechanical disruption of blood vessels and (2) secretion of propermeability factors from adjacent cells.[33] However, additional factors, for example,

detachment of perivascular pericytes, have been described but are poorly understood at the present time.[34,35] The increase in BBB permeability seen in vasogenic edema follows a bimodal time course with peaks at 1 to 3 hours after injury as demonstrated by immunoglobulin G (IgG) immunoreactivity in the brain followed by an increase in microglia activation seen after 5 days after injury.[36,37] Therefore, mechanical disruption of brain blood vessels as evidence by contusions, brain petechiae, and increasing CSF concentrations of plasma-derived proteins, for example, IgG and albumin, results in the initial flux of vasogenic edema at the time of the initial injury. Secretion of propermeability factors, on the other hand, likely accounts for vasogenic edema more delayed in onset, especially in the absence of space-occupying mass lesions, which may lead to avulsion of perforating branches of small vessels.

Studies have suggested that the relative contributions of different mechanisms of vasogenic edema depend on injury severity. For example, studies in high-energy blast wave–induced TBI demonstrate an increase in BBB disruption with blast wave overpressure but found no difference in brain IgG immunoreactivity between the immediate postinjury period and 48 hours later.[38,39] This finding suggests that much of the BBB disruption was mechanical and occurred at the time of injury. In TBI with comparatively milder mechanisms of injury, oxidative stress and inflammatory second messenger cascades make larger contributions to the development of altered BBB permeability, which peaks 6 to 24 hours after injury.[40,41] Furthermore, mild TBI can induce chronic changes to the brain microvasculature that are evident even months after the initial injury.[42]

Studies in preclinical animal models demonstrate induction of expression of the free-radical–generating enzymes nicotinamide adenine dinucleotide phosphate (NADPH) oxidase 1 and inducible nitric oxide synthetase (iNOS) following low-energy brain injury.[38,40] Generation of free radicals in turn leads to microvascular injury, endothelial apoptosis, and disruption of endothelial tight junctional protein complexes. Oxidative stress also leads to increased expression of the degrading enzymes MMPs in perivascular cells and infiltrating or resident inflammatory cells leading to further degradation of endothelial tight junctions, basement membranes, and cell adhesion molecules.[43]

Simultaneously, posttraumatic neuroinflammation converges with oxidant stress on the vascular interface. Multiple cell types, including microglia, infiltrating inflammatory cells, neurons, and ECs, increase expression and subsequent secretion of proinflammatory cytokines, namely, interleukin 1β (IL-1β), IL-6, and tumor necrosis factor α.[44,45] These cytokines induce a proinflammatory state and contribute to BBB disruption through loss of tight junction proteins,[46] increased expression of MMPs,[47] and increased levels of other permeability-increasing molecules, for example, bradykinins and the neuropeptide substance P (SP).[48] Disruption in BBB permeability, increased chemokine/cytokine secretion, and increased inflammatory cell adhesion molecules on brain endothelium lead to further recruitment of inflammatory cells from the systemic circulation.[33,49] Infiltration of peripheral inflammatory cells, such as neutrophils and monocytes, may then lead to further endothelial barrier disruption through generation of reactive oxygen species, proteolytic enzymes, and propagation of inflammatory cascades through secretion of cytokines and chemokines.

Disruption of the BBB leads to nonspecific influx of circulating blood-borne cells, plasma-derived proteins, and other solutes that contribute to neuronal dysfunction and further injury following TBI.[24,25,28,33,50] Nonspecific protein flux into brain interstitial fluid increases oncotic pressure giving rise to brain edema, which may occlude small vessels and give rise to local hypoperfusion.[12,24,28] Many plasma-derived proteins, for example, plasmin, thrombin, fibrin, and erythrocyte-derived free iron, have direct neurotoxic and/or proinflammatory properties.[24,27–29,50] Albumin, in addition to serving as an important determinant of oncotic pressure, increases neuronal irritability and contributes to ictogenesis.[51] Therefore, disruption of the BBB may have several deleterious consequences in addition to the formation of edema following TBI.

Cytotoxic Edema

Cytotoxic edema is defined as intracellular swelling that results from dysfunction of ionic and osmotic flux.[13,14] An inability to maintain cell membrane electrochemical gradients is one common etiologic factor, most often resulting from ischemia or hypoxia. Impaired oxygen and glucose delivery leads to depletion of cellular adenosine triphosphate (ATP) stores, the source of cellular energy. This depletion in turn leads to impaired function of the sodium ion (Na+)/potassium ion (K+) ATPase. Under physiologic conditions, this active transport system normally pumps 3 Na+ out of the cell and 2 K+ into the cell. In the absence of a functional transporter, Na+ cations begin to flow down their electrochemical gradient and accumulate inside of cells.[52,53] Several compensatory mechanisms resist the generation of an osmotic gradient, including the passive diffusion of potassium out of the cell. However, this is overcome by increased influx of negatively charged chloride ions (Cl−) via activation of the SLC26A11 channel, which serves as a voltage-gated Cl− channel when the cell is depolarized.[16] In addition, there is dysfunction in several other cellular cation channels, including acid-sensing ion channels (ASICs), the sulfonylurea receptor 1 (SUR1)-regulated NC_{Ca-ATP} channel (SUR1/Transient receptor potential cation channel subfamily M member 4 [TRPM4]), the NKCC1 channel, and the N-methyl-D-aspartate (NMDA) glutamate receptor channel (**Table 1**).[54–58] An influx of ions into cells increases cell osmolality, and a compensatory movement of free water down its osmotic gradient through specialized channels closely follows and results in cellular swelling.

It is important to note, however, that cell swelling itself does not increase brain volume; cytotoxic edema would be a self-limiting process in the absence of ionic and osmotic fluxes across the BBB.[22,59] Extracellular concentrations of sodium and chloride in the brain interstitial fluid decrease dramatically as these ions move into cells.[52,53] The result is the generation of an osmotic gradient between the vascular compartment and brain interstitial fluid (ISF). This generation is normally mitigated by an intact BBB. However, in brain trauma, disruption of the BBB and/or heightened endothelial permeability contributes to increased influx of circulating molecules, including both ions and water. The NKCC1 secondary active cotransporter and SUR1/TRPM4 channel are expressed on the luminal EC membrane and mediate ion transport into the ECs. Abluminal non–voltage- or ligand-gated sodium channels may then facilitate diffusion of endothelial sodium into the brain interstitial fluid.[60] This diffusion in turn creates a gradient favoring the shift of water from the vasculature into the brain interstitium.

Although water is able to freely diffuse across most tissues in the body, its movement is highly regulated in the central nervous system (CNS) through a family of specialized transmembrane channels known as AQPs.[61] The predominate AQPs of the CNS are AQP-1 and AQP-4.[62,63] AQP-1 is expressed at the apical membrane of the choroid plexus epithelium where it aids in CSF secretion into the ventricles.[64] AQP-4, on the other hand, is located at the basolateral membrane of ventricular ependymal cells and astrocyte foot processes where it facilitates CSF-parenchyma and vascular-parenchyma water transport, respectively.[65] In astrocytes, AQP-4

Table 1
Cation channels involved in the formation of cytotoxic edema

Cation Channel	Permeability	Regulation	Effect in TBI
ASICs	Na+ > Ca2+	It is activated by H+.	Decreased pH associated with ischemia leads to increased Na+ and Ca2+ influx into cells, contributing to edema and cellular injury.
SUR1 regulated NC$_{Ca}$– ATP channel	All inorganic monovalent cations, impermeable to Mg2+ and Ca2+	Channel activity is activated by intracellular Ca2+ and inhibited by intracellular ATP; expression in the CNS is induced following hypoxia or injury.	Decreased intracellular ATP stores in hypoxic cells leads to activation of this channel, resulting in membrane depolarization and excessive intracellular Na+ accumulation.
NKCC1 channel	1 Na+: 1 K+: 2 Cl−	Activity is increased by elevated extracellular K+.	Elevated extracellular K+ from ischemia-related depolarization activates channel, leading to dysregulated Na+ and Cl− influx into cells.
NMDA glutamate receptor channel	Na+, K+, Ca2+	The channel pore opens in response to glutamate or glycine binding coincident with membrane depolarization.	Excessive glutamate release by ischemic neurons leads to unregulated influx of Na+ and Ca2+ through NMDA receptor channels, leading to intracellular accumulation of these ions.

Abbreviation: CNS, central nervous system.

colocalizes with the inwardly rectifying potassium channel Kir4.1, where it is thought to function as a water-potassium transport complex.[63,66] In normal conditions, this facilitates the clearance of K+ and water from synaptic junctions after the neuronal excitation.

Following brain insults, AQP-4 has been implicated in the osmotic shifts that give rise to cerebral edema.[65] As described earlier, injury leads to excessive cellular osmolality and establishes a strong osmotic gradient. This osmotic gradient leads to the passive diffusion of free water through AQP-4 channels found in the astrocyte foot processes surrounding the cerebral vasculature and subsequent astrocyte swelling, the principal cellular source of this type of cellular edema.[32,67]

FUTURE TREATMENT TARGETS

As our understanding of the pathogenesis of cerebral edema in TBI has increased, much research has focused on developing novel antiedema treatments. These new therapies can broadly be categorized as affecting differently molecular pathways that give rise to vasogenic and/or cytotoxic edema (**Table 2**).

Therapies Targeting Vasogenic Edema

Myosin light chain kinase

Myosin light chain kinases (MLCK) and its antagonist myosin light chain phosphatase modulate cytoskeletal contraction and/or rearrangement via phosphorylation or dephosphorylation of the regulatory unit of the myosin light chain, which are expressed in brain ECs.[68] In ECs, MLCK plays an important role in regulating barrier permeability.

Endothelial tight junction proteins, for example, claudin or occludin, are linked to the actin cytoskeleton through adaptor proteins, for example, zonula occludins. Thus, contraction or rearrangement of the actin cytoskeleton modulates endothelial permeability.[69] In preclinical models, expression of MLCK peaks 6 hours following TBI and slowly returns to baseline over 48 hours, a period that coincides with the development of cerebral edema.[70,71] In vitro upregulation of MLCK reduces transendothelial resistance consistent with heightened permeability in response to

Table 2
Potential molecular therapeutic targets for cerebral edema following traumatic brain injury

Protein	Function	Cellular Effect
Vasogenic edema		
MLCK	Modulates cytoskeletal rearrangement	Decreases endothelial tight junction and BBB permeability
GR	Multifunctional transcriptional regulator, includes upregulation of tight junction and adherens junction proteins	Increase endothelial tight and adherens junction proteins
PPAR	Multifunctional nuclear membrane–associated transcription factors, includes downregulation of proinflammatory molecules	Downregulates proinflammatory molecules that increase endothelial permeability, for example, cytokines or chemokines, or degrade tight junction complexes, for example, MMPs
VEGF	Angiogenic factor	Leads to dedifferentiation of brain ECs and loss of barrier properties
MMPs	Proteases that degrade components of the extracellular matrix and endothelial junctional complexes	Increases endothelial permeability through degradation of tight and adherens junctions; destabilizes vascular wall through degradation of vascular basement membrane
SP	Tachykinin promotes protein extravasation and leukocyte adhesion to ECs	Increases endothelial permeability and adhesion molecule expression
Cytotoxic edema targets		
AQP-4	Transmembrane water channels	Regulate brain water transport, predominately in astrocytes
NKCC1 channel	Cotransporter of Na+, K+, and Cl−	Upregulated in brain injury and leads to excessive cellular influx Na+ and Cl−
Vasopressin receptors	Initiate downstream signal transduction, including upregulation of AQP-4	Increase synthesis/release in trauma leads to increased cellular water permeability
SUR1-regulated NC$_{Ca-ATP}$ channel (SUR1/TRPM4)	Associates with and regulates the NCCa-ATP channel: a nonselective cation channel regulated by intracellular ATP and calcium	Upregulated in brain injury and leads to nonspecific cation flux into cells

Abbreviations: GR, glucocorticoid receptor; MLCK, myosin light chain kinase; PPAR, peroxisome proliferator-activated receptor; VEGF, vascular endothelial growth factor.

a myriad of injury factors, including ethanol, methamphetamine, and hypoxia.[69,72–74] Treatment with a pharmacologic inhibitor of MLCK either before or following TBI decreased disruption of the BBB and associated cerebral edema.[70,71] However, the effect of MLCK inhibition on neurologic outcome remains controversial. In a rodent model of closed-head trauma, postinjury treatment with 1-(5-iodonaphthalene-1sulfonyl)-1H-hexahydro-1,4-diazepine hydrochloride (ML-7) resulted in improvements in motor and cognitive function as evidenced by improved performance on the wire hang test and 2 object recognition tests, respectively.[71] However, pretreatment of ML-7 before controlled cortical impact did not influence neurologic severity scoring.[70] Given the significant differences in experimental design, including timing of administration, future studies are needed to further confirm a therapeutic role of MLCK inhibition in the treatment of posttraumatic edema.

Degradation of the glucocorticoid receptor
Glucocorticoids, such as dexamethasone and methylprednisolone, are commonly used to treat neurologic conditions with a disrupted BBB,

including brain tumors and multiple sclerosis.[75,76] Glucocorticoids bind to glucocorticoid receptors (GRs) in cerebrovascular ECs leading to the transcriptional upregulation of the tight and adherens junctional proteins, including claudin, occludin, and vascular endothelial cadherin, while inhibiting MMPs and CNS leukocyte infiltration.[77] Upregulation of tight and adherens junction proteins and downregulation of destabilizing enzymes leads to a restoration of endothelial barrier properties in pathologic conditions. However, glucocorticoid treatment is nonspecific and leads to several potentially deleterious side effects in an injured brain, most notably delayed wound healing and hyperglycemia. As a result, glucocorticoids have not been convincingly shown to improve outcomes in patients with ischemic stroke or TBI[78,79]; high-dose methylprednisolone treatment is contraindicated in moderate to severe TBI as it is associated with increased mortality.[80] Therefore, the potentially beneficial BBB restorative properties of glucocorticoid therapy are offset by the negative systemic consequences of steroid therapy.

One potential mechanism that may explain this phenomenon is the proteasomal degradation or post-translational modifications of GRs in response to brain injury.[81] For example, in hypoxic conditions, brain ECs lose barrier properties that are unable to be restored with glucocorticoids alone. Treatment with these cells with bortezomib, a pharmacologic proteasome inhibitor, restores the probarrier effects of glucocorticoid therapy.[82] Treatment with bortezomib and dexamethasone similarly led to less edema while restoring endothelial occludin levels and BBB integrity than dexamethasone alone in mice following controlled cortical impact. This treatment was associated with less neuronal damage following brain trauma.[81] Whether these results may be replicated in other experimental TBI models remains to be seen, and whether adjuvant therapy may help augment the response to steroids in the injured brain warrants further investigation.

Peroxisome proliferator-activated receptor

Peroxisome proliferator-activated receptors (PPARs) are nuclear membrane–associated transcription factors that function as nuclear receptors that may be pharmacologically targeted by the fenofibrates and thiazolidinediones, including pioglitazone and rosiglitazone.[83] Three different isotypes (α, β/δ, and γ) are differentially expressed in different organ systems throughout the body, with all 3 being expressed in the CNS.[84] These receptors are activated via a dimerization with retinoid-X receptors, which in turn modulate expression of an array of different proteins with several different phenotypic outcomes, including the downregulation of the proinflammatory transcription factors, such as activator protein 1 (AP-1), signal transducer and activator of transcription protein family (STAT), nuclear factor of activated T-cells (NFAT), and nuclear factor kappa-light-chain-enhancer of activated B cells (NF-κB).[15]

The antiinflammatory role of PPAR has led to attention from the TBI community as a possible therapeutic target; pharmacologic agents targeting this pathway, such as fenofibrates or the thiazolidinediones pioglitazone and rosiglitazone, have been applied to several preclinical models. For example, administration of fenofibrate, an agonist of PPARα, reduced brain edema, expression of the inflammatory adhesion molecule intercellular adhesion molecule 1 (ICAM-1), and neurologic deficits in a rat lateral fluid percussion TBI model.[85] At a molecular level, fenofibrate reduced expression of iNOS, cyclooxygenase 2, and MMP-9 as well as markers of oxidant stress.[86] Fenofibrate may, therefore, protect endothelial tight junctions through downregulation of the degradation enzyme MMP-9 and oxidative endothelial injury. In other injury models, such as oxygen glucose deprivation, fenofibrate was shown to have a protective effect on endothelial BBB function.[87] However, the molecular mechanisms of this protection were not described.

Additional studies have begun to explore whether potentiation of PPARγ signaling with treatment of pioglitazone or rosiglitazone may confer benefit in preclinical models of TBI. Collectively, these studies have demonstrated that treatment results in a reduction in lesion size, microglial activation, proinflammatory mediator expression, and neuronal apoptosis while increasing performance on posttraumatic measures of cognition.[88,89] However, the influence on edema and BBB permeability has yet to be studied in the context of treatment with pioglitazone or rosiglitazone. In vitro studies have demonstrated that rosiglitazone altered endothelial expression of the GTPases Rac1 and RhoA, which play a pivotal role in endothelial cytoskeletal rearrangements and inflammatory cell transmigration across the BBB without influencing tight junction protein level.[90] Whether a similar relationship holds true in TBI is unclear, and future studies are needed to better understand PPAR agonism and how it influences posttraumatic brain edema and BBB function.

In vivo experiments examining the effect of pioglitazone in the setting of TBI demonstrated improved cognitive function after injury, reduced lesion size, and lower levels of microglial activation when compared with controls.[88] Similarly, treatment with rosiglitazone showed similar neuroprotective effects with the addition of reduced proinflammatory gene expression, decreased apoptotic neurons, and increased antioxidant enzymes.[89]

Vascular endothelial growth factor

Vascular endothelial growth factor (VEGF) is a potent angiogenic factor essential to initial brain vasculogenesis as well as sprouting angiogenesis, which is responsible for vascular remodeling in both physiologic conditions and in response to brain injury and pathologic states, such as brain tumors, stroke, and neurodegeneration.[91,92] VEGF and VEGF receptors are upregulated by the transcription factors hypoxia-inducible factor (HIF)-1 and HIF-2, both of which become highly expressed in the setting of brain ischemia. VEGF leads to dedifferentiation of brain ECs, which assume a leaky and highly proliferative phenotype. The mechanisms through which VEGF induces disruption of the BBB are numerous and affect both paracellular and transcellular pathways. These mechanisms include acquisition of endothelial fenestrae, increased endothelial pinocytosis and bulk flow transcytosis, and increased size of the interendothelial space with downregulation of the tight junction proteins claudin-5, occludin, and zonula occludin-1.[92,93]

Following TBI, there is an increase in VEGF thought to contribute to reparative mechanisms to restore blood flow to injured brain parenchyma.[94,95] This increase may come at a cost of leaky immature vasculature, which is prone to rupture and contributes to posttraumatic edema.[96,97] Experiments using a rat cold-injury model of brain edema showed that antagonism of the VEGF receptor significantly reduced brain water content in a dose-dependent fashion and reduced vascular permeability.[98] Other investigators using in vivo ischemia/reperfusion injury and venous infarction models found that sequestration or antagonism of VEGF reduced radiologically defined brain edema.[99,100] However, post-TBI treatment with exogenous VEGF may increase neurogenesis, decrease lesion volume, and improve functional outcomes in mice following closed head injury.[101] This information highlights that VEGF influences not only the vasculature but also neuronal health and repair. Thus, targeting VEGF may have both beneficial and deleterious consequences in the posttraumatic setting.

Matrix metalloproteinases

MMPs are a family of neutral proteases that cleave components of the extracellular matrix and are important for wound healing, development, and inflammation.[102,103] Within the CNS, MMPs are closely associated with the neurovascular unit where they serve to regulate the extracellular matrix that contributes to the BBB. MMPs have been shown to degrade tight junction and basal lamina proteins, thereby contributing to the development of increased BBB permeability and vasogenic edema.[47,104] In the CNS, ECs express MMP-9; pericytes express MMP-9 and MMP-3; and astrocytes express MMP-2 constitutively.[102] Following TBI, there is an upregulation in MMP expression and activation, which persists from postinjury day 1 to day 7; higher concentrations are found in human CSF.[105–107] Genetic knockout of MMP-9 reduces lesions sizes, lessens BBB disruption, as well as limits the degradation of zonae occludens-1, the adaptor protein that links tight junctions to the cytoskeleton, when compared with wild-type mice following TBI.[108]

Given this evidence, multiple reports with favorable results have investigated a potential role for pharmacologic inhibition of MMPs immediately following TBI. For example, treatment with a specific inhibitor of gelatinases (MMP-2 and MMP-9) known as SB-3CT reduced lesion volume, dendritic and neuronal degeneration, and microglial activation and astrogliosis while improving sensorimotor and cognitive deficits following controlled cortical impact in mice.[106] In rats, treatment with SB-3CT ameliorated cognitive deficits and hippocampal neuronal loss following fluid percussive injury.[109] A water-soluble derivative of SB-3CT was more recently shown to have a similar effect in reducing lesion volume following TBI.[110] In models of chronic neurodegeneration and subarachnoid hemorrhage, treatment with SB-3CT similarly increased endothelial barrier properties via protection of tight junctional proteins and components of the vascular basement membrane. These changes were associated with and thought to contribute to a protection of neuronal structure and function.[104] Therefore, inhibition of MMPs may have both acute and chronic protective benefits in preserving endothelial BBB properties and may thereby promote neuronal health and repair following TBI.

Substance P

SP is a member of the tachykinin family of kinins along with calcitonin gene–related peptide (CGRP) and neurokinin A. Tachykinins are released by both central and peripheral endings of sensory neurons and function as neurotransmitters. They bind to tachykinin receptors and are key mediators of neurogenic inflammation, with SP primarily binding to the neurokinin 1 (NK1) receptor.[111] Although many members of the kinin family are known to be involved in many aspects of the physiology of neurogenic inflammation, CGRP mediates vasodilation and SP is primarily responsible for enhancing plasma protein extravasation and leukocyte adhesion to ECs.[111,112] It has recently been recognized that neurogenic inflammation plays a role in the development of vasogenic edema.[113] Further studies found that perivascular SP immunoreactivity increases in the perivascular space following TBI, thereby suggesting that SP, not other neuropeptides, might be responsible for the neurogenic inflammation seen following TBI.[114]

Research examining SP inhibition following TBI has shown promising results. A study using a rat model of TBI found that inhibition of the NK1 receptor with N-acetyl-L-tryptophan 30 minutes after injury attenuated vascular permeability and edema formation as well as improved motor and cognitive outcomes.[115] More recently, it was shown that the addition of a lipophilic trifluoromethyl benzyl ester group to N-acetyl-L-tryptophan to improve membrane permeability of the drug extends efficacy in TBI from 5 to 12 hours after injury.[116] Studies using models of ischemic stroke have similarly shown efficacy of NK1 inhibition on BBB permeability, edema formation, infarct size, and neurologic function.[117] Taken together, these results put forward SP inhibition as a potentially neuroprotective therapeutic for TBI.

Cytotoxic Edema Targets

Aquaporins

AQPs play a key role in maintaining brain-water homeostasis, mediating the flux of water at the interface between the cerebral vasculature and both brain parenchyma and the CSF producing choroid plexus.[63] AQP-4 is localized at the astrocyte foot processes and plays a vital molecular role in the pathogenesis of the glial swelling seen in cytotoxic edema following a myriad of brain injuries, including TBI, brain ischemia, hydrocephalus, water intoxication, and bacterial abscesses.[118] In vitro studies in cultured astrocytes demonstrated a 7.1-fold reduction in osmotic water permeability in AQP-4–deficient cells.[67] Similar findings were demonstrated in organotypic slice preparations in $Aqp4^{-/-}$ mice confirming that AQP-4 is the primary route for water transport in astrocytes.[17] Experimental models of cryogenic brain injury, an injury associated with predominantly vasogenic edema, have suggested that AQP-4 may a play a role in the resolution of vasogenic edema in addition to its well-established role in cytotoxic edema.[119]

Following TBI, expression of AQPs is increased in both in vitro and in vivo models of experimental brain injury,[120,121] thus, making it an attractive therapeutic target in TBI. In human subjects, several single nucleotide polymorphisms in AQP-4 are associated with poor functional outcomes following TBI.[122] Preclinical studies in experimental TBI models have shown promising preliminary results. For example, antibody-mediated inhibition of AQP-4 demonstrated a statistically significant reduction in brain water content and neuronal death while improving neurobehavioral outcomes following weight-drop closed-head injury in rats.[121] In juvenile rats, similar protective results were observed following controlled cortical impact with local infusion of small-interfering RNA targeting AQP-4.[123] More recently, controlled cortical impact in $Aqp4^{-/-}$ mice demonstrated reductions in total brain water and ICP when compared with $Aqp4^{+/+}$ mice without differences in BBB permeability. These reductions were associated with milder improvements in neurologic outcomes than have been observed in other injury models with purely cytotoxic injury.[118] This finding led the investigators to conclude that concurrent vasogenic edema may mitigate the potential benefit of AQP inhibition in TBI. Whether treatment with BBB restorative therapy in tandem with AQP inhibition improves outcomes remains to be tested, and future studies are needed to better delineate the role of aquaporin-targeted therapy in TBI.

NKCC1

The NKCC channel is an electroneutral cotransporter of Na+, K+, and Cl−, which is expressed in 2 different isoforms: NKCC1 and NKCC2. NKCC1 is ubiquitously expressed, whereas NKCC2 is found exclusively within the kidney.[124] Within the CNS, the NKCC1 isoform is expressed by glia, neurons, endothelium, and choroid plexus epithelial cells.[125] This cotransporter uses the electrochemical gradient established by the Na+/K+ -ATPase to transport 1 Na+, 1 K+, and 2 Cl− ions across the plasma membrane and into cells. Thus, the NKCC1 is an important regulator of intracellular osmolality and by extension cellular volume.[124]

NKCC1 activity is upregulated following various forms of ischemic and traumatic brain injury.[55,126] During ischemia or hypoxia, NKCC1 contributes to excessive Na+ and Cl− influx into cells increasing cellular osmolality and leading to the development of cytotoxic edema. In TBI, upregulation and increased phosphorylation contribute to increased activity of the NKCC1 transporter.[55,126] In vitro treatment of cultured astrocytes with bumetanide, an inhibitor of NKCC1, or small interfering RNA silencing reduced astro-cytic swelling following barotrauma.[55] To date, no in vivo studies targeting NKCC1 in TBI have been performed. Other models of brain injury, such as experimental middle cerebral artery oc-clusion, have demonstrated a 70% reduction in brain water content with bumetanide-mediated NKCC1 inhibition.[127] Whether similar protective effects may be observed following TBI remains to be determined.

Vasopressin receptors

Arginine vasopressin (AVP) is a neuropeptide hor-mone that regulates plasma osmolality. In addition to peripheral targets, AVP binds to and activates V1 receptors within the CNS, activating down-stream signal transduction in several cell types, including decreases in water permeability of CSF-producing ependymal cells, reduced CSF production, changes in water permeability of as-trocytes, and changes in AQP-4 expression.[128] Following TBI, AVP synthesis is upregulated both within the hypothalamus, namely, within the para-ventricular and supraoptic nuclei, and locally near the traumatic lesion.[129,130] Selection inhibition of the vasopressin V1a receptor has shown prom-ising results in TBI rodent models. Treatment with a small molecule selective V1a receptor antagonist SR 49059 lessened ICP, brain water content, and gliosis while restoring extracellular sodium concentration of brain ISF following focal cortical contusion induced by controlled cortical impact in rats.[131,132] These changes were associ-ated with decreased AQP4 expression in perile-sional astrocytes offering potential mechanistic insights.[131,132] More recently, an independent group demonstrated that intracerebroventricular administration, but not systemic administration, of SR49059 decreased brain edema, posttrau-matic ICP, and secondary contusion expansion in mice following controlled cortical impact (CCI).[133] Further works are needed to better char-acterize these effects in other TBI models.

Sulfonylurea receptor 1–regulated NC_{Ca}– adenosine triphosphate channel

Sulfonylurea receptors (SURs) are integral mem-brane proteins and belong to the ATP binding cassette family of transmembrane proteins. SURs are not ion transport channels but rather associates with a heterologous pore forming units to form ion channels.[58] In the CNS, SUR1 associates with and regulates the function of the NC_{Ca-ATP} channel, a nonselective cation channel regulated by intracel-lular ATP and calcium.[134] The SUR1-regulated NC_{Ca-ATP} channel (SUR1/TRPM4) is not constitu-tively expressed and is upregulated in a variety of brain injury states, including TBI, stroke, and brain tumors.[58,135] ATP normally inhibits SUR1/TRPM4 flux. Following brain injury, ATP depletion leads to opening of the SUR1/TRPM4 channel, which in turn leads to membrane depolarization, blebbing, and swelling.[54,58]

Pharmacologic inhibition of the SUR1/TRPM4 with the sulfonylurea glibenclamide, also known as glyburide, reduces the development of cyto-toxic brain edema in multiple animal models of brain injury.[58,135] In vitro studies have shown reduction in membrane blebbing and cellular swelling in isolated astrocytes following ATP deple-tion.[134] In models of cerebral ischemia, such as middle cerebral occlusion, glibenclamide treat-ment led to approximately 50% reductions in cere-bral edema, infarct volume, and mortality when compared with vehicle-treated rodents.[136] Retro-spective cohort analyses have also demonstrated improved outcomes in diabetic patients treated with sulfonylurea medications following ischemic stroke.[137,138] More recently, these results have been extended to TBI. In rats undergoing CCI, SUR1/TRPM4 was shown to be upregulated within 3 hours following injury, predominantly within brain capillaries. Treatment with glibenclamide or small interfering RNA targeting SUR1 treatment leads to significant reductions in the progressive second-ary hemorrhage of the contused brain. Noted re-ductions in capillary fragmentation and size of the necrotic lesion and improvements on neurobeha-vioral function, as assayed by vertical exploration or rearing, were observed.[139] An independent group demonstrated reductions in posttraumatic edema and confirmed reductions in contusion size and subsequent evolution but failed to find dif-ferences in ICP or biochemical measures, including lactate, pyruvate, and glutamate or changes in mo-tor function, as assessed by beam walking, over the 7 days of study.[140] The source of the discrep-ancies between these studies is unclear and may reflect differences in experimental design or outcome parameters. Additional studies are needed in other TBI models to either confirm or refute these findings.

These promising results from animal studies prompted the glyburide advantage in malignant edema and stroke-pilot (GAMES-Pilot) trial.[137,138] A phase I study confirmed the safety of intrave-nous glyburide administered as a bolus dose fol-lowed by 3-day infusion. The investigators have since initiated a multicenter, prospective, open-label phase IIa trial that completed data collection in June 2012.[141] A secondary analysis of GAMES-Pilot subjects compared with controls from the Echoplanar Imaging Thrombolytic Evaluation Trial (EPITHET) and Multi Modal Imaging: MRI

(MMI-Mri) trial showed improvement in functional measures as well as a trend toward lower mortality among the intervention group, although the study lacked power to demonstrate efficacy.[141] A subsequent case-control study using the GAMES-Pilot subjects demonstrated that intravenous glyburide was associated with reduced surrogate markers of vasogenic edema (namely T2 fluid-attenuated inversion recovery intensity on MRI, apparent diffusion coefficient values, and MMP-9 levels) when compared with historical controls.[142] Given these strong preliminary results, the GAMES-RP trial (phase II) is currently underway to better elucidate the potential efficacy of glyburide pharmacotherapy in ischemic stroke. A similar approach has recently been implemented to investigate the role of glyburide treatment in TBI in a phase II trial with completion of data collection in March 2015.[143] Whether glyburide therapy will show benefit in human patients with TBI remains to be seen.

SUMMARY

Cerebral edema is a dangerous secondary consequence of TBI and is associated with significant morbidity and mortality. In clinical practice, treatment of cerebral edema is limited to hyperosmolar therapy and, if refractory, surgical decompression, such as hemicraniectomy. Although effective in reducing ICP, these interventions lack the ability to modify the underlying pathologic processes that give rise and/or propagate cerebral edema with rare exception. For the purposes of this article, vasogenic and cytotoxic edema are presented separately. However, following brain injury, development of cerebral edema is less finite with multiple points of convergence between vasogenic and cytotoxic components. Continued research should focus on the overlap of vasogenic and cytotoxic pathways and the better delineation of the relative contributions of each process to derive therapies of maximal potential benefit. Whether dual therapies targeting vasogenic and cytotoxic pathways may provide synergistic and/or additive benefit also remains to be seen.

Recent advances in preclinical models of TBI have begun to shed light on prospective molecular targets that may slow and/or reverse cerebral edema and its deleterious sequelae. The heterogeneous nature of TBI-related injury and associated mechanisms of edema will likely present formidable barriers to translation of many of these compounds. Despite the preliminary nature of many of these results, TBI remains a public health epidemic with inappropriately high morbidity and mortality. Further investment and research into disease-modifying agents, with an emphasis on the development of cerebral edema, is warranted to, it is hoped, improve patient outcomes and lessen the person and societal burden of TBI.

REFERENCES

1. Manley GT, Maas AI. Traumatic brain injury: an international knowledge-based approach. JAMA 2013;310:473–4.
2. Menon DK, Schwab K, Wright DW, et al. Position statement: definition of traumatic brain injury. Arch Phys Med Rehabil 2010;91:1637–40.
3. Faul M, Xu L, Wald MM, et al. Traumatic brain injury in the United States: emergency department visits, hospitalizations and deaths, 2002-2006. Atlanta (GA): Centers for Disease Control and Prevention, National Center for Injury; 2010.
4. Langlois JA, Rutland-Brown W, Wald MM. The epidemiology and impact of traumatic brain injury: a brief overview. J Head Trauma Rehabil 2006;21: 375–8.
5. Maas AI, Stocchetti N, Bullock R. Moderate and severe traumatic brain injury in adults. Lancet Neurol 2008;7:728–41.
6. Rosenfeld JV, Maas AI, Bragge P, et al. Early management of severe traumatic brain injury. Lancet 2012;380:1088–98.
7. Masel BE, DeWitt DS. Traumatic brain injury: a disease process, not an event. J Neurotrauma 2010; 27:1529–40.
8. Xiong Y, Mahmood A, Chopp M. Animal models of traumatic brain injury. Nat Rev Neurosci 2013;14: 128–42.
9. Stocchetti N, Maas AI. Traumatic intracranial hypertension. N Engl J Med 2014;370:2121–30.
10. Kim DJ, Czosnyka Z, Kasprowicz M, et al. Continuous monitoring of the Monro-Kellie doctrine: is it possible? J Neurotrauma 2012;29:1354–63.
11. Sheth KN, Stein DM, Aarabi B, et al. Intracranial pressure dose and outcome in traumatic brain injury. Neurocrit Care 2013;18:26–32.
12. Stocchetti N, Maas AI. Traumatic intracranial hypertension. N Engl J Med 2014;371:972.
13. Klatzo I. Pathophysiological aspects of brain edema. Acta Neuropathol 1987;72:236–9.
14. Marmarou A. A review of progress in understanding the pathophysiology and treatment of brain edema. Neurosurg Focus 2007;22:E1.
15. Thal SC, Neuhaus W. The blood-brain barrier as a target in traumatic brain injury treatment. Arch Med Res 2014;45:698–710.
16. Rungta RL, Choi HB, Tyson JR, et al. The cellular mechanisms of neuronal swelling underlying cytotoxic edema. Cell 2015;161:610–21.

17. Thrane AS, Rappold PM, Fujita T, et al. Critical role of aquaporin-4 (AQP4) in astrocytic Ca2+ signaling events elicited by cerebral edema. Proc Natl Acad Sci U S A 2011;108:846–51.

18. Beaumont A, Fatouros P, Gennarelli T, et al. Bolus tracer delivery measured by MRI confirms edema without blood-brain barrier permeability in diffuse traumatic brain injury. Acta Neurochir Suppl 2006; 96:171–4.

19. Marmarou A. Pathophysiology of traumatic brain edema: current concepts. Acta Neurochir Suppl 2003;86:7–10.

20. Marmarou A, Signoretti S, Fatouros PP, et al. Predominance of cellular edema in traumatic brain swelling in patients with severe head injuries. J Neurosurg 2006;104:720–30.

21. Hudak AM, Peng L, Marquez de la Plata C, et al. Cytotoxic and vasogenic cerebral oedema in traumatic brain injury: assessment with FLAIR and DWI imaging. Brain Inj 2014;28:1602–9.

22. Beaumont A, Marmarou A, Hayasaki K, et al. The permissive nature of blood brain barrier (BBB) opening in edema formation following traumatic brain injury. Acta Neurochir Suppl 2000;76:125–9.

23. Stocchetti N, Colombo A, Ortolano F, et al. Time course of intracranial hypertension after traumatic brain injury. J Neurotrauma 2007;24:1339–46.

24. Winkler EA, Bell RD, Zlokovic BV. Central nervous system pericytes in health and disease. Nat Neurosci 2011;14:1398–405.

25. Zlokovic BV. The blood-brain barrier in health and chronic neurodegenerative disorders. Neuron 2008; 57:178–201.

26. Winkler EA, Sengillo JD, Bell RD, et al. Blood-spinal cord barrier pericyte reductions contribute to increased capillary permeability. J Cereb Blood Flow Metab 2012;32:1841–52.

27. Winkler EA, Sagare AP, Zlokovic BV. The pericyte: a forgotten cell type with important implications for Alzheimer's disease? Brain Pathol 2014;24:371–86.

28. Zlokovic BV. Neurovascular pathways to neurodegeneration in Alzheimer's disease and other disorders. Nat Rev Neurosci 2011;12:723–38.

29. Bell RD, Winkler EA, Sagare AP, et al. Pericytes control key neurovascular functions and neuronal phenotype in the adult brain and during brain aging. Neuron 2010;68:409–27.

30. Abbott NJ, Ronnback L, Hansson E. Astrocyte-endothelial interactions at the blood-brain barrier. Nat Rev Neurosci 2006;7:41–53.

31. Iliff JJ, Wang M, Liao Y, et al. A paravascular pathway facilitates CSF flow through the brain parenchyma and the clearance of interstitial solutes, including amyloid beta. Sci Transl Med 2012;4: 147ra111.

32. Manley GT, Fujimura M, Ma T, et al. Aquaporin-4 deletion in mice reduces brain edema after acute water intoxication and ischemic stroke. Nat Med 2000;6:159–63.

33. Chodobski A, Zink BJ, Szmydynger-Chodobska J. Blood-brain barrier pathophysiology in traumatic brain injury. Transl Stroke Res 2011;2:492–516.

34. Dore-Duffy P, Owen C, Balabanov R, et al. Pericyte migration from the vascular wall in response to traumatic brain injury. Microvasc Res 2000;60:55–69.

35. Zehendner CM, Sebastiani A, Hugonnet A, et al. Traumatic brain injury results in rapid pericyte loss followed by reactive pericytosis in the cerebral cortex. Sci Rep 2015;5:13497.

36. Readnower RD, Chavko M, Adeeb S, et al. Increase in blood-brain barrier permeability, oxidative stress, and activated microglia in a rat model of blast-induced traumatic brain injury. J Neurosci Res 2010;88:3530–9.

37. Tanno H, Nockels RP, Pitts LH, et al. Breakdown of the blood-brain barrier after fluid percussive brain injury in the rat. Part 1: distribution and time course of protein extravasation. J Neurotrauma 1992;9:21–32.

38. Shetty AK, Mishra V, Kodali M, et al. Blood brain barrier dysfunction and delayed neurological deficits in mild traumatic brain injury induced by blast shock waves. Front Cell Neurosci 2014;8:232.

39. Yeoh S, Bell ED, Monson KL. Distribution of blood-brain barrier disruption in primary blast injury. Ann Biomed Eng 2013;41:2206–14.

40. Abdul-Muneer PM, Schuetz H, Wang F, et al. Induction of oxidative and nitrosative damage leads to cerebrovascular inflammation in an animal model of mild traumatic brain injury induced by primary blast. Free Radic Biol Med 2013;60:282–91.

41. Elder GA, Gama Sosa MA, De Gasperi R, et al. Vascular and inflammatory factors in the pathophysiology of blast-induced brain injury. Front Neurol 2015;6:48.

42. Gama Sosa MA, De Gasperi R, Janssen PL, et al. Selective vulnerability of the cerebral vasculature to blast injury in a rat model of mild traumatic brain injury. Acta Neuropathol Commun 2014;2:67.

43. Tang X, Zhong W, Tu Q, et al. NADPH oxidase mediates the expression of MMP-9 in cerebral tissue after ischemia-reperfusion damage. Neurol Res 2014;36:118–25.

44. Alves JL. Blood-brain barrier and traumatic brain injury. J Neurosci Res 2014;92:141–7.

45. Brown GC, Neher JJ. Inflammatory neurodegeneration and mechanisms of microglial killing of neurons. Mol Neurobiol 2010;41:242–7.

46. Bolton SJ, Anthony DC, Perry VH. Loss of the tight junction proteins occludin and zonula occludens-1 from cerebral vascular endothelium during

neutrophil-induced blood-brain barrier breakdown in vivo. Neuroscience 1998;86:1245–57.

47. Rosenberg GA, Yang Y. Vasogenic edema due to tight junction disruption by matrix metalloproteinases in cerebral ischemia. Neurosurg Focus 2007;22:E4.

48. Walker K, Perkins M, Dray A. Kinins and kinin receptors in the nervous system. Neurochem Int 1995;26:1–16 [discussion: 17–26].

49. Szmydynger-Chodobska J, Fox LM, Lynch KM, et al. Vasopressin amplifies the production of proinflammatory mediators in traumatic brain injury. J Neurotrauma 2010;27:1449–61.

50. Winkler EA, Sengillo JD, Sagare AP, et al. Blood-spinal cord barrier disruption contributes to early motor-neuron degeneration in ALS-model mice. Proc Natl Acad Sci U S A 2014;111:E1035–42.

51. Seiffert E, Dreier JP, Ivens S, et al. Lasting blood-brain barrier disruption induces epileptic focus in the rat somatosensory cortex. J Neurosci 2004; 24:7829–36.

52. Mori K, Miyazaki M, Iwase H, et al. Temporal profile of changes in brain tissue extracellular space and extracellular ion (Na($+$), K($+$)) concentrations after cerebral ischemia and the effects of mild cerebral hypothermia. J Neurotrauma 2002;19: 1261–70.

53. Stiefel MF, Tomita Y, Marmarou A. Secondary ischemia impairing the restoration of ion homeostasis following traumatic brain injury. J Neurosurg 2005;103:707–14.

54. Chen M, Simard JM. Cell swelling and a nonselective cation channel regulated by internal Ca2+ and ATP in native reactive astrocytes from adult rat brain. J Neurosci 2001;21:6512–21.

55. Jayakumar AR, Panickar KS, Curtis KM, et al. Na-K-Cl cotransporter-1 in the mechanism of cell swelling in cultured astrocytes after fluid percussion injury. J Neurochem 2011;117:437–48.

56. Lu KT, Wu CY, Cheng NC, et al. Inhibition of the Na+ -K+ -2Cl- -cotransporter in choroid plexus attenuates traumatic brain injury-induced brain edema and neuronal damage. Eur J Pharmacol 2006;548:99–105.

57. Shohami E, Biegon A. Novel approach to the role of NMDA receptors in traumatic brain injury. CNS Neurol Disord Drug Targets 2014;13:567–73.

58. Simard JM, Woo SK, Schwartzbauer GT, et al. Sulfonylurea receptor 1 in central nervous system injury: a focused review. J Cereb Blood Flow Metab 2012;32:1699–717.

59. Kahle KT, Simard JM, Staley KJ, et al. Molecular mechanisms of ischemic cerebral edema: role of electroneutral ion transport. Physiology (Bethesda) 2009;24:257–65.

60. Simard JM, Kahle KT, Gerzanich V. Molecular mechanisms of microvascular failure in central nervous system injury–synergistic roles of NKCC1 and SUR1/TRPM4. J Neurosurg 2010;113:622–9.

61. Verkman AS, Anderson MO, Papadopoulos MC. Aquaporins: important but elusive drug targets. Nat Rev Drug Discov 2014;13:259–77.

62. Verkman AS, Yang B, Song Y, et al. Role of water channels in fluid transport studied by phenotype analysis of aquaporin knockout mice. Exp Physiol 2000;85(Spec No):233S–41S.

63. Zador Z, Bloch O, Yao X, et al. Aquaporins: role in cerebral edema and brain water balance. Prog Brain Res 2007;161:185–94.

64. Oshio K, Song Y, Verkman AS, et al. Aquaporin-1 deletion reduces osmotic water permeability and cerebrospinal fluid production. Acta Neurochir Suppl 2003;86:525–8.

65. Bloch O, Manley GT. The role of aquaporin-4 in cerebral water transport and edema. Neurosurg Focus 2007;22:E3.

66. Nagelhus EA, Mathiisen TM, Ottersen OP. Aquaporin-4 in the central nervous system: cellular and subcellular distribution and coexpression with KIR4.1. Neuroscience 2004;129:905–13.

67. Solenov E, Watanabe H, Manley GT, et al. Sevenfold-reduced osmotic water permeability in primary astrocyte cultures from AQP-4-deficient mice, measured by a fluorescence quenching method. Am J Physiol Cell Physiol 2004;286:C426–32.

68. Ishmael JE, Lohr CV, Fischer K, et al. Localization of myosin II regulatory light chain in the cerebral vasculature. Acta Histochem 2008;110:172–7.

69. Shen Q, Rigor RR, Pivetti CD, et al. Myosin light chain kinase in microvascular endothelial barrier function. Cardiovasc Res 2010;87:272–80.

70. Luh C, Kuhlmann CR, Ackermann B, et al. Inhibition of myosin light chain kinase reduces brain edema formation after traumatic brain injury. J Neurochem 2010;112:1015–25.

71. Rossi JL, Todd T, Bazan NG, et al. Inhibition of myosin light-chain kinase attenuates cerebral edema after traumatic brain injury in postnatal mice. J Neurotrauma 2013;30:1672–9.

72. Haorah J, Heilman D, Knipe B, et al. Ethanol-induced activation of myosin light chain kinase leads to dysfunction of tight junctions and blood-brain barrier compromise. Alcohol Clin Exp Res 2005;29:999–1009.

73. Kuhlmann CR, Tamaki R, Gamerdinger M, et al. Inhibition of the myosin light chain kinase prevents hypoxia-induced blood-brain barrier disruption. J Neurochem 2007;102:501–7.

74. Ramirez SH, Potula R, Fan S, et al. Methamphetamine disrupts blood-brain barrier function by induction of oxidative stress in brain endothelial cells. J Cereb Blood Flow Metab 2009;29: 1933–45.

75. Filippini G, Brusaferri F, Sibley WA, et al. Cortico-steroids or ACTH for acute exacerbations in multiple sclerosis. Cochrane Database Syst Rev 2000;(4):CD001331.

76. Ryken TC, McDermott M, Robinson PD, et al. The role of steroids in the management of brain metastases: a systematic review and evidence-based clinical practice guideline. J Neurooncol 2010;96: 103–14.

77. Salvador E, Shityakov S, Forster C. Glucocorticoids and endothelial cell barrier function. Cell Tissue Res 2014;355:597–605.

78. Alderson P, Roberts I. Corticosteroids for acute traumatic brain injury. Cochrane Database Syst Rev 2005;(1):CD000196.

79. Sandercock PA, Soane T. Corticosteroids for acute ischaemic stroke. Cochrane Database Syst Rev 2011;(9):CD000064.

80. Bratton SL, Chestnut RM, Ghajar J, et al. Guidelines for the management of severe traumatic brain injury. XV. Steroids. J Neurotrauma 2007; 24(Suppl 1):S91–5.

81. Thal SC, Schaible EV, Neuhaus W, et al. Inhibition of proteasomal glucocorticoid receptor degradation restores dexamethasone-mediated stabilization of the blood-brain barrier after traumatic brain injury. Crit Care Med 2013;41:1305–15.

82. Kleinschnitz C, Blecharz K, Kahles T, et al. Glucocorticoid insensitivity at the hypoxic blood-brain barrier can be reversed by inhibition of the proteasome. Stroke 2011;42:1081–9.

83. Stahel PF, Smith WR, Bruchis J, et al. Peroxisome proliferator-activated receptors: "key" regulators of neuroinflammation after traumatic brain injury. PPAR Res 2008;2008:538141.

84. Moreno S, Farioli-Vecchioli S, Ceru MP. Immunolocalization of peroxisome proliferator-activated receptors and retinoid X receptors in the adult rat CNS. Neuroscience 2004;123:131–45.

85. Besson VC, Chen XR, Plotkine M, et al. Fenofibrate, a peroxisome proliferator-activated receptor alpha agonist, exerts neuroprotective effects in traumatic brain injury. Neurosci Lett 2005;388:7–12.

86. Chen XR, Besson VC, Palmier B, et al. Neurological recovery-promoting, anti-inflammatory, and anti-oxidative effects afforded by fenofibrate, a PPAR alpha agonist, in traumatic brain injury. J Neurotrauma 2007;24:1119–31.

87. Mysiorek C, Culot M, Dehouck L, et al. Peroxisome-proliferator-activated receptor-alpha activation protects brain capillary endothelial cells from oxygen-glucose deprivation-induced hyperpermeability in the blood-brain barrier. Curr Neurovasc Res 2009;6:181–93.

88. Sauerbeck A, Gao J, Readnower R, et al. Pioglitazone attenuates mitochondrial dysfunction, cognitive impairment, cortical tissue loss, and inflammation following traumatic brain injury. Exp Neurol 2011; 227:128–35.

89. Yi JH, Park SW, Brooks N, et al. PPARgamma agonist rosiglitazone is neuroprotective after traumatic brain injury via anti-inflammatory and anti-oxidative mechanisms. Brain Res 2008;1244:164–72.

90. Zhu D, Wang Y, Singh I, et al. Protein S controls hypoxic/ischemic blood-brain barrier disruption through the TAM receptor Tyro3 and sphingosine 1-phosphate receptor. Blood 2010;115: 4963–72.

91. Nag S, Manias JL, Stewart DJ. Pathology and new players in the pathogenesis of brain edema. Acta Neuropathol 2009;118:197–217.

92. Storkebaum E, Quaegebeur A, Vikkula M, et al. Cerebrovascular disorders: molecular insights and therapeutic opportunities. Nat Neurosci 2011;14: 1390–7.

93. Carmeliet P, Jain RK. Molecular mechanisms and clinical applications of angiogenesis. Nature 2011;473:298–307.

94. Dore-Duffy P, Wang X, Mehedi A, et al. Differential expression of capillary VEGF isoforms following traumatic brain injury. Neurol Res 2007; 29:395–403.

95. Shore PM, Jackson EK, Wisniewski SR, et al. Vascular endothelial growth factor is increased in cerebrospinal fluid after traumatic brain injury in infants and children. Neurosurgery 2004;54:605–11 [discussion: 611–2].

96. Chodobski A, Chung I, Kozniewska E, et al. Early neutrophilic expression of vascular endothelial growth factor after traumatic brain injury. Neuroscience 2003;122:853–67.

97. Hirose T, Matsumoto N, Tasaki O, et al. Delayed progression of edema formation around a hematoma expressing high levels of VEGF and mmp-9 in a patient with traumatic brain injury: case report. Neurol Med Chir (Tokyo) 2013;53:609–12.

98. Koyama J, Miyake S, Sasayama T, et al. Effect of VEGF receptor antagonist (VGA1155) on brain edema in the rat cold injury model. Kobe J Med Sci 2007;53:199–207.

99. Kimura R, Nakase H, Tamaki R, et al. Vascular endothelial growth factor antagonist reduces brain edema formation and venous infarction. Stroke 2005;36:1259–63.

100. van Bruggen N, Thibodeaux H, Palmer JT, et al. VEGF antagonism reduces edema formation and tissue damage after ischemia/reperfusion injury in the mouse brain. J Clin Invest 1999;104:1613–20.

101. Thau-Zuchman O, Shohami E, Alexandrovich AG, et al. Vascular endothelial growth factor increases neurogenesis after traumatic brain injury. J Cereb Blood Flow Metab 2010;30:1008–16.

102. Nag S, Kapadia A, Stewart DJ. Review: molecular pathogenesis of blood-brain barrier breakdown

in acute brain injury. Neuropathol Appl Neurobiol 2011;37:3–23.

103. Rosenberg GA. Matrix metalloproteinases in neuro-inflammation. Glia 2002;39:279–91.

104. Bell RD, Winkler EA, Singh I, et al. Apolipoprotein E controls cerebrovascular integrity via cyclophilin A. Nature 2012;485:512–6.

105. Grossetete M, Phelps J, Arko L, et al. Elevation of matrix metalloproteinases 3 and 9 in cerebrospinal fluid and blood in patients with severe traumatic brain injury. Neurosurgery 2009;65:702–8.

106. Hadass O, Tomlinson BN, Gooyit M, et al. Selective inhibition of matrix metalloproteinase-9 attenuates secondary damage resulting from severe traumatic brain injury. PLoS One 2013;8:e76904.

107. Hayashi T, Kaneko Y, Yu S, et al. Quantitative analyses of matrix metalloproteinase activity after traumatic brain injury in adult rats. Brain Res 2009; 1280:172–7.

108. Asahi M, Asahi K, Jung JC, et al. Role for matrix metalloproteinase 9 after focal cerebral ischemia: effects of gene knockout and enzyme inhibition with BB-94. J Cereb Blood Flow Metab 2000;20: 1681–9.

109. Jia F, Yin YH, Gao GY, et al. MMP-9 inhibitor SB-3CT attenuates behavioral impairments and hippocampal loss after traumatic brain injury in rat. J Neurotrauma 2014;31:1225–34.

110. Lee M, Chen Z, Tomlinson BN, et al. Water-soluble MMP-9 inhibitor reduces lesion volume after severe traumatic brain injury. ACS Chem Neurosci 2015;6: 1658–64.

111. Vink R, van den Heuvel C. Substance P antagonists as a therapeutic approach to improving outcome following traumatic brain injury. Neurotherapeutics 2010;7:74–80.

112. Donkin JJ, Vink R. Mechanisms of cerebral edema in traumatic brain injury: therapeutic developments. Curr Opin Neurol 2010;23:293–9.

113. Nimmo AJ, Cernak I, Heath DL, et al. Neurogenic inflammation is associated with development of edema and functional deficits following traumatic brain injury in rats. Neuropeptides 2004;38:40–7.

114. Zacest AC, Vink R, Manavis J, et al. Substance P immunoreactivity increases following human traumatic brain injury. Acta Neurochir Suppl 2010; 106:211–6.

115. Donkin JJ, Nimmo AJ, Cernak I, et al. Substance P is associated with the development of brain edema and functional deficits after traumatic brain injury. J Cereb Blood Flow Metab 2009;29:1388–98.

116. Donkin JJ, Cernak I, Blumbergs PC, et al. A substance P antagonist reduces axonal injury and improves neurologic outcome when administered up to 12 hours after traumatic brain injury. J Neurotrauma 2011;28:217–24.

117. Turner RJ, Helps SC, Thornton E, et al. A substance P antagonist improves outcome when administered 4 h after onset of ischaemic stroke. Brain Res 2011; 1393:84–90.

118. Yao X, Uchida K, Papadopoulos MC, et al. Mildly reduced brain swelling and improved neurological outcome in aquaporin-4 knockout mice following controlled cortical impact brain injury. J Neurotrauma 2015;32:1458–64.

119. Papadopoulos MC, Manley GT, Krishna S, et al. Aquaporin-4 facilitates reabsorption of excess fluid in vasogenic brain edema. FASEB J 2004; 18:1291–3.

120. Ding JY, Kreipke CW, Speirs SL, et al. Hypoxia-inducible factor-1alpha signaling in aquaporin upregulation after traumatic brain injury. Neurosci Lett 2009;453:68–72.

121. Shenaq M, Kassem H, Peng C, et al. Neuronal damage and functional deficits are ameliorated by inhibition of aquaporin and HIF1alpha after traumatic brain injury (TBI). J Neurol Sci 2012; 323:134–40.

122. Dardiotis E, Paterakis K, Tsivgoulis G, et al. AQP4 tag single nucleotide polymorphisms in patients with traumatic brain injury. J Neurotrauma 2014; 31:1920–6.

123. Fukuda AM, Adami A, Pop V, et al. Posttraumatic reduction of edema with aquaporin-4 RNA interference improves acute and chronic functional recovery. J Cereb Blood Flow Metab 2013;33: 1621–32.

124. Chen H, Luo J, Kintner DB, et al. Na(+)-dependent chloride transporter (NKCC1)-null mice exhibit less gray and white matter damage after focal cerebral ischemia. J Cereb Blood Flow Metab 2005;25:54–66.

125. Watanabe M, Fukuda A. Development and regulation of chloride homeostasis in the central nervous system. Front Cell Neurosci 2015;9:371.

126. Lu KT, Cheng NC, Wu CY, et al. NKCC1-mediated traumatic brain injury-induced brain edema and neuron death via Raf/MEK/MAPK cascade. Crit Care Med 2008;36:917–22.

127. Yan Y, Dempsey RJ, Flemmer A, et al. Inhibition of Na(+)-K(+)-Cl(-) cotransporter during focal cerebral ischemia decreases edema and neuronal damage. Brain Res 2003;961:22–31.

128. Ameli PA, Ameli NJ, Gubernick DM, et al. Role of vasopressin and its antagonism in stroke related edema. J Neurosci Res 2014;92:1091–9.

129. Huang WD, Pan J, Xu M, et al. Changes and effects of plasma arginine vasopressin in traumatic brain injury. J Endocrinol Invest 2008;31:996–1000.

130. Szmydynger-Chodobska J, Zink BJ, Chodobski A. Multiple sites of vasopressin synthesis in the injured brain. J Cereb Blood Flow Metab 2011;31: 47–51.

131. Filippidis AS, Liang X, Wang W, et al. Real-time monitoring of changes in brain extracellular sodium and potassium concentrations and intracranial pressure after selective vasopressin-1a receptor inhibition following focal traumatic brain injury in rats. J Neurotrauma 2014;31:1258–67.

132. Marmarou CR, Liang X, Abidi NH, et al. Selective vasopressin-1a receptor antagonist prevents brain edema, reduces astrocytic cell swelling and GFAP, V1aR and AQP4 expression after focal traumatic brain injury. Brain Res 2014;1581:89–102.

133. Krieg SM, Sonanini S, Plesnila N, et al. Effect of small molecule vasopressin V1a and V2 receptor antagonists on brain edema formation and secondary brain damage following traumatic brain injury in mice. J Neurotrauma 2015;32:221–7.

134. Chen M, Dong Y, Simard JM. Functional coupling between sulfonylurea receptor type 1 and a nonselective cation channel in reactive astrocytes from adult rat brain. J Neurosci 2003;23:8568–77.

135. Walcott BP, Kahle KT, Simard JM. Novel treatment targets for cerebral edema. Neurotherapeutics 2012;9:65–72.

136. Simard JM, Chen M, Tarasov KV, et al. Newly expressed SUR1-regulated NC(Ca-ATP) channel mediates cerebral edema after ischemic stroke. Nat Med 2006;12:433–40.

137. Kunte H, Busch MA, Trostdorf K, et al. Hemorrhagic transformation of ischemic stroke in diabetics on sulfonylureas. Ann Neurol 2012;72:799–806.

138. Kunte H, Schmidt S, Eliasziw M, et al. Sulfonylureas improve outcome in patients with type 2 diabetes and acute ischemic stroke. Stroke 2007;38:2526–30.

139. Simard JM, Kilbourne M, Tsymbalyuk O, et al. Key role of sulfonylurea receptor 1 in progressive secondary hemorrhage after brain contusion. J Neurotrauma 2009;26:2257–67.

140. Zweckberger K, Hackenberg K, Jung CS, et al. Glibenclamide reduces secondary brain damage after experimental traumatic brain injury. Neuroscience 2014;272:199–206.

141. Sheth KN, Kimberly WT, Elm JJ, et al. Pilot study of intravenous glyburide in patients with a large ischemic stroke. Stroke 2014;45:281–3.

142. Kimberly WT, Battey TW, Pham L, et al. Glyburide is associated with attenuated vasogenic edema in stroke patients. Neurocrit Care 2014;20:193–201.

143. Diaz-Arrastia R, Kochanek PM, Bergold P, et al. Pharmacotherapy of traumatic brain injury: state of the science and the road forward: report of the Department of Defense Neurotrauma Pharmacology Workgroup. J Neurotrauma 2014;31:135–58.

Hypothermia in Traumatic Brain Injury

Aminul I. Ahmed, MA (Cantab), MD, PhD*, M. Ross Bullock, MD, PhD, W. Dalton Dietrich, PhD

KEYWORDS

- Hypothermia • Traumatic brain injury • Neuroprotection • Intracranial pressure

KEY POINTS

- Mild to moderate hypothermia reduces the intracranial pressure (ICP).
- Randomized control trials for short-term hypothermia indicate no benefit in outcome after severe traumatic brain injury.
- Longer-term hypothermia could be of benefit by reducing ICP, and ongoing studies may determine this.

INTRODUCTION

Introduction and History

The use of therapeutic hypothermia in clinical medicine has become widely established in the management of cardiac arrest and neonatal hypoxia, whereas the body of evidence in stroke, spinal cord injury, and traumatic brain injury (TBI) remains an ongoing area of active research and discussion.[1,2] Some of the original laboratory studies for TBI used crude methods of cooling, and to temperatures regarded as extreme by current standards. For instance, Rosomoff[3] induced a "closed head injury" in 2 groups of mongrel dogs either at normothermia or at 25°C body temperature, by pouring liquid air into a cylinder in contact with the dura. The hypothermic dogs survived 5 times longer than the normothermic dogs, and this was accompanied by reduced brain swelling. Again, in the laboratory, surface cooling of uninjured dogs to 28°C to 30°C led to a drop in the cerebrospinal fluid (CSF) pressure.[4] Concurrently, several remarkable clinical studies reported instances of the effect of cooling in patients following TBI. Perhaps the first was by Fay,[5] who described therapeutic cooling of the human brain after cerebral trauma as early as 1941, in which he cooled the brain using local irrigation of ice-cold fluids into the cranial vault or cooled systemically using a refrigeration blanket. Some anecdotes that he reported indicate serendipitous, yet remarkable improvement of the patient with cooling (for example, see page 254 of his seminal paper). Around the same time, in a cohort of 30 patients with severe TBI who were cooled, 17 of them survived, which was a large number in the 1950s.[6] To determine the mechanisms that may underlie this improvement, in a controlled study in a small number of patients, the CSF pressure was reduced following hypothermia.[7] These initial groundbreaking studies laid the foundation for hypothermia research in the context of severe TBI and now include the more recent and numerous preclinical mechanistic studies, along with early clinical and more recently larger randomized control trials (RCTs) in an effort to determine whether therapeutic hypothermia is of benefit following severe TBI.

Basic Science Studies

In rodent studies, following a lateral fluid percussion injury, rats undergoing induced hypothermia did better in terms of survival and behavior.[8–10]

Disclosure Statement: The authors have nothing to disclose.
Miami Project to Cure Paralysis, Lois Pope Life Center, University of Miami, 1095 Northwest, 14th Terrace, Miami, FL 33136, USA
* Corresponding author. Clinical Experimental Sciences, University Hospitals Southampton, University of Southampton, LD83, South Academic Block, Tremona Road, Southampton SO16 6YD, United Kingdom.
E-mail address: a.ahmed@soton.ac.uk

neurosurgery.theclinics.com

The mechanisms by which this occurs in animal models are multifactorial but include the prevention of secondary brain injury by reducing the excitotoxic, oxidative, and inflammatory effect, by targeting ischemia-reperfusion, and by minimizing cortical depolarization.[11] Hypothermia decreases cerebral metabolic rate and alters release of excitatory neurotransmitters following injury.[12,13] Other mechanisms also include attenuated proinflammatory cytokines, reduced free radicals, and excitotoxic substances.[13,14] Lowering the temperature after TBI has a protective effect on hypoxia-induced cell death.[15–17] Hypothermia also prevents the disruption of the blood brain barrier following injury.[18] Cooling induces a reduction in brain metabolism by 5% per 1°C reduction in core temperature, leading to vasoconstriction and reduced cerebral blood volume, hence a decrease in intracranial pressure (ICP).[19] Moreover, after-injury hypothermia leads to a reduction of chemically induced seizures and spreading depolarizations,[20] and this hypothermia-dependent reduction in seizures has also been reported clinically in TBI patients.[21] Perhaps critically, if the rate of rewarming is too fast, the benefits of reducing the core temperature are lost.[22] With this mechanistic knowledge of the benefits of hypothermia, numerous clinical studies have been undertaken to demonstrate if this treatment modality is ultimately of benefit in the severely injured TBI patient.

TREATMENT OPTIONS
Literature Review

Overview of clinical trials
Clinical trials of hypothermia have 2 broad aims: first, to control the ICP, and second, to provide neuroprotection. As a consequence, the mortality and morbidity outcome determines whether the treatment regimen instigated is of clinical benefit. In general terms, ICP control has been more widely studied in the Far East, whereas primary neuroprotection has been the focus of western clinical trials. The initial western trials involved small patient numbers up to 80. In an early trial, with moderate hypothermia between 32°C and 33°C for 48 hours, a trend toward a better Glasgow Outcome Score (GOS) with a reduction in seizures was observed.[23] In a similar trial, with the same target temperature but for 24 hours, the ICP and cerebral blood flow were lower, and a similar trend toward an improved outcome was observed.[24] In a follow-up study, similar improvements in GOS were observed in patients with a Glasgow Coma Score (GCS) of between 5 and 7, but this difference in GOS was insignificant by 1 year.[25] To evaluate

the effect of mild hypothermia (34°C) on ICP in severely head-injured patients, Shiozaki and colleagues[26] in Japan determined that ICP was significantly reduced and cerebral perfusion pressure was increased in those with hypothermia. Hypothermia was continued for at least 2 days, or until it was thought not to be effective. Similarly, reducing the temperature to 35°C resulted in ICP control and improved cerebral perfusion pressure (CPP) in TBI patients, while also reducing metabolism and energy expenditure but maintaining hemodynamic stability.[27] In summary, these small studies were the foundation of larger RCTs to determine the efficacy of hypothermia in the TBI patient.

Short-term hypothermia
With the small case control studies suggesting a benefit of hypothermia in the severely injured TBI patient, the argument for larger RCTs for short-term hypothermia led to several trials in both adult and pediatric populations. The National Acute Brain Injury: Hypothermia (NABIS:H) study was an RCT that had the premise of a neuroprotective strategy so the patients in the treatment group were cooled for 48 hours after injury.[28] The target temperature was 33°C, and the patients were rewarmed at 48 hours irrespective of their ICP. There was no difference in outcome (GOS at 6 months) between the cooled and normothermic groups, although there were significant intercenter differences. The most experienced centers had greater success, using faster cooling times from injury and avoiding hypotension and hypovolemia[29] in the hypothermia group. With these differences between centers, NABIS:H II attempted to address the criticisms of NABIS:H.[30] There were 6 dedicated centers, where patients were rapidly cooled using ice saline within 4 hours of injury. Again, the target temperature was 33°C with rewarming after 48 hours, and the primary outcome was the GOS at 6 months. The trial was terminated early because there was no difference to the null hypothesis, and these 2 studies have been interpreted to suggest that short-term hypothermia does not improve outcome nor provide neuroprotection in TBI. Interestingly, the hypothermia group had more patients with raised ICP and may be in part due to rebound ICP problems because hypothermia was only 48 hours, with ICP problems usually occurring after this during the at-risk swelling phase. Subgroup analysis of the surgical group in which patients had evacuation of an intracerebral hematoma suggested that hypothermia was of benefit, although the number of patients was small (28 surgical cases in which 15 had hypothermia therapy and

did better overall as a cohort). A similar RCT from Japan instigated hypothermia for 48 hours before rewarming over 3 days in severe TBI patients.[31] Importantly, all patients in the study had ICPs that were low (less than 25 mm Hg) before randomization. Again there was no difference in clinical outcome at 3 months between the hypothermic and normothermic groups. In the pediatric population, the instigation of short-term hypothermia again demonstrates no benefit. For example, the Cool Kids trial in which hypothermia (32°C–33°C) for 48 to 72 hours followed by slow rewarming was stopped early due to absence of any trend toward treatment benefit when looking at the 3-month pediatric GOS.[32] Similarly, an even shorter cooling period of 24 hours to 33°C in the pediatric TBI population demonstrated no improvement in the Pediatric Cerebral Performance Score at 6 months, and in fact, showed a trend toward an increase in mortality with hypothermia.[33] Clearly, based on these trials, the argument for short-term hypothermia was not justified, and therefore, attention was focused toward extending the length of hypothermia beyond the 48-hour time period.

Long-term hypothermia

A recently published trial, Eurotherm 3235, examined the hypothesis that titrated hypothermia treatments raised ICP in TBI patients and demonstrated a decrease in the ICP with hypothermia,[34] but was closed for recruitment early. The trial results demonstrated that hypothermia, a stage 2 treatment in the tiered management of a severe head injury patient, was associated with worse outcomes in terms of GOS-E compared with patients in which hypothermia was not instigated.[35] Critically, in this study, hypothermia was used instead of other stage 2 measures such as osmotherapy, which were only introduced if hypothermia failed to control ICP greater than 20 mm Hg. Also in this trial, hypothermia was maximal at day 3, after which the patients were warmed back to normothermia, and half the patients went to stage 3 treatment with either thiopentone coma or decompressive craniectomy. A similar Japanese trial, the B-HYPO study, where patients were cooled for 3 days to 32 to 34°C before rewarming, was again stopped early due to no observable difference in the GOS at 6 months.[36] Rather than using medium-term hypothermia for the immediate benefits of neuroprotection, longer periods of hypothermia, beyond 3 days, improved ICP control. In the severe TBI cohort with a GCS of 8 or less, hypothermia to 33°C to 35°C for between 3 and 14 days led to decreased mortality compared with the normothermic control group.[37]

This decrease in mortality may have been because the long-term hypothermia reduced the ICP and swelling during the critical swelling phase. The same group compared short-term (2 days) versus long-term (average of 5 days) hypothermia in patients with TBI with mass effect and midline shift.[38] The outcomes were improved in the patients with prolonged hypothermia, and they also observed that rebound intracranial hypertension often occurs with shorter periods of hypothermia. Currently, an ongoing trial may add to the evidence to demonstrate benefit in long-term cooling. The POLAR-RCT (NCT00987688) is an Australasian trial to determine if early prophylactic sustained hypothermia has outcome benefit; patients will be cooled for between 3 and 7 days to 33°C. Similarly, the LTH-1 trial (NCT01886222)[39] is a Chinese study to determine if cooling to 34°C to 35°C for between 5 and 14 days leads to improved GOS at 6 months. With longer periods of hypothermia, cytotoxic edema and intracellular cascades of neurotoxicity may be attenuated.[40] Cerebral edema peaks between 3 to 5 days; therefore, the long-term hypothermia may overcome the rebound intracranial hypertension observed in the short-term cooling studies.

Hypothermia with surgical lesions

Following the NABIS:H trials, a pooled meta-analysis indicated a benefit for hypothermia in patients with a surgical hematoma or acute subdural hematoma requiring evacuation.[41] The rationale may be due to a high proportion of acute subdural hematoma patients getting either cortical spreading depolarizations or hyperemia, and hence, cooling is able to target both. Consequently, the HOPES (HypOthermia for Patients requiring Evacuation of Subdural hematoma) trial is currently recruiting to determine if early cooling, regardless of timing of surgery, is of benefit in this specific subdural hematoma TBI population (NCT02064959). Moreover, in a small randomized trial, cooling after a craniotomy for TBI led to a favorable outcome at 1 year.[42]

Summary papers

With a large body of clinical evidence for the use of cooling in severe TBI, several systematic reviews and meta-analyses have pooled data in an attempt to clarify the evidence base for therapeutic hypothermia. Reviewing the effect of hypothermia on ICP, all but 1 of 15 studies demonstrated a decrease in ICP.[2] Similarly, comparing 11 prospective RCTs, mild hypothermia was associated with lowering the ICP.[43] In a review of 12 trials with more than 1000 patients, McIntyre and colleagues[18] concluded that the evidence suggested a benefit of mild to moderate hypothermia in severe TBI with a reduction in risk of both death (relative reduction, RR 19%) and poor neurologic outcome (RR 22%). It also suggested that a longer period of cooling, greater than 48 hours, might be beneficial because 9 studies with short-term hypothermia had no difference in outcome, whereas 3 long-term hypothermia studies demonstrated benefit. A similar finding demonstrated better mortality outcome from 12 studies; however, if the 4 short-term studies (48 hours of cooling or less) were taken out, there was no difference in outcome[44] (**Table 1**).

Several further systematic reviews come to differing conclusions based on the selection of available evidence for the use of cooling in TBI. Several reviews do not support the use of hypothermia.[12,45,46] This goes against the review by McIntyre and colleagues[18] that states there is a benefit in the RR of hypothermia, even more so with prolonged hypothermia. In support of this later review, Crossley and colleagues[47] analyzed 20 RCTs with almost 2000 patients, similarly concluding an RR reduction in both mortality and outcome. When accounting for studies with low bias, this RR was greater. Interestingly, the incidence of pneumonia, one of the recognized risks of hypothermia, was not significantly different. In summary, although the review articles do come to differing conclusions, when dissecting out longer-term hypothermia beyond 3 days, the evidence to support this becomes more convincing.

Guidelines

Based on the current evidence for the use of hypothermia in severe TBI, the Brain Trauma Foundation (BTF) guidelines from 2007[48] are the most widely used guide to management for TBI. The latest 2016 BTF recommendations are due to be published imminently, but the 2007 guidelines suggest not to use hypothermia as standard of care, but to be used by experienced clinicians. The information is based on 6 RCTs,[48] the conclusion of which is that hypothermia in severe TBI is likely to have a favorable neurologic outcome and may have a chance of reducing mortality if hypothermia is maintained greater than 48 hours.

Based on the data, the BTF gives a level 3 recommendation:

- Hypothermia does not reduce mortality. Preliminary data suggest that it may if hypothermia is maintained for more than 48 hours.
- Hypothermia is associated with better GOS.

Following on from these BTF recommendations, the above evidence provides further points for consideration that include:

- The depth of hypothermia: The target temperature should be titrated against ICP; 35°C to 35.5°C treats raised ICP and maintains CPP, and there is no compromise of cardiac function.[27] Temperatures lower than 35°C may reduce brain tissue oxygenation,[49] but overall the target temperature will need to be individualized.
- The duration of hypothermia: This depends on the severity of injury. The duration should be greater than 48 hours and continue until the peak period of swelling and subsequent intracranial hypertension (3–5 days) subside.
- Rate of rewarming: Fast rewarming not only loses any benefit of hypothermia but makes things worse.[50] Moreover, there is a rebound raised ICP if rewarming is too rapid.[51] Therefore, a rate of rewarming no more than 0.1°C to 0.2°C per hour should be used.
- Mass lesions: Patients with a focal mass lesion following TBI may respond to hypothermia better than a more diffuse injury.

With the above considerations, future guidelines should incorporate hypothermia in a tiered system of ICP management of the severely injured TBI patient. These guidelines should ideally be part of a standardized treatment algorithm that includes clear protocols for inducing cooling. **Boxes 1** and **2** demonstrate 2 examples of algorithms from 2 large level 1 trauma centers: Jackson Memorial Hospital, Miami, Florida, USA and Wessex Neurological Centre, Southampton, Hampshire, UK.

Treatment Table

The options for cooling include surface and endovascular routes. Surface cooling was used in many early studies and includes the use of ice packs, cooling blankets, and helmets. These items tend to cool more slowly, but are associated with fewer severe complications. Newer gel pads that conduct heat better have been recently introduced. Endovascular cooling (such as the use of Coolgard) uses a femoral vein balloon catheter and is more efficient and faster to get to the target temperature. It can be used in the conscious patient, avoids shivering, and allows tighter temperature control to prevent overshoot hypothermia. Conversely, venous catheters are invasive, and the costs for cooling are high. Less common techniques include ice-cold saline infusion, which can be used at the roadside,[52] the use of fans, and ice-cold gastric lavage.[53]

Hyperthermia

Whether active cooling is instigated in TBI patients or not, most importantly, hyperthermia

Table 1

Relative risk of mortality from short-term and long-term cooling compared with standard treatment in severe traumatic brain injury

Review: Hypothermia TBI
Comparison: 01 Hypothermia vs. Control
Outcome: 01 Mortality

Study or sub-category	Hypothermia n/N	Control n/N	RR (random) 95% CI	Weight %	RR (random) 95% CI
01 Short-term cooling strategy					
Clifton 1993	8/23	8/22		4.13	0.96 [0.44, 2.10]
Hirayama 1994	4/12	5/10		2.50	0.67 [0.24, 1.83]
Marion 1997	9/39	10/42		4.12	0.97 [0.44, 2.13]
Clifton 2001	53/190	48/178		23.11	1.03 [0.74, 1.44]
Subtotal (95% CI)	264	252		33.86	0.98 [0.75, 1.30]
Total events: 74 (Hypothermia), 71 (Control)					
Test for heterogeneity: Chi² = 0.66, df = 3 (P = .88), I² = 0%					
Test for overall effect: Z = 0.11 (P = .91)					
02 Long-term/goal-directed cooling strategy					
Aibiki 2000	1/12	3/10		0.58	0.28 [0.03, 2.27]
Jiang 2000	11/43	20/44		7.02	0.56 [0.31, 1.03]
Chen 2001	3/30	8/30		1.70	0.38 [0.11, 1.28]
Yan 2001	13/24	16/20		13.95	0.68 [0.44, 1.04]
Zhi 2003	51/198	72/198		28.47	0.71 [0.52, 0.96]
Qiu 2005	11/43	22/43		7.41	0.50 [0.28, 0.90]
Smrcka 2005	5/35	11/37		2.83	0.48 [0.19, 1.24]
Liu 2006	6/21	12/23		4.19	0.55 [0.25, 1.20]
Subtotal (95% CI)	406	405		66.14	0.62 [0.51, 0.76]
Total events: 101 (Hypothermia), 164 (Control)					
Test for heterogeneity: Chi² = 3.16, df = 7 (P = .87), I² = 0%					
Test for overall effect: Z = 4.74 (P < .00001)					
Total (95% CI)	670	657		100.00	0.73 [0.62, 0.85]
Total events: 175 (Hypothermia), 235 (Control)					
Test for heterogeneity: Chi² = 10.87, df = 11 (P = .45), I² = 0%					
Test for overall effect: Z = 3.92 (P < .0001)					

0.1 0.2 0.5 1 2 5 10

Favours treatment   Favours control

From Fox JL, Vu EN, Doyle-Waters M, et al. Prophylactic hypothermia for traumatic brain injury: a quantitative systematic review. CJEM 2010;12(4):360; with permission.

Box 1
Treatment protocol for intracranial pressure management at Jackson Memorial Hospital Neurosurgical Intensive Care Unit

Intracranial pressure management protocol: Jackson Memorial Hospital WW8 Neurosurgical Intensive Care Unit (NSICU)

Targets: Aim is to optimize brain perfusion and avoid secondary damage CPP 60 to 70; ICP less than 20; temperature less than 37°C; CVP 6 to 10.

Maintain CPP with fluids and pressors as needed.

Stage 1

- Position: Head up 30° to 45°
- Sedation: Propofol, 40 μm/kg/min titrated to RASS −2
- Analgesia: opiates—fentanyl infusion, 100 μg/h
- Ventilation: normocarbia—Pco_2: 34 to 36 mm Hg
- Temp: normothermia: 36 to 37.5°C
- CSF drainage: Vent ventricular drain for 5 minutes at a time if ICP greater than 20 for greater than 5 minutes (if possible)

Stage 2

- Osmotherapy: Mannitol 20% bolus 1 g/kg then 0.5 g/kg × 4 to 6 bolus doses/24 h or until plasma osm 320/L. Continue into subsequent stages.

Stage 3[a]

- Neuromuscular paralysis with cisatracurium or vecuronium to TOF 2/4
- Switch sedation to benzodiazepine infusion: Midazolam–0.5 to 0.1 mg/kg/h
- Mild hyperventilation: Pco_2: 32 to 35 mm Hg

Stage 4[a]

- Hypothermia: @ 34 to 35°C, use "Arctic sun" surface system (Arctic Sun Medivance, Louisville, CO), or Coolgard catheter (ZOLL Medical Corporation, Chelmsford, MA)

Stage 5[a]

- Decompressive craniectomy

Stage 6[a]

- Burst suppression: Barbiturate sedation—pentobarbital: loading dose over 30 minutes is 10 mg/kg followed by 1 mg/kg/h; may reload with 5 mg/kg as needed and titrate drip up to 3 mg/kg/h
- Stop benzodiazepine infusion

Tiered therapy for temperature regulation is shown in Stage 4.
   Obtain computed tomographic head scan if ICP spikes greater than 25 suddenly and sustained more than 5 minutes.
   [a] NSGY/NSICU Attending must be contacted at this stage.
Abbreviations: CVP, central venous pressure; osm, osmolarity; NSGY, neurosurgery; TOF, train of four ratios; RASS, richmond agitation-sedation scale; WW8, west wing 8.
Courtesy of Jackson Memorial Hospital, Miami, FL, USA; with permission.

---

should be avoided in all TBI patients[27,54]; this notion is supported by rodent studies.[55,56] Hyperthermia has been shown to occur in up to 93% of the time in TBI patients admitted for 2 weeks or more.[57] In a case control study, induced normothermia, and therefore, prevention of a fever, reduced the number of ICP spikes greater than 25 mm Hg,[58] although no randomized placebo controlled trials for very

mild hypothermia/normothermia are currently published.[59]

COMPLICATIONS

There are many recognized complications of induced hypothermia[60–62]:

- Pneumonias and infections

Box 2
Treatment protocol for intracranial pressure management at Wessex Neurologic Centre Neurological Intensive Care Unit

Wessex Neurological Centre, Southampton, UK
Levels of intracranial pressure management

At all stages, consider evacuation of intracranial hematoma.

- Level 1: Sedation and optimization
  - Adequate sedation with midazolam and morphine
  - Maintain $Pao_2 \geq 13$ kPa, target $Paco_2$ 4.5 to 5.0 kPa
  - If ICP greater than 20 mm Hg, aim for Na greater than 140 mmol/L
  - Target CPP of 60 mm Hg
  - *Avoid pyrexia*
  - Neuromuscular blockade (pharmacologic paralysis)
- Level 2: External ventricular drain placement
- *Level 3: Cool to 35°C*

  Cooling reduces cerebral metabolic rate by 6% for each 1°C and will usually reduce ICP. Insert femoral cooling line.

- *Level 4: Cool to 34°C*

  Cooling to 34°C should lower cerebral metabolic rate further; however, it may be associated with more complications.

- Level 5: Thiopentone coma or decompressive craniectomy

  Thiopentone coma

  Decompressive craniectomy

Tiered therapy for temperature regulation is shown in italic. For more information, please visit www. neuroicu.org.uk.
  Courtesy of Wessex Neurological Centre, Southampton, Hampshire, UK; with permission.

- Hypokalemia, arrhythmias, reduced cardiac output
- Shivering if surface cooling resulting in increased oxygen consumption
- Line infection and deep vein thrombosis in endovascular cooling
- Reduced liver function, bleeding diathesis, thrombocytopenia
- Hyperglycemia

SUMMARY

- Short-term hypothermia does not improve outcome in severe TBI.
- Long-term hypothermia may be of benefit.
- Patients with focal mass lesions may benefit from hypothermia, although evidence is limited.
- Hypothermia should be instigated as part of a staged treatment protocol.
- Cooling should be finely controlled, and rewarming should be slow to avoid rebound intracranial hypertension.

REFERENCES

1. Bernard SA, Gray TW, Buist MD, et al. Treatment of comatose survivors of out-of-hospital cardiac arrest with induced hypothermia. N Engl J Med 2002; 346(8):557–63.
2. Marion D, Bullock MR. Current and future role of therapeutic hypothermia. J Neurotrauma 2009; 26(3):455–67.
3. Rosomoff HL. Experimental brain injury during hypothermia. J Neurosurg 1959;16(2):177–87.
4. Lund LO, Beckwitt HJ, Grover RF, et al. Effect of hyperventilation, hypothermia and urea on circulation and cerebrospinal fluid pressure in the dog. (2). Anesthesiology 1965;26:45–8.
5. Fay T. Early experiences with local and generalized refrigeration of the human brain. J Neurosurg 1959; 16(3):239–59 [discussion: 259–60].
6. Sedzimir CB. Therapeutic hypothermia in cases of head injury. J Neurosurg 1959;16(4):407–14.
7. Lundberg N, Troupp H, Lorin H. Continuous recording of the ventricular-fluid pressure in patients with severe acute traumatic brain injury. A preliminary report. J Neurosurg 1965;22(6):581–90.
8. Clifton GL, Jiang JY, Lyeth BG, et al. Marked protection by moderate hypothermia after experimental traumatic brain injury. J Cereb Blood Flow Metab 1991;11(1):114–21.
9. Dietrich WD. The importance of brain temperature in cerebral injury. J Neurotrauma 1992;9(Suppl 2): S475–85.
10. Bramlett HM, Green EJ, Dietrich WD, et al. Posttraumatic brain hypothermia provides protection from sensorimotor and cognitive behavioral deficits. J Neurotrauma 1995;12(3):289–98.
11. Urbano LA, Oddo M. Therapeutic hypothermia for traumatic brain injury. Curr Neurol Neurosci Rep 2012;12(5):580–91.
12. Sydenham E, Roberts I, Alderson P. Hypothermia for traumatic head injury. Cochrane Database Syst Rev 2009;(2):CD001048.
13. Polderman KH. Induced hypothermia and fever control for prevention and treatment of neurological injuries. Lancet 2008;371(9628):1955–69.

14. Dietrich WD, Bramlett HM. The evidence for hypothermia as a neuroprotectant in traumatic brain injury. Neurotherapeutics 2010;7(1):43–50.

15. Busto R, Dietrich WD, Globus MY, et al. Small differences in intraischemic brain temperature critically determine the extent of ischemic neuronal injury. J Cereb Blood Flow Metab 1987;7(6):729–38.

16. Bramlett HM, Dietrich WD, Green EJ, et al. Chronic histopathological consequences of fluid-percussion brain injury in rats: effects of post-traumatic hypothermia. Acta Neuropathol 1997;93(2):190–9.

17. Dietrich WD, Alonso O, Busto R, et al. Post-traumatic brain hypothermia reduces histopathological damage following concussive brain injury in the rat. Acta Neuropathol 1994;87(3):250–8.

18. McIntyre LA, Fergusson DA, Hebert PC, et al. Prolonged therapeutic hypothermia after traumatic brain injury in adults: a systematic review. JAMA 2003;289(22):2992–9.

19. Finkelstein RA, Alam HB. Induced hypothermia for trauma: current research and practice. J Intensive Care Med 2010;25(4):205–26.

20. Atkins CM, Truettner JS, Lotocki G, et al. Post-traumatic seizure susceptibility is attenuated by hypothermia therapy. Eur J Neurosci 2010;32(11): 1912–20.

21. Hartings JA, Watanabe T, Bullock MR, et al. Spreading depolarizations have prolonged direct current shifts and are associated with poor outcome in brain trauma. Brain 2011;134(Pt 5):1529–40.

22. Povlishock JT, Wei EP. Posthypothermic rewarming considerations following traumatic brain injury. J Neurotrauma 2009;26(3):333–40.

23. Clifton GL, Allen S, Barrodale P, et al. A phase II study of moderate hypothermia in severe brain injury. J Neurotrauma 1993;10(3):263–71 [discussion: 273].

24. Marion DW, Obrist WD, Carlier PM, et al. The use of moderate therapeutic hypothermia for patients with severe head injuries: a preliminary report. J Neurosurg 1993;79(3):354–62.

25. Marion DW, Penrod LE, Kelsey SF, et al. Treatment of traumatic brain injury with moderate hypothermia. N Engl J Med 1997;336(8):540–6.

26. Shiozaki T, Sugimoto H, Taneda M, et al. Effect of mild hypothermia on uncontrollable intracranial hypertension after severe head injury. J Neurosurg 1993;79(3):363–8.

27. Tokutomi T, Morimoto K, Miyagi T, et al. Optimal temperature for the management of severe traumatic brain injury: effect of hypothermia on intracranial pressure, systemic and intracranial hemodynamics, and metabolism. Neurosurgery 2003;52(1):102–11 [discussion: 111–2].

28. Clifton GL, Miller ER, Choi SC, et al. Lack of effect of induction of hypothermia after acute brain injury. N Engl J Med 2001;344(8):556–63.

29. Chesnut RM, Marshall LF, Klauber MR, et al. The role of secondary brain injury in determining outcome from severe head injury. J Trauma 1993;34(2):216–22.

30. Clifton GL, Valadka A, Zygun D, et al. Very early hypothermia induction in patients with severe brain injury (the National Acute Brain Injury Study: Hypothermia II): a randomised trial. Lancet Neurol 2011; 10(2):131–9.

31. Shiozaki T, Hayakata T, Taneda M, et al. A multicenter prospective randomized controlled trial of the efficacy of mild hypothermia for severely head injured patients with low intracranial pressure. Mild Hypothermia Study Group in Japan. J Neurosurg 2001;94(1):50–4.

32. Adelson PD, Wisniewski SR, Beca J, et al. Comparison of hypothermia and normothermia after severe traumatic brain injury in children (Cool Kids): a phase 3, randomised controlled trial. Lancet Neurol 2013;12(6):546–53.

33. Hutchison JS, Ward RE, Lacroix J, et al. Hypothermia therapy after traumatic brain injury in children. N Engl J Med 2008;358(23):2447–56.

34. Flynn LM, Rhodes J, Andrews PJ. Therapeutic hypothermia reduces intracranial pressure and partial brain oxygen tension in patients with severe traumatic brain injury: preliminary data from the Eurotherm3235 Trial. Ther Hypothermia Temp Manag 2015;5(3):143–51.

35. Andrews PJ, Sinclair HL, Rodriguez A, et al. Hypothermia for intracranial hypertension after traumatic brain injury. N Engl J Med 2015;373(25):2403–12.

36. Maekawa T, Yamashita S, Nagao S, et al. Prolonged mild therapeutic hypothermia versus fever control with tight hemodynamic monitoring and slow rewarming in patients with severe traumatic brain injury: a randomized controlled trial. J Neurotrauma 2015;32(7):422–9.

37. Jiang J, Yu M, Zhu C. Effect of long-term mild hypothermia therapy in patients with severe traumatic brain injury: 1-year follow-up review of 87 cases. J Neurosurg 2000;93(4):546–9.

38. Jiang JY, Xu W, Li WP, et al. Effect of long-term mild hypothermia or short-term mild hypothermia on outcome of patients with severe traumatic brain injury. J Cereb Blood Flow Metab 2006;26(6):771–6.

39. Lei J, Gao G, Mao Q, et al. Rationale, methodology, and implementation of a nationwide multicenter randomized controlled trial of long-term mild hypothermia for severe traumatic brain injury (the LTH-1 trial). Contemp Clin Trials 2015;40:9–14.

40. Kramer C, Freeman WD, Larson JS, et al. Therapeutic hypothermia for severe traumatic brain injury: a critically appraised topic. Neurologist 2012;18(3): 173–7.

41. Clifton GL. A review of clinical trials of hypothermia treatment for severe traumatic brain injury. Ther Hypothermia Temp Manag 2011;1(3):143–9.

42. Qiu W, Zhang Y, Sheng H, et al. Effects of therapeutic mild hypothermia on patients with severe traumatic brain injury after craniotomy. J Crit Care 2007;22(3):229–35.

43. Schreckinger M, Marion DW. Contemporary management of traumatic intracranial hypertension: is there a role for therapeutic hypothermia? Neurocrit Care 2009;11(3):427–36.

44. Fox JL, Vu EN, Doyle-Waters M, et al. Prophylactic hypothermia for traumatic brain injury: a quantitative systematic review. CJEM 2010;12(4):355–64.

45. Sandestig A, Romner B, Grande PO. Therapeutic hypothermia in children and adults with severe traumatic brain injury. Ther Hypothermia Temp Manag 2014;4(1):10–20.

46. Alderson P, Gadkary C, Signorini DF. Therapeutic hypothermia for head injury. Cochrane Database Syst Rev 2004;(4):CD001048.

47. Crossley S, Reid J, McLatchie R, et al. A systematic review of therapeutic hypothermia for adult patients following traumatic brain injury. Crit Care 2014;18(2): R75.

48. Bullock MR, Povlishock JT. Guidelines for the management of severe traumatic brain injury. Editor's commentary. J Neurotrauma 2007;24(Suppl 1). 2 p preceding S1.

49. Gupta AK, Al-Rawi PG, Hutchinson PJ, et al. Effect of hypothermia on brain tissue oxygenation in patients with severe head injury. Br J Anaesth 2002; 88(2):188–92.

50. Suehiro E, Ueda Y, Wei EP, et al. Posttraumatic hypothermia followed by slow rewarming protects the cerebral microcirculation. J Neurotrauma 2003;20(4): 381–90.

51. Thompson HJ, Kirkness CJ, Mitchell PH. Hypothermia and rapid rewarming is associated with worse outcome following traumatic brain injury. J Trauma Nurs 2010;17(4):173–7.

52. Polderman KH, Rijnsburger ER, Peerdeman SM, et al. Induction of hypothermia in patients with various types of neurologic injury with use of large volumes of ice-cold intravenous fluid. Crit Care Med 2005;33(12):2744–51.

53. Inamasu J, Nakatsukasa M, Suzuki M, et al. Therapeutic hypothermia for out-of-hospital cardiac arrest: an update for neurosurgeons. World Neurosurg 2010;74(1):120–8.

54. Sakurai A, Atkins CM, Alonso OF, et al. Mild hyperthermia worsens the neuropathological damage associated with mild traumatic brain injury in rats. J Neurotrauma 2012;29(2):313–21.

55. Dietrich WD, Alonso O, Halley M, et al. Delayed posttraumatic brain hyperthermia worsens outcome after fluid percussion brain injury: a light and electron microscopic study in rats. Neurosurgery 1996; 38(3):533–41 [discussion: 541].

56. Dietrich WD, Bramlett HM. Hyperthermia and central nervous system injury. Prog Brain Res 2007;162: 201–17.

57. Kilpatrick MM, Lowry DW, Firlik AD, et al. Hyperthermia in the neurosurgical intensive care unit. Neurosurgery 2000;47(4):850–5 [discussion: 855–6].

58. Puccio AM, Fischer MR, Jankowitz BT, et al. Induced normothermia attenuates intracranial hypertension and reduces fever burden after severe traumatic brain injury. Neurocrit Care 2009;11(1):82–7.

59. Saxena M, Andrews PJ, Cheng A. Modest cooling therapies (35 degrees C to 37.5 degrees C) for traumatic brain injury. Cochrane Database Syst Rev 2008;(3):CD006811.

60. Polderman KH. Mechanisms of action, physiological effects, and complications of hypothermia. Crit Care Med 2009;37(7 Suppl):S186–202.

61. Sadaka F, Veremakis C. Therapeutic hypothermia for the management of intracranial hypertension in severe traumatic brain injury: a systematic review. Brain Inj 2012;26(7–8):899–908.

62. Gebauer CM, Knuepfer M, Robel-Tillig E, et al. Hemodynamics among neonates with hypoxic-ischemic encephalopathy during whole-body hypothermia and passive rewarming. Pediatrics 2006; 117(3):843–50.

Seizures and the Role of Anticonvulsants After Traumatic Brain Injury

Lara L. Zimmermann, MD[a],*, Ramon Diaz-Arrastia, MD, PhD[b],
Paul M. Vespa, MD[a]

KEYWORDS

- Traumatic brain injury • Seizure • Nonconvulsive seizure • Posttraumatic seizure
- Status epilepticus • Continuous electroencephalography • Metabolic crisis • Secondary brain injury

KEY POINTS

- As commonly defined, early posttraumatic seizures occur within 7 days of injury, whereas late posttraumatic seizures occur more than 7 days after injury and define posttraumatic epilepsy (PTE).
- Early posttraumatic seizures are not benign and are associated with increased intracranial pressure, metabolic crisis, brain atrophy, and worse outcomes.
- The use of continuous electroencephalography in patients with moderate or severe traumatic brain injury should be the standard of care because of the high incidence of seizures and resultant secondary brain injury in this population.
- Antiepileptic drug prophylaxis is indicated within 7 days of injury to decrease the incidence of early posttraumatic seizures, but does not prevent PTE.
- The risk of developing PTE is strongly related to the severity of head injury and is highest in the first 2 years after traumatic brain injury.

INTRODUCTION

Posttraumatic seizures are a common complication of traumatic brain injury (TBI), occurring in more than 20% of patients in the intensive care unit (ICU)[1] and in 25% to 50% of patients chronically. At a time when the injured brain is critically sensitive to secondary insults, posttraumatic seizures result in secondary brain injury caused by increased intracranial pressure (ICP) and metabolic crisis and are associated with worse patient outcomes. Most posttraumatic seizures in the ICU are nonconvulsive and therefore continuous electroencephalography (cEEG) monitoring in patients with moderate or severe brain injury is essential (**Fig. 1**). This article reviews the current data on the incidence of posttraumatic seizures, both in the ICU and after hospital discharge. The latest literature showing the malignant consequences of early posttraumatic seizures, including increased ICP and metabolic crisis, is reviewed. Seizure prophylaxis, indications for starting antiepileptic drug (AED) treatment, and the duration of treatment after posttraumatic seizures are discussed. The recommended management of status epilepticus (SE) is described. In addition, important counseling points, including the period of highest risk for developing posttraumatic epilepsy (PTE), are provided.

DEFINITIONS

Posttraumatic seizures are commonly classified as:

1. Immediate seizures: occurring less than 24 hours after injury
2. Early seizures: occurring 24 hours to 7 days after injury

[a] Department of Neurosurgery, Ronald Reagan UCLA Medical Center, 757 Westwood Plaza, Suite 6236, Los Angeles, CA 90095, USA; [b] Center for Neuroscience and Regenerative Medicine, Uniformed Services University of the Health Sciences, Rockville, MD, USA
* Corresponding author.
E-mail address: Zimmermann.Lara.L@gmail.com

Neurosurg Clin N Am 27 (2016) 499–508
http://dx.doi.org/10.1016/j.nec.2016.06.001
1042-3680/16/© 2016 Elsevier Inc. All rights reserved.

neurosurgery.theclinics.com

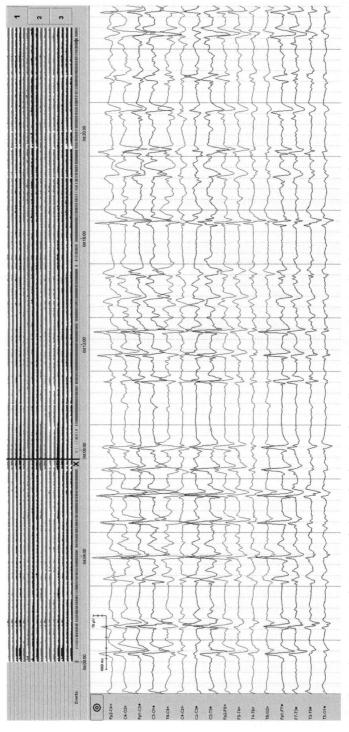

Fig. 1. Sixteen-channel continuous electroencephalography showing frontally predominant generalized periodic epileptiform discharges at time point X in a patient with nonconvulsive status epilepticus. (*Above*) Quantitative electroencephalography showing the percentage alpha variability over 24 hours.

3. Late seizures: occurring more than 7 days after injury and constituting the diagnosis of PTE

TBI severity is most commonly defined as:

1. Mild TBI: Glasgow Coma Scale (GCS) 13 to 15, loss of consciousness for less than 30 minutes, and negative brain imaging
2. Moderate TBI: GCS 9 to 12, loss of consciousness 30 minutes to 24 hours, and either positive or negative brain imaging
3. Severe TBI: GCS 3 to 8; loss of consciousness for more than 24 hours; and with contusion, hematoma, or skull fracture

POSTTRAUMATIC SEIZURES IN NEUROSCIENCE INTENSIVE CARE UNIT PATIENTS

Seizures are common in ICU patients both with and without acute brain injury.[1–7] Seizures in the ICU are most frequently focal onset with secondary generalization and are typically nonconvulsive. In a seminal article, Vespa and colleagues[1] (1999) prospectively studied 94 patients with moderate to severe TBI for a mean of 7 days after brain injury and reported an incidence of electrographic seizures of 22%, with most (52%) showing nonconvulsive seizures.[1] Ronne-Engstrom and colleagues[8] (2006) retrospectively reviewed cEEG in 70 patients with TBI and found that 33% developed seizures, which occurred on average 74 hours after initial injury. Claassen and colleagues[3] (2004) studied a mixed population of ICU patients with acute brain injury, including intracerebral hemorrhage, subarachnoid hemorrhage, and ischemic stroke, using cEEG and detected a 19% incidence of seizures, with most (92%) exclusively nonconvulsive.

Published risk factors for early convulsive seizures include severity of head injury, younger age, acute intracerebral hematoma, acute subdural hematoma, diffuse cerebral edema, intracranial metal fragment retention, depressed/linear skull fractures, and chronic alcoholism.[9,10] However, it is important to recognize that these risk factors were identified in studies that used witnessed convulsive seizures as the primary end point; therefore, they likely do not accurately reflect risk factors for early posttraumatic nonconvulsive seizures, which are more common than early convulsive seizures.

The incidence of early posttraumatic seizures in children has recently been published. O'Neill and colleagues[11] (2015) prospectively studied 144 children with mild, moderate, or severe TBI who underwent cEEG monitoring and identified seizures in 30% of them. Of these children, 94% had nonconvulsive seizures, including 40% with exclusively nonconvulsive seizures. Children less than 2.4 years of age (odds ratio [OR], 8.7) and children with abusive head trauma (OR, 6.0) were at significantly increased risk for seizures.[11]

Given the high incidence of nonconvulsive seizures in patients with acute brain injury or unexplained coma, the Neurocritical Care Society International Multidisciplinary Consensus Conference on Multimodality Monitoring recommends that electroencephalography (EEG) "should be considered in all patients with acute brain injury and unexplained and persistent altered consciousness and in comatose intensive care unit patients without an acute primary brain condition who have an unexplained impairment of mental status."[7]

EARLY POSTTRAUMATIC SEIZURES ARE NOT BENIGN

Early posttraumatic seizures cause secondary brain injury by eliciting a pathophysiologic response at a time when the brain is most vulnerable and are associated with worse outcomes. Early posttraumatic seizures may lead to secondary brain injury through a variety of mechanisms, including cerebral metabolic crisis,[12–14] increased intracranial pressure,[15] and cerebral edema,[16] and are associated with brain atrophy.[17]

Cerebral microdialysis directly measures brain metabolism by sampling extracellular tissue for metabolites, including lactate, pyruvate, glycerol, and glucose. Metabolic crisis describes a state of reduced oxidative metabolism, increased glucose consumption, and an impaired redox state of the brain. It is operationally defined as an increased lactate/pyruvate ratio (LPR) combined with decreased extracellular glucose level. Metabolic crisis occurs frequently after TBI and is a strong independent predictor of poor outcome at 6 months.[18] Stein and colleagues[18] examined 89 patients with moderate or severe TBI and found that 74% of patients experienced metabolic crisis during the first 72 hours after injury. Metabolic crisis occurs despite adequate hemodynamic resuscitation and controlled ICP. The duration of metabolic crisis was significantly longer in patients who had a poor functional outcome. Metabolic crisis occurs independently of brain ischemia after severe TBI.[19]

The cause of metabolic crisis is not known, but early posttraumatic seizures are clearly associated with cerebral metabolic distress. Seizures are associated with increased extracellular glutamate[12] at levels known to induce cell death and swelling. Seizures are also associated with increased levels of extracellular glycerol,[13] which is an end product of phospholipid breakdown. Increased extracellular glycerol level likely reflects cell membrane disruption from seizure-induced excitotoxicity.

Vespa and colleagues[15] (2007) showed that early posttraumatic nonconvulsive seizures and SE result in prolonged increases in ICP and metabolic crisis. The investigators analyzed continuous EEG and microdialysis data from 10 patients with moderate or severe TBI and seizures or SE and 10 matched controls for 7 days after injury. Electrographic seizures were associated with episodic and prolonged increase in ICP and LPR beyond postinjury hour 100.[15] Seizure-induced excitotoxicity and metabolic crisis are two likely mechanisms underlying the observation that seizures after brain hemorrhage are independently associated with increased brain edema and midline shift.[16] A rodent model of TBI showed ipsilateral hippocampal atrophy with loss of CA3 and CA4 pyramidal neurons after hippocampal activation and seizures.[20] Early posttraumatic nonconvulsive seizures are also associated with hippocampal atrophy at 6 months in humans.[17] Together, these studies show that early posttraumatic nonconvulsive seizures are harmful secondary insults to the recently traumatized brain.

Metabolic crisis cannot be entirely explained by seizures as detected by continuous EEG monitoring. The incidence of electrographic seizures in TBI is between 21% and 25% but the incidence of metabolic crisis exceeds 70%.[18] Therefore, Vespa and colleagues[14] (2016) studied 34 patients with severe TBI who underwent multimodal monitoring with scalp EEG, depth electrode, and cerebral microdialysis. The incidence of seizures and periodic discharges as detected by surface or depth EEG was 61.8%. Importantly, epileptiform activity was solely detectable on depth EEG in 42.9% of patients.

The investigators also found that periodic discharges, which did not meet formal criteria for seizures, as well as seizures were significantly associated with metabolic crisis.[14] These data suggest that early posttraumatic seizures may be even more common than previously reported and that periodic discharges are also harmful to the posttraumatic brain.

IMPAIRED PERCENTAGE ALPHA VARIABILITY IS ASSOCIATED WITH POOR OUTCOME AFTER TRAUMATIC BRAIN INJURY

Traditional prognostic variables in TBI include age, GCS, pupil reactivity, early hypotension, hypoxia, and computed tomography (CT) severity scores.[21] As reviewed earlier, early posttraumatic seizures cause secondary brain injury and are associated with worse outcomes. Quantitative EEG is also useful to predict outcome after TBI. Vespa and colleagues[22] performed continuous EEG monitoring in 89 patients with moderate or severe TBI

and examined the quantitative EEG parameter percentage alpha variability (PAV), defined as the percentage variability of the alpha rhythm (8–12 Hz) across time. They showed that a low PAV (≤ 0.1) is highly predictive of poor outcome or death at 30 days and a high PAV (>0.2) is predictive of a good outcome at 6 months.[23] The anatomic and physiologic basis for PAV is not completely understood, but the thalamus is recognized as a central regulator of the alpha rhythm and PAV is thought to be a marker of thalamocortical pacemaker activity. Support for this comes from data showing that injury to the thalamus, basal ganglia, or diffuse edema predicts low PAV.[23] Disruption of the thalamocortical circuit may be one explanation for persistent coma after brain injury. Although quantitative EEG is useful to predict outcome after TBI, continuous EEG has not yet proved useful to predict PTE in a given patient. EEG predictors of PTE is an area of active research.

POSTTRAUMATIC EPILEPSY
Epidemiology and Risk Factors for Posttraumatic Epilepsy

PTE is defined as recurrent, spontaneous seizures that occur more than 7 days after brain injury. PTE accounts for 20% of symptomatic epilepsy in the general population and 5% of all epilepsy (Hauser and colleagues,[24] 1993). In a large population-based study from Rochester, Minnesota, head trauma was identified as the cause of epilepsy in about 6% of cases.[25] The risk of developing PTE after TBI is 2% to 25%,[26] and as high as 53% in a military population with penetrating head trauma.[27]

Selected studies on the incidence and risk factors for PTE are discussed later.

Annegers and colleagues[28] (1998) published a retrospective population-based study of 4541 children and adults with TBI in Olmsted County, Minnesota, from 1935 to 1984. The probability of developing unprovoked seizures 5 years after TBI was 0.7% after mild TBI, 1.2% after moderate TBI, and 10% after severe TBI. A cohort of patients with 30-year follow-up showed that the cumulative probability of developing seizures within 30 years after TBI was 2.1% after mild TBI, 4.2% after moderate TBI, and 16.7% after severe TBI. After considering the expected incidence of epilepsy in the general population, the investigators reported an increased risk of developing PTE, with an overall standard incidence ratio of 3.1. They identified an increased risk of PTE with an overall standard incidence ratio of 1.5, 2.9, and 17 for mild, moderate, and severe TBI, respectively. The risk of epilepsy after mild TBI was no greater than in the general population after 5 years.

Englander and colleagues[29] (2003) published a prospective observational study of 647 patients, aged greater than or equal to 16 years, with moderate or severe TBI who were followed for up to 2 years. The cumulative risk of developing a late posttraumatic seizure was 10.2% at 2 years. Of these, 63.6% had a first late posttraumatic seizure within 6 months of injury, 80.3% within 12 months of injury, and 92.4% within 18 months of injury. The cumulative incidence of PTE at 2 years was 8% for mild TBI, 24% for moderate TBI, and 16.8% for severe TBI.

Angeleri and colleagues[30] (1999) prospectively studied 137 adults with TBI and reported an incidence of PTE (defined as at least 2 unprovoked seizures between 2 and 12 months postinjury) of 13.1% at 1 year.

Asikainen and colleagues[31] (1999) studied 490 patients with TBI who were admitted to a rehabilitation and reemployment program and followed for greater than or equal to 5 years. Therefore, this sample excluded patients who were so severely disabled or who recovered so fully that they were not candidates for or in need of rehabilitation services. The incidence of unprovoked late seizures was 25.3% with mean follow-up 12 years.

Ferguson and colleagues[32] (2010) performed a population-based study of 2118 adolescent and adult patients hospitalized for TBI who were followed for 3 years after discharge. The cumulative incidence of PTE was 9.1% over 3 years. The incidence was 2.2% in the first year, 4.1% in the second year, and 3.1% in the third year postinjury. Patients with severe TBI were at higher risk for developing PTE compared with mild or moderate TBI. The cumulative incidence of PTE at 3 years by TBI severity was 4.4% for mild TBI, 7.6% for moderate TBI, and 13.6% for severe TBI.

Risk Factors for Posttraumatic Epilepsy

There is a strong relationship between TBI severity and the risk of developing PTE, as discussed earlier. Patients with mild, moderate, and severe TBI have a 1.4-fold, 4-fold, and 29-fold increased risk of developing epilepsy, respectively, compared with the general population.[33]

In addition to TBI severity, key risk factors for the development of PTE include skull fracture and intracranial hematoma. Seizures within the first week after TBI may also be a risk factor for PTE.[34]

In the large, population-based study by Annegers and colleagues[28] (1998) discussed earlier, structural risk factors that placed patients at the highest risk for PTE were cerebral contusion (relative risk [RR] = 5) or subdural hematoma (RR = 6) or cerebral contusion plus subdural

hematoma (RR = 12). Additional risk factors significant in multivariate analysis included prolonged coma and linear or depressed skull fractures. Note that early seizure was strong risk factor in univariate analysis, but was not significant in multivariate analysis.

In the prospective observational study by Englander and colleagues[29] (2003), discussed earlier, in which 10.2% of patients with moderate or severe TBI developed a PTE, the investigators reported the highest probability for late posttraumatic seizures in patients with biparietal contusions (66%), dural penetration with bone or metal fragments (62.5%), multiple intracranial operations (36.5%), multiple subcortical contusions (33.4%), subdural hematoma with evacuation (28%), midline shift greater than 5 mm (25.8%), or multiple or bilateral cortical contusions (25%). Patients with multiple contusions had a higher cumulative probability for developing PTE than those with a single contusion (8%) or no contusions (6%).

Temkin[35] (2003) followed 783 patients with TBI at high risk for posttraumatic seizures and identified multiple risk factors that put patients at especially high risk for PTE at 2 years. In addition to TBI severity, subdural hematomas large enough to require surgical evacuation were associated with a 44% cumulative incidence of seizures by 2 years. Additional risk factors significant in multivariate analysis included early seizures, prolonged coma, dural penetration, depressed skull fracture not surgically treated, and at least 1 nonreactive pupil.

Genetics may play an important role in the risk of developing PTE. Diaz-Arrastia and colleagues (2003) prospectively collected DNA samples from 106 patients with moderate or severe TBI and followed the patients for 6 months. Twenty percent of the patients had at least 1 posttraumatic seizure within 6 months. The relative risk of posttraumatic seizures with the episilon4 allele was 2.41 (95% confidence interval [CI], 1.15–5.07; $P = .03$).[36] These data suggest that genetic variability in addition to injury severity and other clinical or demographic risk factors may affect the epileptogenic process.

Time Interval to Development of Posttraumatic Epilepsy

The risk of developing PTE after TBI is highest in the first 2 years after injury. Approximately 80% of individuals with PTE experience their first seizure within the first year after injury and more than 90% by the end of the second year.[24,28,29] For patients with mild TBI, there is little to no increased risk of developing PTE beyond 5 years postinjury. However, for patients with moderate or severe TBI the risk does remain increased, albeit much less so, for at least 10 years postinjury,[28] and up to 15% to 20% of patients may have their first seizure after 2 years postinjury.[24]

The time interval between brain injury and the first late posttraumatic seizure may be shorter for children than for adults. In the study discussed earlier by Asikainen and colleagues[31] (1999), 47% of children aged less than or equal to 7 years who developed PTE had their first seizure within 6 months of injury. In children aged 8 to 16 years, only 35% had their first seizure within 1 year and 47.5% had their first seizure 5 years or more after injury. In patients more than 16 years of age, 41% had their first seizure within 1 year, but 26% did not have their first seizure until greater than or equal to 5 years after injury. These data suggest that the process of epileptogenesis may be related to age at the time of injury.

Subtypes of Posttraumatic Epilepsy

PTE is the leading cause of epilepsy with onset in young adulthood. It accounts for approximately 5% of focal epilepsy in the general population and 4% to 5% of all referrals to specialized epilepsy centers. PTE is largely a localization-related epilepsy (>90%) arising from the mesial temporal lobe structures or from focal neocortical scars. However, some patients are diagnosed with idiopathic or generalized epilepsy with onset after TBI.

Gupta and colleagues[37] (2014) retrospectively studied 123 patients with medically refractory PTE referred for video electroencephalography at a single center over a 10-year period. Most of these patients were diagnosed with localization-related epilepsy (93%), of whom 57% had temporal lobe epilepsy, 35% had frontal lobe epilepsy, and 3% each had parietal and occipital lobe epilepsy. Of the patients with temporal lobe epilepsy, approximately 50% were diagnosed with unilateral mesial temporal sclerosis and 4 patients had bilateral mesial temporal sclerosis. Only 1 patient was diagnosed with multifocal epilepsy, but this may have been because of selection bias because patients with known multifocal epilepsy may not have been referred for evaluation. A few patients were diagnosed with primary generalized epilepsy and the investigators postulated that head trauma might have led to expression of an underlying susceptibility in these patients.

MANAGEMENT OF POSTTRAUMATIC SEIZURES
Seizure Prophylaxis

The Brain Trauma Foundation and American Academy of Neurology recommend the use of prophylactic anticonvulsants to decrease the incidence of early posttraumatic seizures within 7 days of TBI.[38,39] These recommendations are based on literature indicating that prophylaxis with phenytoin is effective in decreasing the risk of early posttraumatic seizures, but is probably not effective in decreasing the risk of late posttraumatic seizures or PTE.

In a landmark study by Temkin and colleagues[40] (1990), investigators performed a randomized, double-blind trial to evaluate the effectiveness of phenytoin in preventing PTE in 404 patients with severe TBI. They randomized patients with severe TBI to treatment with phenytoin or placebo for 1 year after injury. Treatment with phenytoin that was started within 1 day of injury significantly reduced the incidence of seizures in the first 7 days after injury (3.6% vs 14.2%; $P<.001$), but did not reduce the risk of posttraumatic seizures.

The effectiveness of valproate to prevent early and late posttraumatic seizures has also been study in a randomized, double-blind trial.[41] One-hundred and thirty-two patients with moderate or severe TBI were randomized to a 1-week course of phenytoin, a 1-month course of valproate, or a 6-month course of valproate and followed for 2 years. Valproate was no better than phenytoin at preventing early seizures and neither drug prevented late seizures. There was a trend toward higher mortality in patients treated with valproate. Therefore, most physicians now use phenytoin rather than valproate for seizure prophylaxis after TBI.

In total, 5 drugs (phenytoin, valproate, phenobarbital, carbamazepine, and magnesium) have been well studied for an antiepileptic effect and none reduced the risk of late posttraumatic seizures.[42]

Because of the risk of potential harmful side effects and drug interactions with phenytoin, some experts tend to use levetiracetam for seizure prophylaxis after TBI. Recently, Szaflarski and colleagues[43] (2010) studied levetiracetam versus phenytoin for seizure prophylaxis in a prospective, randomized trial. Investigators enrolled 52 patients (89% with severe TBI) and monitored them with continuous EEG for 72 hours. There was no difference in the incidence of early seizures, seizures at 6 months, or mortality. Patients treated with levetiracetam had significantly better Disability Rating Scale scores at 6 months. Based on this study, levetiracetam may be an effective alternative to phenytoin for seizure prophylaxis after TBI.

At present, most TBI experts choose to use either phenytoin or levetiracetam for 7 days for seizure prophylaxis after moderate or severe TBI.

Treatment of Early Posttraumatic Seizures

The incidence of early posttraumatic seizures after moderate or severe TBI is 22% and more than half are nonconvulsive.[1] Patients with early convulsive or nonconvulsive posttraumatic seizures should be started on an AED immediately. For patients already optimized on monotherapy, a second drug should be added and so on. Patients who develop posttraumatic SE should be treated according to the SE protocol discussed later. Duration of AED treatment after early posttraumatic seizures is typically at least 3 to 6 months.

Treatment of Late Posttraumatic Seizures or Posttraumatic Epilepsy

The definition of PTE is recurrent, spontaneous seizures that occur more than 1 week after TBI. The incidence of late posttraumatic seizures after moderate or severe TBI is 2% to 25% and is highest in the first 2 years after injury. Patients who experience a late posttraumatic seizure are at very high risk for recurrent seizures. Haltiner and colleagues[44] (1997) studied the risk of a second seizure after a first late posttraumatic seizure in patients with moderate or severe head injury. The rate of seizure recurrence at year 2 was extremely high (86%) in all patients, but slightly lower (73%) in patients who were taking an AED.

Patients should be started on an AED and treated aggressively after a first late posttraumatic seizure because of the very high risk of seizure recurrence. Duration of AED treatment in patients with PTE is typically at least 2 years. Regular follow-up should occur with a neurologist throughout treatment. After 2 years seizure free, it is reasonable to discuss the possibility of tapering antiepileptic therapy slowly over a period of months. It is important to consider the presence of focal neurologic deficits, CT evidence of structural brain disease, and persistent EEG abnormalities because these factors likely increase the risk for recurrent seizures.[10]

Treatment of Posttraumatic Status Epilepticus

SE is defined as the state of recurrent or continuous seizure activity lasting for more than 5 minutes and without return to neurologic baseline (Lowenstein and colleagues,[45] 1999). SE is a neurologic emergency and should be treated aggressively, as outlined in **Table 1**. The longer the seizures persist, the harder it is to stop them.

Table 1
Treatment of SE

Stage	Recommended Treatment
Diagnose SE 0–5 min	Manage ABC, check serum glucose, consider thiamine 200 mg IV
Emergent initial therapy 2–10 min	Lorazepam 4 mg IVP q5–10 min × 2 doses as needed for ongoing seizures. Midazolam 10 mg IM is an alternative if IV access not obtained
Urgent control therapy 10–20 min	Phenytoin 20 mg/kg IV at maximum infusion rate 50 mg/min Or: Fosphenytoin 20 mgPE/kg at maximum infusion rate 150 mg/min Or: Sodium valproate 40 mg/kg IV over 10 min plus an additional 20 mg/kg over 5 min if still seizing Or: Levetiracetam 1–3 g IV at infusion rate 2–5 mg/kg/min
Refractory SE 20–60 min	Continuous IV midazolam, load 0.2 mg/kg; repeat 0.2–0.4 mg/kg boluses every 5 min until seizures stop, up to a maximum of 2 mg/kg Continuous IV dose range: 0.1–2 mg/kg/h Or: Continuous IV propofol: load 1 mg/kg, can repeat 1–2 mg/kg boluses every 3–5 min, not to exceed a total of 4 doses or until seizures stop Continuous IV dose range: 25–150 μg/kg/min If seizures persist, proceed to pentobarbital
Refractory SE > 60 min	Continuous IV pentobarbital: load 5–10 mg/kg Continuous IV dose range: 1–10 mg/kg/h. Traditionally titrated to burst suppression 8–12 Hz

Abbreviations: ABC, airway, breathing, circulation; IM, intramuscular; IV, intravenous; IVP, intravenous push; mgPE, milligrams of phenytoin equivalent.

Initial therapy

Two prospective randomized controlled trials established intravenous (IV) lorazepam as the best initial treatment of SE.[46,47] Recently, it was shown in a double-blind, randomized trial that intramuscular midazolam (10 mg in adults, 5 mg in children) is at least as safe and effective as IV lorazepam for terminating SE in adults and children.[48,49] Based on this literature, IV lorazepam is indicated as initial treatment of SE. Intramuscular midazolam is an effective alternative for patients without IV access.

Following administration of a short-acting benzodiazepine, urgent control therapy with an IV bolus of an AED should be initiated for all patients with SE in order to rapidly attain therapeutic drug levels or stop SE if ongoing.[50]

Treatment of refractory status epilepticus

Refractory SE is defined as continued convulsive or nonconvulsive seizures after treatment with a benzodiazepine plus 1 appropriate AED. At this point, IV bolus followed by a continuous infusion of propofol or midazolam is recommended,[50] as outlined in **Table 1**.

PATIENT COUNSELING

The risk of developing PTE is highest in the first 2 years following TBI but persists for at least 10 years after injury for patients with severe TBI. Patients with posttraumatic seizures should be counseled on the following points:

- Do not drive for 3 to 6 months following complete seizure control. Some states, including California, have mandatory physician reporting to the Department of Public Health for all patients who experience loss of consciousness.
- Avoid working in high places or with dangerous machinery and avoid unsupervised activities (such as swimming or taking a bath) during which a seizure could result in serious injury.
- Women of reproductive age should be asked about their intention to become pregnant and offered preconception counseling and care. Important topics include the teratogenic effects of certain AEDs, reduced efficacy of hormonal contraception, and the importance of folic acid supplementation.

REFERENCES

1. Vespa PM, Nuwer MR, Nenov V, et al. Increased incidence and impact of nonconvulsive and convulsive seizures after traumatic brain injury as detected by continuous electroencephalographic monitoring. J Neurosurg 1999;91(5):750–60.
2. Dennis LJ, Claassen J, Hirsch LJ, et al. Nonconvulsive status epilepticus after subarachnoid hemorrhage. Neurosurgery 2002;51(5):1136–43 [discussion: 1144].
3. Claassen J, Mayer SA, Kowalski RG, et al. Detection of electrographic seizures with continuous EEG monitoring in critically ill patients. Neurology 2004; 62(10):1743–8.
4. Claassen J, Jette N, Chum F, et al. Electrographic seizures and periodic discharges after intracerebral hemorrhage. Neurology 2007;69(13):1356–65.
5. Oddo M, Carrera E, Claassen J, et al. Continuous electroencephalography in the medical intensive care unit. Crit Care Med 2009;37(6):2051–6.
6. Kamel H, Betjemann JP, Navi BB, et al. Diagnostic yield of electroencephalography in the medical and surgical intensive care unit. Neurocrit Care 2013;19(3):336–41.
7. Claassen J, Vespa P. Electrophysiologic monitoring in acute brain injury. Neurocrit Care 2014;21(Suppl 2):S129–47.
8. Ronne-Engstrom E, Winkler T. Continuous EEG monitoring in patients with traumatic brain injury reveals a high incidence of epileptiform activity. Acta neurologica Scandinavica 2006;114(1):47–53.
9. Frey LC. Epidemiology of posttraumatic epilepsy: a critical review. Epilepsia 2003;44(Suppl 10):11–7.
10. Ding K, Gupta PK, Diaz-Arrastia R. Frontiers in neuroscience epilepsy after traumatic brain injury. In: Laskowitz D, Grant G, editors. Translational research in traumatic brain injury. Boca Raton (FL): CRC Press/Taylor and Francis Group; 2016.
11. O'Neill BR, Handler MH, Tong S, et al. Incidence of seizures on continuous EEG monitoring following traumatic brain injury in children. J Neurosurg Pediatr 2015;16(2):167–76.
12. Vespa P, Prins M, Ronne-Engstrom E, et al. Increase in extracellular glutamate caused by reduced cerebral perfusion pressure and seizures after human traumatic brain injury: a microdialysis study. J Neurosurg 1998;89(6):971–82.
13. Vespa P, Martin NA, Nenov V, et al. Delayed increase in extracellular glycerol with post-traumatic electrographic epileptic activity: support for the theory that seizures induce secondary injury. Acta Neurochir Suppl 2002;81:355–7.
14. Vespa P, Tubi M, Claassen J, et al. Metabolic crisis occurs with seizures and periodic discharges after brain trauma. Ann Neurol 2016;79(4):579–90.
15. Vespa PM, Miller C, McArthur D, et al. Nonconvulsive electrographic seizures after traumatic brain injury result in a delayed, prolonged increase in intracranial pressure and metabolic crisis. Crit Care Med 2007;35(12):2830–6.
16. Vespa PM, O'Phelan K, Shah M, et al. Acute seizures after intracerebral hemorrhage: a factor in progressive

midline shift and outcome. Neurology 2003;60(9): 1441–6.

17. Vespa PM, McArthur DL, Xu Y, et al. Nonconvulsive seizures after traumatic brain injury are associated with hippocampal atrophy. Neurology 2010;75(9): 792–8.

18. Stein NR, McArthur DL, Etchepare M, et al. Early cerebral metabolic crisis after TBI influences outcome despite adequate hemodynamic resuscitation. Neurocrit Care 2012;17(1):49–57.

19. Vespa P, Bergsneider M, Hattori N, et al. Metabolic crisis without brain ischemia is common after traumatic brain injury: a combined microdialysis and positron emission tomography study. J Cereb Blood Flow Metab 2005;25(6):763–74.

20. Zanier ER, Lee SM, Vespa PM, et al. Increased hippocampal CA3 vulnerability to low-level kainic acid following lateral fluid percussion injury. J Neurotrauma 2003;20(5):409–20.

21. Panczykowski DM, Puccio AM, Scruggs BJ, et al. Prospective independent validation of IMPACT modeling as a prognostic tool in severe traumatic brain injury. J Neurotrauma 2012;29(1):47–52.

22. Vespa PM, Boscardin WJ, Hovda DA, et al. Early and persistent impaired percent alpha variability on continuous electroencephalography monitoring as predictive of poor outcome after traumatic brain injury. J Neurosurg 2002;97(1):84–92.

23. Hebb MO, McArthur DL, Alger J, et al. Impaired percent alpha variability on continuous electroencephalography is associated with thalamic injury and predicts poor long-term outcome after human traumatic brain injury. J Neurotrauma 2007;24(4): 579–90.

24. Agrawal A, Timothy J, Pandit L, et al. Post-traumatic epilepsy: an overview. Clin Neurol Neurosurg 2006; 108(5):433–9.

25. Hauser WA, Annegers JF, Kurland LT. Incidence of epilepsy and unprovoked seizures in Rochester, Minnesota: 1935-1984. Epilepsia 1993;34(3): 453–68.

26. Garga N, Lowenstein DH. Posttraumatic epilepsy: a major problem in desperate need of major advances. Epilepsy Curr 2006;6(1):1–5.

27. Salazar AM, Jabbari B, Vance SC, et al. Epilepsy after penetrating head injury. I. Clinical correlates: a report of the Vietnam Head Injury Study. Neurology 1985;35(10):1406–14.

28. Annegers JF, Hauser WA, Coan SP, et al. A population-based study of seizures after traumatic brain injuries. N Engl J Med 1998;338(1):20–4.

29. Englander J, Bushnik T, Duong TT, et al. Analyzing risk factors for late posttraumatic seizures: a prospective, multicenter investigation. Arch Phys Med Rehabil 2003;84(3):365–73.

30. Angeleri F, Majkowski J, Cacchio G, et al. Posttraumatic epilepsy risk factors: one-year prospective study after head injury. Epilepsia 1999;40(9): 1222–30.

31. Asikainen I, Kaste M, Sarna S. Early and late posttraumatic seizures in traumatic brain injury rehabilitation patients: brain injury factors causing late seizures and influence of seizures on long-term outcome. Epilepsia 1999;40(5):584–9.

32. Ferguson PL, Smith GM, Wannamaker BB, et al. A population-based study of risk of epilepsy after hospitalization for traumatic brain injury. Epilepsia 2010;51(5):891–8.

33. Herman ST. Epilepsy after brain insult: targeting epileptogenesis. Neurology 2002;59(9 Suppl 5):S21–6.

34. Lowenstein DH. Epilepsy after head injury: an overview. Epilepsia 2009;50(Suppl 2):4–9.

35. Temkin NR. Risk factors for posttraumatic seizures in adults. Epilepsia 2003;44(Suppl 10):18–20.

36. Diaz-Arrastia R, Gong Y, Fair S, et al. Increased risk of late posttraumatic seizures associated with inheritance of APOE epsilon4 allele. Archives of neurology 2003;60(6):818–22.

37. Gupta PK, Sayed N, Ding K, et al. Subtypes of posttraumatic epilepsy: clinical, electrophysiological, and imaging features. J Neurotrauma 2014;31(16): 1439–43.

38. Chang BS, Lowenstein DH. Practice parameter: antiepileptic drug prophylaxis in severe traumatic brain injury: report of the Quality Standards Subcommittee of the American Academy of Neurology. Neurology 2003;60(1):10–6.

39. Bratton SL, Chestnut RM, Ghajar J, et al. Guidelines for the management of severe traumatic brain injury. XIII. Antiseizure prophylaxis. J Neurotrauma 2007; 24(Suppl 1):S83–6.

40. Temkin NR, Dikmen SS, Wilensky AJ, et al. A randomized, double-blind study of phenytoin for the prevention of post-traumatic seizures. N Engl J Med 1990;323(8):497–502.

41. Temkin NR, Dikmen SS, Anderson GD, et al. Valproate therapy for prevention of posttraumatic seizures: a randomized trial. J Neurosurg 1999;91(4):593–600.

42. Temkin NR. Preventing and treating posttraumatic seizures: the human experience. Epilepsia 2009; 50(Suppl 2):10–3.

43. Szaflarski JP, Sangha KS, Lindsell CJ, et al. Prospective, randomized, single-blinded comparative trial of intravenous levetiracetam versus phenytoin for seizure prophylaxis. Neurocrit Care 2010;12(2): 165–72.

44. Haltiner AM, Temkin NR, Dikmen SS. Risk of seizure recurrence after the first late posttraumatic seizure. Arch Phys Med Rehabil 1997;78(8):835–40.

45. Lowenstein DH, Bleck T, Macdonald RL. It's time to revise the definition of status epilepticus. Epilepsia 1999;40(1):120–2.

46. Treiman DM, Meyers PD, Walton NY, et al. A comparison of four treatments for generalized

convulsive status epilepticus. Veterans Affairs Status Epilepticus Cooperative Study Group. N Engl J Med 1998;339(12):792–8.

47. Alldredge BK, Gelb AM, Isaacs SM, et al. A comparison of lorazepam, diazepam, and placebo for the treatment of out-of-hospital status epilepticus. N Engl J Med 2001;345(9): 631–7.

48. Silbergleit R, Durkalski V, Lowenstein D, et al. Intramuscular versus intravenous therapy for prehospital status epilepticus. N Engl J Med 2012;366(7):591–600.

49. Welch RD, Nicholas K, Durkalski-Mauldin VL, et al. Intramuscular midazolam versus intravenous lorazepam for the prehospital treatment of status epilepticus in the pediatric population. Epilepsia 2015; 56(2):254–62.

50. Brophy GM, Bell R, Claassen J, et al. Guidelines for the evaluation and management of status epilepticus. Neurocrit Care 2012;17(1):3–23.

The Role of Multimodal Invasive Monitoring in Acute Traumatic Brain Injury

CrossMark

Christos Lazaridis, MD[a],*, Claudia S. Robertson, MD[b]

KEYWORDS

- Intracranial pressure • Cerebral perfusion pressure • Brain tissue oxygen • Lactate/pyruvate ratio
- Pressure reactivity index • Neuromonitoring

KEY POINTS

- Secondary injury is characterized by a cascade of biochemical, cellular, and molecular events, often compounded by the effects of systemic insults, such as hypotension and hypoxemia.
- ICP, CPP, PRx, CBF, $PbtO_2$, LPR, and electrophysiologic data are parts of an integrated, patient-specific approach.
- Incorporation of patient demographics, brain imaging, and multimodality data can lead to the creation of individualized patient trajectories and physiologic latent states.

INTRODUCTION

This article reviews the role of modalities that directly monitor the brain parenchyma in patients with severe traumatic brain injury (TBI). The physiology monitored involves compartmental and perfusion pressures, tissue oxygenation and metabolism, quantitative blood flow, pressure autoregulation, and electrophysiology. There are several proposed roles for this multimodality monitoring (MMM):

- Track, prevent, and treat the cascade of secondary brain injury (SBI), known to occur after primary TBI at the tissue and cell level.
- Monitor the neurologically injured, often heavily sedated, patient who may have no informative clinical examination. This takes into account the idea that irreversible brain injury may have occurred by the time clinical examination changes are noted at the bedside.
- Integrate clinical examination, neuroimaging, and MMM data into a composite, patient-specific and dynamic picture. Based on this, aim toward targeted management that optimally balances the timing and the benefit/risk ratio of medical-surgical interventions.
- Apply protocolized, pathophysiology-driven intensive care.
- Use as a prognostic marker.
- Understand the pathophysiologic mechanisms involved in SBI to develop preventive and abortive therapies, and to inform future clinical trials.

PATHOPHYSIOLOGIC RATIONALE

Secondary injury is characterized by a cascade of biochemical, cellular, and molecular events, including the endogenous evolution of cerebral damage and the effects of systemic insults, such as hypotension and hypoxemia.[1,2] Based on

None of the authors have conflicts of interest in relation to this article. No funding has been received in relation to this article.

[a] Division of Neurocritical Care, Department of Neurology, Baylor College of Medicine Medical Center, Baylor College of Medicine, McNair Campus, 7200 Cambridge Street, 9th Floor, MS: NB302, Houston, TX 77030, USA;
[b] Department of Neurosurgery, Baylor College of Medicine, One Baylor Plaza, Houston, TX 77030, USA
* Corresponding author.
E-mail address: lazaridi@bcm.edu

Neurosurg Clin N Am 27 (2016) 509–517
http://dx.doi.org/10.1016/j.nec.2016.05.010

experimental TBI models the mechanisms producing SBI can be grouped as (1) those associated with ischemia, excitotoxicity, energy failure, and resultant cell death cascades; (2) secondary cerebral swelling; (3) axonal injury; and (4) inflammation and regeneration.[1] At the core of these mechanisms a resultant tissue hypoxia and/or dysoxia is believed to underlie a state of cellular energy failure.

Oxidative metabolism is based on convective oxygen transport from ambient air to blood capillaries, with hemoglobin and erythrocytes as vehicles; oxygen diffusion from erythrocytes in the capillaries to mitochondria in the cells; and oxygen reduction in the mitochondria via the electron transport chain.[3] Failure in any of these three steps could result in similar clinical manifestations; nevertheless, targeted and differentiated management requires distinguishing the actual mechanisms involved. The main types, causes, and neuromonitoring profiles of tissue hypoxia are summarized in **Table 1**. In clinical practice, it is difficult to determine the exact nature of tissue hypoxia without integration of data from MMM and neuroimaging.[4]

Among the different types of hypoxia, ischemia has long been regarded as the central cause of SBI. Studies in the 1970s demonstrated low cerebral blood flow (CBF) in the first few hours after injury, and postmortem examination of patients with fatal head injuries provided evidence of ischemic necrosis.[5,6] These findings led to management strategies directed at augmenting cerebral perfusion, blood flow, and oxygen delivery. These strategies, however, have not reliably proven to positively impact clinical outcomes, although they are known to potentially carry significant morbidity. The finding of a high rate of acute respiratory distress syndrome in patients treated with hemodynamic augmentation as an anti-ischemia regimen is a prime example.[7,8]

There are further mechanistic objections to the current model of ischemic hypoxia as the predominant mechanism.[9] It seems that except for cases of extremely low cerebral perfusion pressure (CPP) the presence of ischemia, using a variety of techniques, has remained elusive.[5] Recent observations have highlighted alternative mechanisms: dysperfusion hypoxia as a result of increased mean diffusion length from erythrocytes to mitochondria caused by intracellular or interstitial edema,[10] uncoupling hypoxia caused by intrinsic mitochondrial dysfunction,[11] and shunt hypoxia in the forms of capillary transit time heterogeneity and thoroughfare channel shunt flow.[12,13] Increases in capillary transit time heterogeneity were shown to reduce the maximum achievable oxygen extraction fraction (OEF) for a given CBF and tissue oxygen tension. This overview provides the context for the discussion that follows on the different components of MMM.

Table 1
Types of brain hypoxia in TBI

Type	Pathophysiology	Neuromonitoring Profile
Ischemic	Inadequate CBF	↓CBF, ↓PbtO$_2$, ↑LPR (high lactate/low pyruvate), ↑OEF
Low extraction	Low arterial Po$_2$ (hypoxemic hypoxia) Low hemoglobin concentration (anemic hypoxia) Low half-saturation tension P50 (high-affinity hypoxia)	≅CBF, ↓PbtO$_2$, ↑LPR (high lactate/low pyruvate), ≅OEF
Shunt	Arteriovenous shunting (microvascular shunt)	↑CBF, ≅PbtO$_2$, ↑LPR (high lactate/low pyruvate), ↓OEF
Dysperfusion	Diffusion barrier (intracellular or interstitial edema)	≅CBF, ≅PbtO$_2$, ↑LPR (high lactate/low pyruvate), ↓OEF
Uncoupling	Mitochondrial dysfunction	≅CBF, ≅PbtO$_2$, ↑LPR (high lactate/normal pyruvate), ↓OEF
Hypermetabolic	Increased demand	↑CBF, ↓PbtO$_2$, ↑LPR (high lactate/low pyruvate), ↑OEF

Abbreviations: ≅, no change or in either direction; CBF, cerebral blood flow; LPR, lactate/pyruvate ratio; OEF, oxygen extraction fraction; P50, oxygen half-saturation of hemoglobin; PbtO$_2$, partial brain tissue oxygen tension; Po$_2$, arterial oxygen tension.

MODALITIES

Intracranial Pressure and Derived Indices (Pressure Reactivity Index)

Cerebral swelling and accompanying intracranial hypertension contributes to secondary damage in two ways. Intracranial hypertension can compromise cerebral perfusion leading to secondary ischemia; in addition, it can produce the devastating consequences of deformation through herniation syndromes. Intracranial hypertension has been closely linked to adverse outcomes after TBI. In conjunction with optimization of CPP, the control of raised intracranial pressure (ICP) has formed the cornerstone of brain trauma guidelines, and together these have led to a reduction in mortality from TBI.[14] In the absence of randomized controlled trials (RCTs) directly comparing ICP treatment thresholds, the cutoff for treatment had been traditionally set at 20 mm Hg based on observational data.[15] Nevertheless, the Brain Trauma Foundation guidelines had recognized that rather than accepting a generic, absolute ICP threshold, an attempt should be made to individualize thresholds based on patient characteristics, other critical parameters, and on a risk-benefit consideration of treating ICP values.[16]

The recent BEST-TRIP trial compared two management protocols for treatment of severe TBI: one involving ICP monitoring (with a threshold of 20 mm Hg) and the other involving serial computed tomography imaging and neurologic examination. It is beyond the scope of this article to discuss this study in any detail apart from highlighting some points recently made by an international panel of experts. It should be appreciated that this was not a trial of ICP monitoring or the efficacy of such monitoring, and as a consequence the role of ICP monitoring in directing the treatment of established intracranial hypertension cannot be decided based on the data from the BEST TRIP. The primary impact of the trial should be to promote further investigation into understanding the clinical profile of patients who may actually benefit from monitoring, into determining patient-specific ICP thresholds, and in sharpening therapeutic algorithms.[17,18]

How can the main criticisms against the traditional approach to intracranial hypertension be summarized? (1) The ICP threshold set at 20 to 25 mm Hg has resulted from an overall low level of evidence, making the validity of the chosen value questionable. Furthermore, the methods used have not allowed for differentiation between a potentially modifiable therapeutic target and a mere surrogate of injury severity. (2) Absolute thresholds ignore the variability of brain injury

types and host characteristics and responses. They also mandate the same unvarying goal throughout a patient's course. (3) SBI insults, under current paradigms, are treated as unidimensional excursions over a certain number, whereas degree and time range of excursion are not considered. (4) A range of potentially important pathophysiologic variables that describe the relationships among CBF, perfusion pressure, and oxygen delivery/use, and cellular metabolism and mitochondrial state remain unaccounted. (5) The therapeutic interventions that are used carry a price that potentially outweighs the benefits of achieving a fixed ICP goal.[19]

However, continuous ICP monitoring offers the ability to investigate waveform morphology and metrics, potentially expanding the available information from a single number to evaluation of intracranial compliance and pressure-volume compensatory reserve. Continuous ICP can also be used as a surrogate of cerebral blood volume (CBV) (under conditions of a steep pressure-volume curve) and thus when correlated to spontaneous blood pressure fluctuations, offers a window into cerebrovascular pressure autoregulation and reactivity. Cerebrovascular pressure reactivity is defined as the ability of vascular smooth muscle to respond to changes in transmural pressure, and is determined by observing the response of ICP to changes in arterial blood pressure (ABP)[20]; in pressure-reactive conditions, a rise in ABP leads within 5 to 15 seconds to vasoconstriction with reduction of CBV, and ICP decreases; if defective, CBV increases passively and ICP rises. The opposite applies to a reduction in ABP.[21] A computer-aided method has been developed at Cambridge University to calculate and monitor the moving coherence/correlation index between spontaneous slow waves (20–200 seconds) of ABP and ICP. This method derives a pressure reactivity index (PRx) that has values in the range between −1 and +1. A negative or zero value reflects a normally reactive vascular bed, whereas positive values reflect passive, nonreactive vessels. Previous studies have established a significant correlation between PRx and outcome after head injury, including a time-dependent element: if PRx persisted above 0.2 for more than 6 hours, this was usually associated with a fatal outcome.[22–24]

Steiner and colleagues[25] and more recently Aries and colleagues[26] have demonstrated the value of using the PRx in identifying an optimal CPP, under and above which clinical outcome worsens. However, the PRx has also been recently used in defining individualized ICP thresholds. When these patient-specific thresholds were used to quantify individualized intracranial hypertension burden, in the form of ICP dose, were shown to be stronger predictors of 6-month clinical outcome as compared with doses derived from the conventional thresholds of 20 and 25 mm Hg. It is furthermore of note that the absolute doses based on the standard thresholds were larger than the individualized ones. This work suggests that the impact of ICP on clinical outcome is critically linked with the state of cerebrovascular pressure reactivity[27]; pressure-passive conditions add vulnerability in the presence of intracranial hypertension.

Partial Brain Tissue Oxygen Tension

In 1956, Clark[28] described the principles of an electrode that could measure oxygen tension polarographically in blood or tissue. The diffusion of oxygen molecules through an oxygen-permeable membrane into an electrolyte solution causes depolarization at the nearby cathode, starting an electrical current related to the amount of oxygen. These measurements today are performed via the Licox catheter (Integra Neurosciences, San Diego, CA). The probe has a diameter of 0.5 mm, and the measurement area is 5 mm long; clinical experience has shown a run-in time before stable measurements are obtained of less than 2 hours. The catheter requires temperature correction by means of core temperature or, preferably, measurement of brain temperature.

The more interesting question is what is actually measured by the Licox probe? Is partial brain tissue oxygen tension ($PbtO_2$) simply a CBF surrogate? Can it be used as an indicator of the balance between oxygen delivery, demand, and consumption? Although the physiologic significance of $PbtO_2$ is still not fully understood, our working model is as follows: $PbtO_2$ (and the lactate-pyruvate ratio [LPR] for that matter, as discussed later) should not be simplistically viewed as a marker of ischemic hypoxia but rather as a complex measure resulting from the various mechanisms involved in the oxygen delivery-utilization pathway.[4,29] Gupta and colleagues[30] demonstrated that $PbtO_2$ does not represent end-capillary oxygen tension. Subsequently, Menon and colleagues[10] highlighted the importance of diffusion barriers in the oxygen pathway from blood to the mitochondrial respiratory chain; this barrier is localized in the microvasculature with structural substrates of vascular collapse, endothelial swelling, and perivascular edema. Diringer and colleagues[31] found no improvement in the cerebral metabolic rate for oxygen ($CMRO_2$) after normobaric hyperoxia, "disconnecting" $PbtO_2$,

and $CMRO_2$. Finally, Rosenthal and colleagues[32] reinforced the idea that $PbtO_2$ is not closely related to total oxygen delivery or to cerebral oxygen metabolism, and instead identified a parabolic relationship between $PbtO_2$ and the product of CBF and arteriovenous oxygen tension.

Persistently depressed $PbtO_2$ has been linked with poor neurologic outcomes; similarly to the situation with ICP, it is to date unclear if it represents a mere surrogate of injury severity or if it could be a modifiable treatment target with outcome implications. The preliminary step toward answering this question was undertaken in a phase II RCT of the safety and efficacy of brain tissue oxygen monitoring. In the Brain Tissue Oxygen Monitoring in Traumatic Brain Injury (BOOST-2) trial, 110 patients were randomized to treatment based on ICP monitoring alone (goal ICP <20 mm Hg) versus treatment based on ICP (goal <20 mm Hg) and $PbtO_2$ (goal >20 mm Hg). The primary outcome was achieved with a median fraction of time with $PbtO_2$ less than 20 mm Hg of 0.44 in the ICP group and 0.14 in the ICP + $PbtO_2$ group ($P<.00001$). There was no significant difference between adverse events and protocol violations were infrequent. The nonfutility outcome measure was also met, with a nonstatistical trend toward lower mortality and poor outcome at 6-months in the ICP + $PbtO_2$ group. The investigators therefore concluded that a treatment protocol guided by both ICP and $PbtO_2$ reduces the duration of measured brain tissue hypoxia. The findings of this study will help determine the sample size for a phase III RCT.[33]

Microdialysis

Microdialysis is used clinically to estimate extracellular interstitial concentrations of small molecules (a standard 20-kDa nominal molecular weight cutoff membrane recovers glucose, pyruvate, lactate, glycerol, and glutamate), but can also be used to recover much larger molecules, such as inflammatory mediators from the interstitial fluid. The physiologic premise for obtaining tissue metabolic data rests on the assumption that it is critical to know when there is a transition from aerobic to anaerobic metabolism as a sine qua non of energy failure. This is signified by a biochemical pattern of increased lactate production and pyruvate consumption, leading to an increased LPR (thresholds of >25 or >40 have been used). Consequently, the LPR is thought of as a sensitive marker of brain redox state and secondary ischemic injury, and when raised has been associated with unfavorable clinical outcomes.[34]

PET studies have found variable relationships among $CMRO_2$, OEF, and LPR based on the thresholds for ischemia used, timing of monitoring, and probe location.[35,36] Type of tissue hypoxia is also expected to affect the OEF-LPR relationship, because OEF is expected to increase in ischemic and decrease in shunt or diffusion barrier hypoxia.[4] Recent works further demonstrate that an increased LPR may have a wide differential diagnosis.[37] Importantly, energy crisis has been demonstrated to occur in the absence of ischemia or defects in oxygen delivery and on the basis of primary mitochondrial dysfunction.[11,36] A pattern of increased lactate with near normal pyruvate may indicate mitochondrial failure rather than ischemia.[38] Knowledge of the functional status of mitochondria and of the presence of oxygen diffusion barriers is critical in the interpretation of an increased LPR.

Cerebral Blood Flow

Historically, methods measuring CBF involved "one-time" measurements with the use of administered tracer gases and dyes, or thermodilution.[39] Modern neuromonitoring paradigms require that the measurements be continuous and applicable at the bedside. One such technique uses thermal diffusion to measure local CBF; it uses an intraparenchymal probe with a thermistor and a temperature sensor and measures the thermal gradient between the distal thermistor that is heated by 2°C and the proximal temperature sensor and provides a quantified regional CBF measurement in mL/100 g/min.[40] Preliminary small studies have been done to assess its usefulness and reliability in measuring autoregulation combined with ICP, CPP, and PRx and found it to be safe with minimal complications and able to provide assessment of local vascular resistance changes in response to blood pressure and hyperventilation challenges.[41]

A mean value of 18 to 25 mL/100 g/min is considered normal; however, serial changes or trends rather than absolute values may better detect early neurologic deterioration or vasospasm or help assess a response to therapy.[42] Limitations include effects of temperature and hyperthermia, and there are no data correlating with clinical outcomes at this time. Also the limitation of interpreting absolute CBF numbers, outside of extremes, without local oxygenation and metabolic data should be kept in mind. Technical limitations, such as measurement drift, have also been recently described.[43] Examples of MMM in regional ischemia, transient intracranial hypertension, and systemic hypotension are demonstrated in **Figs. 1–3**, respectively.

Electrocorticography

Electrocorticography is an invasive form of electrocardiogram (EEG) monitoring where recording grids and strips are laid on the cortical surface intraoperatively. This technique affords more sensitive readings than surface EEG and allows the detection of self-propagating waves of neural and astrocyte depolarization, known as cortical spreading depression (CSD). These CSD waves lead to depressed spontaneous cortical activity for periods lasting minutes to hours. In experimental models of focal cerebral ischemia, the presence of CSD is associated with vasoconstriction, lesion expansion, and SBI.[44–46] Spreading depolarizations have been also found to correlate with clinical outcome and be predictive of metabolic crisis, increased ICP, vasospasm, and delayed cerebral ischemia.[47] Prolonged depolarizations are thought to reflect poor tissue perfusion and/or neurovascular uncoupling with disturbed flow autoregulation, and correlate with a worse prognosis in patients with TBI.[48,49]

In addition there are some data to suggest that, at least on some occasions, CSD development may be associated with the development of seizures as seen in one human study using subdural electrodes placed along a region of hemorrhage or contusion in TBI patients. The presence of seizures on subdural electrodes was strongly associated with the presence of CSD.[50] The relationship between CSD and seizures remains an intriguing question that it is hoped will be explored in future studies, particularly as intracranial EEG becomes more readily available.[51] The development of single probes able to provide electrophysiologic, oxygen, and neurochemistry data could facilitate exploration of the pathophysiologic interactions and offer significant insight into the mechanisms of SBI.[52]

FUTURE DIRECTIONS

The true value of monitoring may be in understanding mechanisms of injury and in tracking pathophysiologic interactions at the tissue level. Mechanisms of injury can differ among and within patients, offering an individualized approach to management. Better methods of integrating data from multiple monitors and synthesizing the information are still needed. The goal should be less about responding to particular thresholds and more about transitioning from an abnormal to a normal physiologic state.[53] In particular, the promise of neurocritical care bioinformatics may lie in the potential to use advanced analytical techniques on high-resolution multimodal physiologic

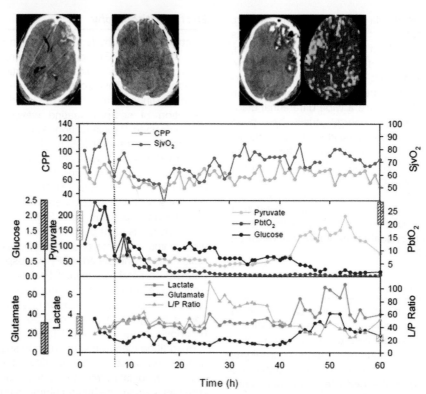

Fig. 1. An example of regional ischemia is depicted. The *upper panel* demonstrates relatively stable CPP and jugular bulb saturation (SjvO₂). The *middle panel* shows a precipitous drop of PbtO₂ with concurrent glucose depletion. In the *lower panel* an accompanying rise in LPR is seen with a later rise in lactate.

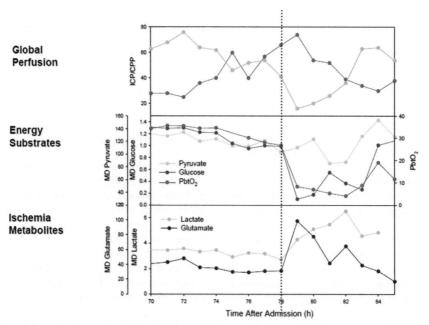

Fig. 2. Multimodality signature of transient intracranial hypertension. As ICP increases and CPP falls, drop in glucose and PbtO₂ can be appreciated with rises in glutamate and lactate. Oxygen and metabolism seem to recover as ICP returns to baseline. MD, microdialysis.

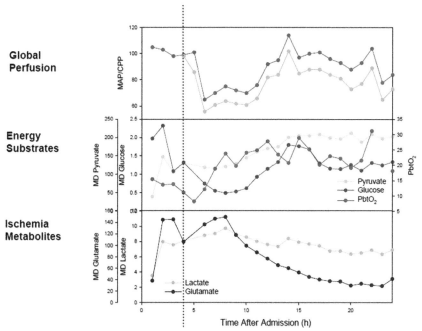

Fig. 3. Effects of transient systemic hypotension. Decreasing mean arterial pressure (MAP) and CPP lead to decreases in PbtO$_2$ and glucose, whereas a spike in glutamate and lactate is appreciated. MD, microdialysis.

data to predict future events, such as elevated ICP or low PbtO$_2$, and thereby provide targets in real time and before irreversible SBI sets in. We have recently shown a highly accurate predictive model for the prediction of intracranial hypertension and brain tissue hypoxia crises using just a few features extracted from the ICP and PbtO$_2$ time series, respectively.[54]

An important caveat in how to evaluate all physiologic monitoring in intensive care pertains to the potential disconnection between obtained data and the clinical interventions that inform them. Furthermore, the lack of adequate information on what is a mere surrogate of injury severity and what is a modifiable target confounds the effort of showing clinical outcome benefit of MMM-guided protocols. Ultimately, the additional consideration of patient demographic information and brain imaging data can lead to the creation of patient-specific trajectories and physiologic latent states, offering a more comprehensive picture in which ICP, CPP, PRx, CBF, PbtO$_2$, LPR, and electrophysiologic data are parts of an integrated, patient-specific approach.

REFERENCES

1. Kochanek PM, Clark RS, Ruppel RA, et al. Biochemical, cellular, and molecular mechanisms in the evolution of secondary damage after severe traumatic brain injury in infants and children: lessons learned from the bedside. Pediatr Crit Care Med 2000;1(1): 4–19.

2. Chesnut RM, Marshall LF, Klauber MR, et al. The role of secondary brain injury in determining outcome from severe head injury. J Trauma 1993;34:216–22.

3. Siggaard-Andersen O, Ulrich A, Gothgen IH. Classes of tissue hypoxia. Acta Anaesthesiol Scand Suppl 1995;107:137–42.

4. Haitsma IK, Maas AI. Advanced monitoring in the intensive care unit: brain tissue oxygen tension [review]. Curr Opin Crit Care 2002;8(2):115–20.

5. Diringer MN, Zazulia AR, Powers WJ. Does Ischemia contribute to energy failure in severe TBI? Transl Stroke Res 2011;2(4):517–23.

6. Graham DI, Adams JH, Doyle D. Ischaemic brain damage in fatal non-missile head injuries. J Neurol Sci 1978;39(2–3):213–34.

7. Robertson C, Valadka A, Hannay H, et al. Prevention of secondary ischemic insults after severe head injury. Crit Care Med 1999;27(10):2086–95.

8. Contant CF, Valadka AB, Gopinath SP, et al. Adult respiratory distress syndrome: a complication of induced hypertension after severe head injury. J Neurosurg 2001;95(4):560–8.

9. Lazaridis C, Andrews C. Brain tissue oxygenation, lactate pyruvate ratio, and cerebrovascular pressure reactivity monitoring in severe TBI: a systematic review and viewpoint. Neurocrit Care 2014;21:345–55.

10. Menon DK, Coles JP, Gupta AK, et al. Diffusion limited oxygen delivery following head injury. Crit Care Med 2004;32:1384–90.

11. Verweij BH, Muizelaar JP, Vinas FC, et al. Impaired cerebral mitochondrial function after traumatic brain injury in humans. J Neurosurg 2000;93(5):815–20.

12. Jespersen SN, Østergaard L. The roles of cerebral blood flow, capillary transit time heterogeneity and oxygen tension in brain oxygenation and metabolism. J Cereb Blood Flow Metab 2012;32:264–77.

13. Bragin DE, Bush RC, Müller WS, et al. High intracranial pressure effects on cerebral cortical microvascular flow in rats. J Neurotrauma 2011;28(5):775–85.

14. Gerber LM, Chiu YL, Carney N, et al. Marked reduction in mortality in patients with severe traumatic brain injury. Clinical article. J Neurosurg 2013;119: 1583–90.

15. Marmarou A, Anderson RL, Ward JD, et al. Impact of ICP instability and hypotension on outcome in patients with severe head trauma. J Neurosurg 1991; 75(Suppl 1):S59–66.

16. Bratton SL, Chestnut RM, Ghajar J, et al. Guidelines for the management of severe traumatic brain injury. VIII. Intracranial pressure thresholds. J Neurotrauma 2007;24(Suppl 1):S55–8 [Erratum appears in J Neurotrauma 2008;25:276–8].

17. Chesnut RM, Temkin N, Carney N, et al. A trial of intracranial-pressure monitoring in traumatic brain injury. N Engl J Med 2012;367:2471–81.

18. Chesnut R, Bleck T, Citerio G, et al. A consensus-based interpretation of the BEST TRIP ICP Trial. J Neurotrauma 2015;32(22):1722–4.

19. Lazaridis C, Czosnyka M. Patient-specific intracranial pressure. Response. J Neurosurg 2014; 120(4):892.

20. Paulson OB, Strandgaard S, Edvinsson L. Cerebral autoregulation. Cerebrovasc Brain Metab Rev 1990;2:161–92.

21. Rosner MJ, Becker DP. Origin and evolution of plateau waves. Experimental observations and a theoretical model. J Neurosurg 1984;60:312–24.

22. Czosnyka M, Smielewski P, Kirkpatrick P, et al. Continuous assessment of the cerebral vasomotor reactivity in head injury. Neurosurgery 1997;41:11–9.

23. Smielewski P, Lavinio A, Timofeev I, et al. ICM+, a flexible platform for investigations of cerebrospinal dynamics in clinical practice. Acta Neurochir Suppl 2008;102:145–51.

24. Lazaridis C, Smielewski P, Steiner LA, et al. Optimal cerebral perfusion pressure: are we ready for it? Neurol Res 2013;35:138–48.

25. Steiner LA, Czosnyka M, Piechnik SK, et al. Continuous monitoring of cerebrovascular pressure reactivity allows determination of optimal cerebral perfusion pressure in patients with traumatic brain injury. Crit Care Med 2002;30:733–8.

26. Aries MJ, Czosnyka M, Budohoski KP, et al. Continuous determination of optimal cerebral perfusion pressure in traumatic brain injury. Crit Care Med 2012;40:2456–63.

27. Lazaridis C, DeSantis SM, Smielewski P, et al. Patient-specific thresholds of intracranial pressure in severe traumatic brain injury. J Neurosurg 2014; 120:893–900.

28. Clark LC. Monitor and control of blood and tissue oxygen tensions. Trans Am Soc Artif Int Org 1956;2: 41–5.

29. Nortje J, Gupta AK. The role of tissue oxygen monitoring in patients with acute brain injury. Br J Anaesth 2006;97:95–106.

30. Gupta AK, Hutchinson PJ, Fryer T, et al. Measurement of brain tissue oxygenation performed using positron emission tomography scanning to validate a novel monitoring method. J Neurosurg 2002; 96(2):263–8.

31. Diringer MN, Aiyagari V, Zazulia AR, et al. Effect of hyperoxia on cerebral metabolic rate for oxygen measured using positron emission tomography in patients with acute severe head injury. J Neurosurg 2007;106(4):526–9.

32. Rosenthal G, Hemphill JC 3rd, Sorani M, et al. Brain tissue oxygen tension is more indicative of oxygen diffusion than oxygen delivery and metabolism in patients with traumatic brain injury. Crit Care Med 2008;36(6):1917–24.

33. Shutter L. For BOOST-2 investigators. Preliminary results of BOOST-2. Oral presentation of breaking clinical trial abstracts presented at Annual Meeting of Neurocritical Care Society. Seattle (WA), September 11–14, 2014. ClinicalTrials.gov NCT00974259.

34. Hutchinson PJ, Jalloh I, Helmy A, et al. Consensus statement from the 2014 International Microdialysis Forum. Intensive Care Med 2015;41(9):1517–28.

35. Hutchinson PJ, Gupta AK, Fryer TF, et al. Correlation between cerebral blood flow, substrate delivery, and metabolism in head injury: a combined microdialysis and triple oxygen positron emission tomography study. J Cereb Blood Flow Metab 2002;22(6): 735–45.

36. Vespa P, Bergsneider M, Hattori N, et al. Metabolic crisis without brain ischemia is common after traumatic brain injury: a combined microdialysis and positron emission tomography study. J Cereb Blood Flow Metab 2005;25(6):763–74.

37. Larach DB, Kofke WA, Le Roux P. Potential nonhypoxic/ischemic causes of increased cerebral interstitial fluid lactate/pyruvate ratio: a review of available literature. Neurocrit Care 2011;15(3): 609–22.

38. Nielsen TH, Schalén W, Ståhl N, et al. Bedside diagnosis of mitochondrial dysfunction after malignant middle cerebral artery infarction. Neurocrit Care 2014;21(1):35–42.

39. Steiner LA, Andrews PJ. Monitoring the injured brain: ICP and CBF. Br J Anaesth 2006;97:26–38.

40. Wajkoczy P, Roth H, Horn P, et al. Continuous monitoring of regional cerebral blood flow: experimental

and clinical validation of a novel thermal diffusion microprobe. J Neurosurg 2000;93:265–74.

41. Rosenthal G, Sanchez-Mejia RO, Phan N, et al. Incorporating a parenchymal thermal diffusion cerebral blood flow probe in bedside assessment of cerebral autoregulation and vasoreactivity in patients with severe traumatic brain injury. J Neurosurg 2011;114(1):62–70.

42. Vajkoczy P, Horn P, Thome C, et al. Regional cerebral blood flow monitoring in the diagnosis of delayed ischemia following aneurysmal subarachnoid hemorrhage. J Neurosurg 2003;98:1227–34.

43. Wolf S, Vajkoczy P, Dengler J, et al. Drift of the Bowman Hemedex® cerebral blood flow monitor between calibration cycles. Acta Neurochir Suppl 2012;114:187–90.

44. Strong AJ, Fabricius M, Boutelle MG, et al. Spreading and synchronous depressions of cortical activity in acutely injured human brain. Stroke 2002; 33:2738–43.

45. Shin HK, Dunn AK, Jones PB, et al. Vasoconstrictive neurovascular coupling during focal ischemic depolarizations. J Cereb Blood Flow Metab 2006;26: 1018–30.

46. Strong AJ, Anderson PJ, Watts HR, et al. Peri-infarct depolarizations lead to loss of perfusion in ischaemic gyrencephalic cerebral cortex. Brain 2007;130: 995–1008.

47. Dreier JP. The role of spreading depression, spreading depolarization and spreading ischemia in neurological disease. Nat Med 2011;17:439–47.

48. Hartings JA, Watanabe T, Bullock MR, et al. Spreading depolarizations have prolonged direct current shifts and are associated with poor outcome in brain trauma. Brain 2011;134:1529–40.

49. Hinzman JM, Andaluz N, Shutter LA, et al. Inverse neurovascular coupling to cortical spreading depolarizations in severe brain trauma. Brain 2014; 137(Pt 11):2960–72.

50. Fabricius M, Fuhr S, Willumsen L, et al. Association of seizures with cortical spreading depression and peri-infarct depolarisations in the acutely injured human brain. Clin Neurophysiol 2008;119:1973–84.

51. Schmitt S, Dichter MA. Electrophysiologic recordings in traumatic brain injury. Handb Clin Neurol 2015;127:319–39.

52. Li C, Limnuson K, Wu Z, et al. Single probe for real-time simultaneous monitoring of neurochemistry and direct-current electrocorticography. Biosens Bioelectron 2015;77(11):62–8.

53. Frontera J, Ziai W, O'Phelan K, et al. Regional brain monitoring in the neurocritical care unit. Neurocrit Care 2015;22(3):348–59.

54. Myers RB, Lazaridis C, Jermaine CM, et al. Predicting intracranial pressure and brain tissue oxygen crises in patients with severe traumatic brain injury. Crit Care Med 2016. [Epub ahead of print].

The Role of Surgical Intervention in Traumatic Brain Injury

Hadie Adams, MD*, Angelos G. Kolias, MRCS,
Peter J. Hutchinson, FRCS SN, PhD

KEYWORDS

- Neurosurgery • Traumatic brain injury • Neurotrauma • Decompressive craniectomy
- Neuromonitoring

KEY POINTS

- The general consensus to optimize the care for severe TBI patients is management at specialized neurotrauma centers with neurosurgical and neurocritical care support and the use of guidelines-based standardized protocols.
- It is important to recognize the heterogeneity of TBI and that the "one-size-fits-all approach" may not always be appropriate for all TBI patients.
- Knowledge synthesis activities in neurotrauma are important to define future research agendas. Advances have influenced neurotrauma as it continues to mature into a distinct subspecialty of neurosurgery.

TRAUMATIC BRAIN INJURY EPIDEMIOLOGY AND CRANIAL SURGERY RATES

In the United States, there were 2.5 million emergency department (ED) visits, hospitalizations, and deaths attributed to traumatic brain injuries (TBI) in 2010 alone, either as an isolated injury or in combination with extracranial injuries.[1] Approximately 2% of those patients (>50,000) died, accounting for approximately 40% of all deaths from acute injuries in the United States.[1] The major causes of TBI-related hospitalizations were falls, assaults, and motor vehicle traffic incidents.[1,2] TBI also remains the most common cause of disability among people younger than 40. An estimated 3.2 million to 5.3 million persons in the United States are living with disabilities acquired from a TBI-related event.[3–5] Since 2007, the number of TBI-related ED visits has increased by

56%.[1] This increase did not apply to TBI-related hospitalizations and deaths. TBI-related crude mortality rates slightly decreased from 18.2 to 17.1 per 100,000 persons from 2007 to 2010.[1] Although the exact cause for this decrease has not been established, it is thought to follow a continued reduction in motor vehicle traffic incidents. In addition, advances in prehospital and neuro–intensive care in specialized trauma centers led to improved care quality and health outcomes for TBI patients.[6] A study conducted using the National Trauma Data Bank (NTDB) found that craniotomies were performed in 3.6% of all head-injured patients.[7] More than 95% of patients with head injuries in the NTDB received conservative/nonoperative management. However, the NTDB included patients with both mild and moderate head injuries, and the absolute number of

P.J. Hutchinson is supported by an NIHR Research Professorship and the NIHR Cambridge BRC.
Division of Neurosurgery, Department of Clinical Neurosciences, Addenbrooke's Hospital, University of Cambridge, Cambridge Biomedical Campus, Cambridge CB2 0QQ, UK
* Corresponding author.
E-mail address: ha356@cam.ac.uk

neurosurgery.theclinics.com

emergency cranial surgical procedures has not been established firmly.[7] It remains important to track these rates to assess practice patterns, implementations of guidelines, and impact on patient outcome.[7-9]

INVASIVE BRAIN MONITORING

Monitoring of intracranial pressure (ICP), clinical neurologic examination, and computed tomography (CT) scanning are currently the primary methods to guide treatment of patients with TBI during neurointensive care.[10,11] Unconscious or unstable patients are often sedated, therefore, limiting the utility of clinical examinations. In these cases, ICP monitoring is traditionally used to guide management to maintain adequate cerebral perfusion and oxygenation and avoid secondary injuries.[11,12] The BEST TRIP study provided evidence that patients may be treated without ICP monitoring.[13] However, the Brain Trauma Foundation guidelines and a recent consensus conference held in Milan recommend ICP monitoring in salvageable severe TBI patients with abnormal CT finding (mass lesions, swelling, herniation, or compressed basal cisterns).[11,14]

Measurement of ICP can be done in several ways. Many consider intraventricular catheters as the gold standard method of ICP monitoring.[11] This method allows both measurement of ICP and the possibility to treat raised ICP via drainage of cerebrospinal fluid (CSF). Intraventricular catheters can be connected with fluid-coupled catheter to an external strain gauge or available with an integrated micro strain gauge or fiber-optic–tipped catheter. As with all intraventricular catheters, there is chance of drain-related infections that increase the longer a catheter is in place.[15-17] In addition, in a trauma setting it can be technically challenging to insert an intraventricular catheter in a patient with cerebral edema, midline shift, or small/compressed ventricles.[18]

Intraparenchymal ICP monitoring devices use fiber-optic catheters to measure the ICP without CSF diversion. Compared with intraventricular catheters, parenchymal monitors are a less-invasive alternative to measure ICP and carry a lower risk of infection and hemorrhage.[19-21] However, this method does not allow CSF drainage for therapeutic purposes. There are varying reports on the drift of parenchymal monitors, although this drift is not deemed a clinical concern.[11,22-24] Subdural, subarachnoid, and epidural monitors are also described and are currently considered less accurate than intraventricular or intraparenchymal devices.[11] In TBI cases with mass lesions, it has been known that ICP is not transmitted equally throughout the

intracranial space. Studies suggest that expanding mass lesions are associated with ICP gradients, in particular, acute subdural hematomas.[25] Greater than 10–mm Hg differences have been described between hemispheres. Further research is needed to define the optimal ICP measurement location to guide ICP management for these cases.

Multimodality neuromonitoring, including ICP, partial pressure of oxygen, and cerebral microdialysis can provide a more comprehensive monitoring of the injured brain than ICP monitoring alone.[10,12,26] These methods allow individualized management of secondary cerebral insults targeting patient-specific pathophysiology. Current cranial access devices enable multiple catheters and sensors to be transmitted into the brain parenchyma, to allow for ICP, cerebral microdialysis (monitoring of chemistry of the extracellular space), and partial pressure of oxygen (monitoring of cerebral oxygen metabolism) catheters to be monitored continuously at the bed-side.[27]

EVACUATION OF INTRACRANIAL HEMATOMAS

The role of surgery in traumatic intracranial hematomas is to prevent irreversible brain injury or death caused by hematoma expansion, increased ICP, and herniation of the brain.[28-30] An initial assessment of neurologic deficits, pupil abnormalities, degree of midline shift, hematoma volume, and the presence/severity of associated trauma are required to determine the necessity for emergency cranial surgery. For neurosurgeons, one of the most complicated decisions is whether moderate-sized mass lesions should be evacuated or observed. On one hand, surgical intervention might be unnecessary; on the other hand, neurologic deterioration with possible secondary insults to the brain may negatively impact the patient's outcome. Current guidelines and recommendations are available but principally drawn up by experts and the (limited) evidence that is available.[28-30]

Epidural Hematomas

Epidural hematomas (EDH) usually develop in young adults after traffic-related accidents, falls, and assaults.[29] In TBI patients, the incidence of surgical and nonsurgical EDH cases has been estimated between 2.7% to 4%.[29] EDH are thought to result from a direct blow to head and are usually found on the same side impacted by the blow. Typically, the source of bleeding is arterial after a trauma to the sphenoid or temporal bone with subsequent tearing of the middle meningeal artery and hematoma formation in the middle of the cranial fossa. EDH may also occur in the frontal, occipital, and vertex regions and are usually associated with the anterior ethmoidal artery, transverse or sigmoid sinuses, and superior sagittal sinus, respectively. EDH originating from venous sources are thought to expand more slowly compared with their arterial counterparts.[31] EDH specific mortality has been described to be around 10% in adult patients.[29] The role of surgery is to prevent irreversible brain injury or death caused by hematoma expansion, increased ICP, and herniation of the brain. Patients presenting with (progressive) focal neurologic signs or symptoms or hematoma growth must be considered as emergency cases. Evidence and expert-based recommendations for evacuations of EDH are surgery for all adult patients with a hematoma volume greater than 30 cm^3 (>30 mL) regardless of the Glasgow Coma Scale (GCS) score and comatose patients (GCS <9) with pupillary abnormalities.[29] Evacuation should be performed through a craniotomy window fashioned according to the location of the hematoma, providing adequate access to the hematoma margins. If the brain appears tight, it is important to inspect the subdural space for additional clots. When the bone flap is replaced, several tenting sutures should be placed to minimize the epidural space. Bone flaps are not generally left out for isolated EDH with no parenchymal injuries. Close observation and conservative management are appropriate for patients with no focal neurologic deficits, with a small hematoma (<30 cm^3), a clot thickness less than 15 mm, and midline shift less than 5 mm on imaging.[29]

Acute Subdural Hematomas

Acute subdural hematomas (aSDH) usually develop from motor vehicle accidents (MVA), falls, or assaults.[28] In younger patients (18–40 years), 56% of the aSDH were caused by MVA and only 12% were caused by falls. Unlike the young patients, those 65 years and older had, in 22% of the cases, an MVA and 56% had a fall.[28] Unlike EDH, the source of bleeding is usually venous caused by torn bridging veins under acceleration conditions, with arterial bleeding sources reported for approximately 20% to 30% of aSDH cases.[32,33] Mortality rates for aSDH patients requiring surgery is between 15% and 60%.[28,34–39] Evidence and expert-based recommendations for evacuations of aSDH are surgery for all adult patients with a hematoma thickness greater than 10 mm, midline shift greater than 5 mm, GCS score decreased by ≥2 points from injury to hospital admission, or patients presenting with pupillary abnormalities.[28] Because advanced age has been associated with increased

rates of adverse outcome, age should be taken into account when deciding to perform surgery. TBI patients presenting with an aSDH frequently have significant parenchymal injury and swelling on imaging.[28,38,40] Patients with aSDH that require surgery to remove the clot are treated either with a craniotomy or a decompressive craniectomy (DC). However, there is often uncertainty as to whether the bone flap should be replaced.[41] The RESCUE-ASDH trial is currently recruiting aSDH patients and aims to compare craniotomy versus DC for adult patients undergoing evacuation of an aSDH.[42] The results of this trial will inform surgical decision making in the management of aSDH patients. Close observation and conservative management is appropriate for patients that are neurologically stable and have hematoma thickness less than 10 mm, midline shift less than 5 mm, no pupillary abnormalities, and no intracranial hypertension on ICP monitoring.[28] Conservatively managed aSDH resolve gradually and are usually absorbed over weeks although in elderly patients may turn into a chronic subdural hematoma.

Traumatic Intracerebral Hemorrhage

Traumatic intracerebral hemorrhage (ICH) is also referred to as *traumatic intraparenchymal hemorrhage* and *(hemorrhagic) contusion*. Posttraumatic contusions are usually multiple and are located in the basal surface of the frontal and temporal lobes.[30] In the acute stages, the ICH consists of a (semi-)liquid mass of blood with surrounding edema. These mass lesions evolve over days and change consistency while edema begins to recede. Mortality secondary to traumatic ICH is related to the location and size of the lesion(s).[30] Surgical interventions are aimed at preventing secondary damage, brainstem compression, and herniation of the brain. Unfortunately, the only trial investigating the role of early surgery versus initial conservative treatment to anticipate and prevent secondary damage in traumatic ICH was halted early.[43,44] Although the evidence is limited because of the low sample size resulting from premature termination, it appears that the STITCH(Trauma) Trial observed reduced mortality with early surgery.[44] However, patients in this trial were mostly recruited in resource-limited settings in which ICP monitoring was not usually available. Current evidence and expert-based recommendations for evacuations of traumatic ICH involving the cerebral hemispheres recommend surgery for patients with focal lesions and the following indications: progressive neurologic deterioration, medically refractory raised ICP, a hematoma volume greater than 50 cm^3 (>50 mL), GCS score of 6 to

8 in a patient with a frontal or temporal hemorrhage greater than 20 cm^3 (>20 mL) with either midline shift of greater than 5 mm, or cisternal compression on CT scan.[30] Patients with diffuse injuries developing medically refractory posttraumatic cerebral edema and intracranial hypertension may be considered for a bifrontal DC within 48 hours of injury.[30] DCs may also be considered for patients with refractory intracranial hypertension and diffuse injuries with clinical and radiographic evidence for transtentorial herniation. Evacuation of a traumatic ICH in the posterior fossa is recommended when there is evidence of neurologic dysfunction/deterioration and significant mass effect on the basal cisterns, fourth ventricle, or signs of obstructive hydrocephalus.[45] Intensive monitoring and serial imaging are appropriate for patients with no focal neurologic deficits and nonsignificant mass effect on imaging.

DECOMPRESSIVE CRANIECTOMY IN TRAUMATIC BRAIN INJURY

Management of refractory raised ICP after severe TBI consist of medical and surgical treatments.[46,47] DC is generally considered a surgical treatment of diffuse brain swelling or expanding contusions/hematomas refractory to medical treatment and impending herniation.[48,49] In recent years, the role of DC has been discussed as a primary treatment in the acute phase, leaving out the bone flap after evacuation of a mass lesion or as a second- or third-tier therapeutic measure for diffuse brain injury and edema, commonly named *secondary* or *protocol-driven* DC. The expansion of a swollen brain outside the skull can potentially lead to a reduction in ICP and risk of herniation. The physiologic improvements described in severe TBI patients after DC, include improvement in brain tissue oxygenation, cerebral perfusion, and neurochemistry.[50–55] The risk of complications should also be considered, as early or delayed complications can occur after DC.[48] Expansion of (contralateral) mass lesions, wound infections and healing problems, subdural or subgaleal collections, hydrocephalus, syndrome of the trephined, and complication related to the subsequent cranioplasty have been recognized as DC-related complications.[56–58] Because the risk of severe disability and death in severe TBI remains relatively high, several trials have explored the use of DC to improve patient outcomes.[42,59,60] However, defining the indications, timing, techniques, and optimal outcome measures for DC is difficult, and good-quality evidence linking efficacy to outcome is lacking.[48]

Decompressive Craniectomy Methods

Decompressive craniectomy is an umbrella term for a group of procedures in which part of the skull is removed. In severe TBI, the most frequently described DC procedures in adults are bifrontal DC and unilateral frontotemporoparietal craniectomy, also termed *hemi(spherical)-craniectomy* or *unilateral DC.*[48,61,62] For unilateral conditions with midline shift and (potential) swelling (eg, aSDH with parenchymal injuries), a hemicraniectomy can be useful. Evidence and expert-based recommendations for adequate hemi-craniectomies suggest that the bone flap should be large with a minimum anteroposterior diameter of 11 to 12 cm[40,63] to achieve an adequate reduction of ICP and reduce the risk of transcalvarial herniation that is associated with parenchymal injuries at the bone edge.[64,65] Bifrontal DC is a treatment option for diffuse (bihemispheric) injuries with medically refractory intracranial hypertension.[48] A bifrontal DC extends from the floor of the anterior cranial fossa to the coronal suture posteriorly and to the temporal floor bilaterally. A widely opened dura mater is required to allow the brain to sufficiently expand. Different techniques are described for the dura (left open with onlay of hemostatic material, pericranium, or temporalis fascia or closure with dural expansion grafts)[66–68] and sagittal sinus sectioning or sparing.[49] Reports also describe bilateral hemicraniectomies as an approach for patients with diffuse injuries, although an improvement over the bifrontal DC approach has not been investigated.[62] For patients with temporal lesions or edema causing brainstem compression, extension of the DC to the floor of the middle cranial fossa is essential.

Evidence Base for Decompressive Craniectomy in Traumatic Brain Injury

The DECRA trial failed to find an improvement in functional outcome by performing early bifrontal DC over medical management for patients with diffuse TBI.[59] The study found that patients treated with DC had shorter duration of ventilation and length of stay in the intensive care unit. The RESCUEicp trial aimed to examine the clinical and cost effectiveness of secondary DC (unilateral or bifrontal DC) for severe TBI patients with refractory intracranial hypertension as a last-tier therapy. The target sample size of 400 patients was achieved, and the study is currently in the analysis/write-up phase, results are expected in 2016.[60] In contrast to the aforementioned trials, the RESCUE-ASDH trial is an ongoing randomized trial comparing primary unilateral DC with craniotomy (bone flap out vs bone flap replaced) for patients with aSDH.[42] Information from these studies will define the role of secondary and primary DC in future TBI treatment guidelines. Based on the current available evidence, neurosurgeons and neurointensivists must weigh the potential risks and benefits faced by their individual patients when deciding to perform a DC.

EXTERNAL VENTRICULAR DRAINAGE IN TRAUMATIC BRAIN INJURY

External ventricular drainage not only allows for measurement of ICP but also drainage of CSF at the bedside to control increased ICP.[11] This method is fast, minimally invasive, and effective for patients with intracranial hypertension even without hydrocephalus.[69] However, this procedure also carries certain risks and potential complications.[15–17] Complications of external ventricular drain (EVD) placement include the risk of infection, increasing with the length of drainage, and the risk of hemorrhages, increased by posttraumatic clotting derangements. Image guidance can facilitate safe placement of the catheter in TBI patients with diffuse brain swelling that often have small ventricles. Optical and electromagnetic neuronavigation systems can be used, with the latter not requiring rigid pinning cranial fixation.[70] There is no class I evidence on the use of EVD as a first-tier or second-tier intervention in severe TBI patients, and there is also clinical uncertainty regarding continuous drainage of CSF (open EVD system) versus intermittent opening as necessary to drain CSF (closed EVD system).[71] Although the latter method would allow for real-time measurement of ICP, it can potentially expose patients to elevations of ICP between drainage periods. The theoretic benefit of an open EVD system is tighter and stable ICP control; however, there is a risk of overdraining with potential subsequent collapse of the ventricles.

SURGICAL MANAGEMENT OF SKULL FRACTURES

Skull fractures most frequently involve the parietal bone, followed by the temporal, occipital, and frontal bones.[72] TBI patients usually present with linear fractures and less frequently with depressed and skull base fractures. The force of the trauma to the skull required to cause fractures is significant; therefore, patients are at significant risk of underlying brain injury. Evidence and expert-based recommendations for skull fractures are elevation and washout for patients with open skull fractures depressed more than the thickness of the cranium or more than 5 mm below the adjacent inner

table.[73] The rationale is reducing the risk of infection for these cases with early surgery, especially in the presence of dural tears, pneumocephalus, frontal sinus involvement, or contaminated wounds. Emergent surgery is also indicated for fractures with an underlying (expanding) hematoma. Elevation of the fracture also improves cosmesis for cases of significant displacement of the bone. Reconstruction can usually be achieved by using the bone fragments; if this is not feasible, implants can be used to cover the skull defect.[74] Antibiotics are usually administered to patients with open skull fractures; currently routine prophylaxis for all skull fractures is not supported by the available evidence.[73,75,76]

POSTTRAUMATIC CEREBROSPINAL FLUID LEAKS

It is estimated that CSF leaks occur in approximately 2% of TBI patients.[77–79] Fractures carrying a high risk of CSF leaks are those involving the frontal or ethmoidal sinuses and the temporal bone.[78,80] Most CSF leaks are self-limiting and resolve spontaneously within days.[77,81,82] Surgical interventions are aimed at reducing the symptoms and risk of infection in cases of persistent CSF leaks/fistulas. Studies report infection rates between 7% and 30% for TBI patients with CSF leaks, with each day of leakage increasing the risk of ascending intracranial infection.[77,83–87] Lumbar drainage is recognized as a treatment option for TBI patient with CSF leaks while also facilitating a route to administer intrathecal fluorescein for diagnostic purposes.[85,88] In addition, lumbar drains are used to relieve CSF pressure after surgical repairs to increase the success rate. The relative importance of antibiotic prophylaxis and the selection of the "true" high-risk candidates remain to be defined.[89] However, the Centers for Disease Control and Prevention recommend either the pneumococcal conjugate vaccine or the pneumococcal polysaccharide vaccine for patients with CSF leaks.[90]

POSTTRAUMATIC HYDROCEPHALUS

Posttraumatic hydrocephalus (PTH) is a complication of TBI, and studies have found clinical improvement after permanent CSF diversion.[91] Patients who had TBI and are under active follow-up care are usually monitored for PTH, which can present as worsening neurologic status or lack of improvement. It is important to recognize and treat PTH, as it could impact morbidity and mortality if left untreated.[92–94] The incidence of PTH is reported to range between 0.7% and 51.4%.[91,95,96] However, it is often difficult to determine whether ventriculomegaly observed after TBI is related to atrophy or hydrocephalus; computerized CSF infusion studies can be useful in distinguishing between the 2 processes.[97,98] Selection of patients benefiting from permanent CSF diversion is important, as shunting is also associated with significant complications. No clear guidelines exist for PTH treatment; however, adjustable or flow-regulated ventriculo-peritoneal shunts are most commonly described as the preferred choice of shunting to reduce the risk of overdrainage. PTH is reported to be a relative contraindication to endoscopic third-ventriculostomy[99]; however, this notion has been challenged by others.[100] It is difficult to predict the response of CSF diversion in PTH, as these patients often have comorbidities and significant underlying brain injury. Studies also suggest that DC is a risk factor for hydrocephalus,[48,96] whereas others do not support this hypothesis.[101] Hydrocephalus has been described in TBI patients undergoing DC, ranging in case series between 0% and 88.2%.[102] It is thought that CSF malabsorption or obstructed flow are the cause of post-DC hydrocephalus. However, the current case series are limited by their design and heterogeneity of criteria used to diagnose hydrocephalus.

CRANIOPLASTY

Cranioplasty is the surgical reconstruction of a bone defect after a previous operation, usually DC or owing to a skull injury. A cranioplasty is usually recommended for protection of the underlying brain that is left vulnerable to damage with a skull defect and also for cosmetic issues that might have psychological and social consequences for the patient.[48] The cranioplasty can also facilitate neurologic rehabilitation and may also improve neurologic function, as observed in patients with syndrome of the trephined.[103–106] However, this procedure is associated with challenging complications; the most discussed are wound healing problems and implant-related infections.[107–109] Complications can also be specific to the type of material chosen, for example, resorption of the bone with autologous bone. The wide range of techniques, graft materials (autologous bone, metal or synthetic), and timing of reconstruction (1–12 months) discussed in the literature reflects the lack of consensus and good-quality evidence to guide neurosurgeons when planning cranial reconstruction.[106,110–115] There is also controversy in relation to timing; performing the cranioplasty too early can risk infections or the development of devitalized autograft. In cases of an (suspected) infected area, it is important to wait a certain amount of time (as long as 1 year) to avoid infection of the implant. Also, it is not clear if early

reconstruction can improve the neurologic recovery of TBI patients.[106,110–112,114,115]

SUMMARY

The general consensus to optimize the care for severe TBI patients is management at specialized neurotrauma centers with neurosurgical and neurocritical care support and the use of guidelines-based standardized protocols. Over the last decade, significant efforts have been made to define neurotrauma treatment guidelines. This progress reflects the effort that has been made to examine the evidence that is available to us together with widely held expert opinions. It is, however, important to recognize the heterogeneity of TBI and that the "one-size-fits-all approach" may not always be appropriate for these patients. Knowledge synthesis activities in neurotrauma are important to define future research agendas. Clinical and research advances have influenced neurotrauma as it continues to mature into a distinct subspecialty of neurosurgery.

REFERENCES

1. Centers for Disease Control and Prevention. Traumatic Brain Injury in the United States: Epidemiology and Rehabilitation, Congress Report 2014. Atlanta (GA): National Center for Injury Prevention and Control; Division of Unintentional Injury Prevention; 2015. Available at: http://www.cdc.gov/traumaticbraininjury/pdf/tbi_report_to_congress_epi_and_rehab-a.pdf.
2. Corrigan JD, Selassie AW, Orman JA. The epidemiology of traumatic brain injury. J Head Trauma Rehabil 2010;25(2):72–80.
3. Thurman DJ, Alverson C, Dunn KA, et al. Traumatic brain injury in the United States: a public health perspective. J Head Trauma Rehabil 1999;14(6):602–15.
4. Selassie AW, Zaloshnja E, Langlois JA, et al. Incidence of long-term disability following traumatic brain injury hospitalization, United States, 2003. J Head Trauma Rehabil 2008;23(2):123–31.
5. Zaloshnja E, Miller T, Langlois JA, et al. Prevalence of long-term disability from traumatic brain injury in the civilian population of the United States, 2005. J Head Trauma Rehabil 2008;23(6):394–400.
6. Rosenfeld JV, Maas AI, Bragge P, et al. Early management of severe traumatic brain injury. Lancet 2012;380(9847):1088–98.
7. Esposito TJ, Reed RL 2nd, Gamelli RL, et al. Neurosurgical coverage: essential, desired, or irrelevant for good patient care and trauma center status. Ann Surg 2005;242(3):364–70 [discussion: 370–4].

8. Shafi S, Barnes SA, Millar D, et al. Suboptimal compliance with evidence-based guidelines in patients with traumatic brain injuries. J Neurosurg 2014;120(3):773–7.

9. Alali AS, Fowler RA, Mainprize TG, et al. Intracranial pressure monitoring in severe traumatic brain injury: results from the American College of Surgeons Trauma Quality Improvement Program. J Neurotrauma 2013;30(20):1737–46.

10. Le Roux P, Menon DK, Citerio G, et al. Consensus summary statement of the International Multidisciplinary Consensus Conference on Multimodality Monitoring in Neurocritical Care: a statement for healthcare professionals from the Neurocritical Care Society and the European Society of Intensive Care Medicine. Intensive Care Med 2014;40(9): 1189–209.

11. Brain Trauma Foundation - Guidelines for the Management of Severe Traumatic Brain Injury 3rd Edition. 2007. Available at: https://www.braintrauma. org/uploads/06/06/Guidelines_Management_2007w_ bookmarks_2.pdf. Accessed February 29, 2016.

12. Valadka AB, Robertson CS. Surgery of cerebral trauma and associated critical care. Neurosurgery 2007;61(Suppl 1):203–20 [discussion: 220–1].

13. Chesnut RM, Temkin N, Carney N, et al. A trial of intracranial-pressure monitoring in traumatic brain injury. N Engl J Med 2012;367(26):2471–81.

14. Stocchetti N, Picetti E, Berardino M, et al. Clinical applications of intracranial pressure monitoring in traumatic brain injury: report of the Milan consensus conference. Acta Neurochir 2014; 156(8):1615–22.

15. Study APE, Mayhall CG, Archer NH, et al. Ventriculostomy-Related Infections. N Engl J Med 1984; 310(9):553–9.

16. Holloway KL, Barnes T, Choi S, et al. Ventriculostomy infections: the effect of monitoring duration and catheter exchange in 584 patients. J Neurosurg 1996;85(3):419–24.

17. Lozier AP, Sciacca RR, Romagnoli MF, et al. Ventriculostomy-related infections: a critical review of the literature. Neurosurgery 2008;62(Suppl 2):688–700.

18. Ghajar J. Intracranial pressure monitoring techniques. New Horiz 1995;3(3):395–9.

19. Bekar A, Doğan Ş, Abaş F, et al. Risk factors and complications of intracranial pressure monitoring with a fiberoptic device. J Clin Neurosci 2009; 16(2):236–40.

20. Ostrup RC, Luerssen TG, Marshall LF, et al. Continuous monitoring of intracranial pressure with a miniaturized fiberoptic device. J Neurosurg 1987; 67(2):206–9.

21. Bochicchio M, Latronico N, Zappa S, et al. Bedside burr hole for intracranial pressure monitoring performed by intensive care physicians. A 5-year experience. Intensive Care Med 1996;22(10):1070–4.

22. Zacchetti L, Magnoni S, Di Corte F, et al. Accuracy of intracranial pressure monitoring: systematic review and meta-analysis. Crit Care 2015;19:420.

23. Poca MA, Sahuquillo J, Arribas M, et al. Fiberoptic intraparenchymal brain pressure monitoring with the Camino V420 monitor: reflections on our experience in 163 severely head-injured patients. J Neurotrauma 2002;19(4):439–48.

24. Piper I, Barnes A, Smith D, et al. The Camino intracranial pressure sensor: is it optimal technology? An internal audit with a review of current intracranial pressure monitoring technologies. Neurosurgery 2001;49(5):1158–64 [discussion: 1164–5].

25. Chambers IR, Kane PJ, Signorini DF, et al. Bilateral ICP monitoring: its importance in detecting the severity of secondary insults. In: Marmarou A, Bullock R, Avezaat C, et al, editors. Intracranial pressure and neuromonitoring in brain injury: Proceedings of the Tenth International ICP Symposium, Williamsburg, Virginia, May 25–29, 1997. Vienna: Springer Vienna; 1998. p. 42–3.

26. Makarenko S, Griesdale DE, Gooderham P, et al. Multimodal neuromonitoring for traumatic brain injury: a shift towards individualized therapy. J Clin Neurosci 2016;26:8–13.

27. Hutchinson PJ, Hutchinson DB, Barr RH, et al. A new cranial access device for cerebral monitoring. Br J Neurosurg 2000;14(1):46–8.

28. Bullock MR, Chesnut R, Ghajar J, et al. Surgical management of acute subdural hematomas. Neurosurgery 2006;58(Suppl 3):S16–24 [discussion: Si–iv].

29. Bullock MR, Chesnut R, Ghajar J, et al. Surgical management of acute epidural hematomas. Neurosurgery 2006;58(Suppl 3):S7–15 [discussion Si–iv].

30. Bullock MR, Chesnut R, Ghajar J, et al. Surgical management of traumatic parenchymal lesions. Neurosurgery 2006;58(3):S25–46.

31. Ropper AH, Samuels MA, Klein J. Adams and Victor's principles of neurology. 10th edition. McGraw-Hill Education; 2014.

32. Gennarelli TA, Thibault LE. Biomechanics of acute subdural hematoma. J Trauma Acute Care Surg 1982;22(8):680–6.

33. Maxeiner H, Wolff M. Pure subdural hematomas: a postmortem analysis of their form and bleeding points. Neurosurgery 2007;61(Suppl 1):267–72 [discussion: 272–3].

34. Hatashita S, Koga N, Hosaka Y, et al. Acute subdural hematoma: severity of injury, surgical intervention, and mortality. Neurol Med Chir (Tokyo) 1993;33(1):13–8.

35. Haselsberger K, Pucher R, Auer LM. Prognosis after acute subdural or epidural haemorrhage. Acta Neurochir 1988;90(3–4):111–6.

36. Koc RK, Akdemir H, Oktem IS, et al. Acute subdural hematoma: outcome and outcome prediction. Neurosurg Rev 1997;20(4):239–44.

37. Ryan CG, Thompson RE, Temkin NR, et al. Acute traumatic subdural hematoma: current mortality and functional outcomes in adult patients at a Level I trauma center. J Trauma Acute Care Surg 2012; 73(5):1348–54.

38. Zumkeller M, Behrmann R, Heissler HE, et al. Computed tomographic criteria and survival rate for patients with acute subdural hematoma. Neurosurgery 1996;39(4):708–12 [discussion: 712–3].

39. Servadei F, Nasi MT, Cremonini AM, et al. Importance of a reliable admission Glasgow Coma Scale score for determining the need for evacuation of posttraumatic subdural hematomas: a prospective study of 65 patients. J Trauma 1998; 44(5):868–73.

40. Li LM, Kolias AG, Guilfoyle MR, et al. Outcome following evacuation of acute subdural haematomas: a comparison of craniotomy with decompressive craniectomy. Acta Neurochir 2012;154(9): 1555–61.

41. Kolias AG, Belli A, Li LM, et al. Primary decompressive craniectomy for acute subdural haematomas: results of an international survey. Acta Neurochir 2012;154(9):1563–5.

42. Protocol 14PRT/6944:Randomised Evaluation of Surgery with Craniectomy for patients Undergoing Evacuation of Acute Subdural Haematoma (RESCUE-ASDH) - ISRCTN87370545. 2015. Available at: http://www.thelancet.com/doi/story/10.1016/html.2015.08.14.2280. Accessed February 29, 2016.

43. Gregson BA, Rowan EN, Mitchell PM, et al. Surgical trial in traumatic intracerebral hemorrhage (STITCH(Trauma)): study protocol for a randomized controlled trial. Trials 2012;13:193.

44. Mendelow AD, Gregson BA, Rowan EN, et al. Early Surgery versus Initial Conservative Treatment in Patients with Traumatic Intracerebral Hemorrhage (STITCH[Trauma]): the first randomized trial. J Neurotrauma 2015;32(17):1312–23.

45. Bullock MR, Chesnut R, Ghajar J, et al. Surgical management of posterior fossa mass lesions. Neurosurgery 2006;58(Suppl 3):S47–55 [discussion Si–iv].

46. Stocchetti N, Zanaboni C, Colombo A, et al. Refractory intracranial hypertension and "second-tier" therapies in traumatic brain injury. Intensive Care Med 2008;34(3):461–7.

47. American College of Surgeons - TQIP best practices in the managment of traumatic brain injury. 2015. Available at: https://www.facs.org/quality-programs/trauma/tqip/best-practice. Accessed February 29, 2016.

48. Kolias AG, Kirkpatrick PJ, Hutchinson PJ. Decompressive craniectomy: past, present and future. Nat Rev Neurol 2013;9(7):405–15.

49. Bohman LE, Schuster JM. Decompressive craniectomy for management of traumatic brain injury: an update. Curr Neurol Neurosci Rep 2013; 13(11):392.

50. Lazaridis C, Czosnyka M. Cerebral blood flow, brain tissue oxygen, and metabolic effects of decompressive craniectomy. Neurocrit Care 2012; 16(3):478–84.

51. Stiefel MF, Heuer GG, Smith MJ, et al. Cerebral oxygenation following decompressive hemicraniectomy for the treatment of refractory intracranial hypertension. J Neurosurg 2004;101(2):241–7.

52. Jaeger M, Dengl M, Meixensberger J, et al. Effects of cerebrovascular pressure reactivity-guided optimization of cerebral perfusion pressure on brain tissue oxygenation after traumatic brain injury. Crit Care Med 2010;38(5):1343–7.

53. Ho CL, Wang CM, Lee KK, et al. Cerebral oxygenation, vascular reactivity, and neurochemistry following decompressive craniectomy for severe traumatic brain injury. J Neurosurg 2008;108(5): 943–9.

54. Yamakami I, Yamaura A. Effects of decompressive craniectomy on regional cerebral blood flow in severe head trauma patients. Neurol Med Chir (Tokyo) 1993;33(9):616–20.

55. Bor-Seng-Shu E, Figueiredo EG, Amorim RL, et al. Decompressive craniectomy: a meta-analysis of influences on intracranial pressure and cerebral perfusion pressure in the treatment of traumatic brain injury. J Neurosurg 2012;117(3):589–96.

56. Stiver SI. Complications of decompressive craniectomy for traumatic brain injury. Neurosurg Focus 2009;26(6):E7.

57. Flint AC, Manley GT, Gean AD, et al. Post-operative expansion of hemorrhagic contusions after unilateral decompressive hemicraniectomy in severe traumatic brain injury. J Neurotrauma 2008;25(5): 503–12.

58. Nalbach SV, Ropper AE, Dunn IF, et al. Craniectomy-associated Progressive Extra-Axial Collections with Treated Hydrocephalus (CAPECTH): redefining a common complication of decompressive craniectomy. J Clin Neurosci 2012;19(9): 1222–7.

59. Cooper DJ, Rosenfeld JV, Murray L, et al. Decompressive craniectomy in diffuse traumatic brain injury. N Engl J Med 2011;364(16):1493–502.

60. Hutchinson PJ, Corteen E, Czosnyka M, et al. Decompressive craniectomy in traumatic brain injury: the randomized multicenter RESCUEicp study (www.RESCUEicp.com). Acta Neurochir Suppl 2006; 96:17–20.

61. Kjellberg RN, Prieto A Jr. Bifrontal decompressive craniotomy for massive cerebral edema. J Neurosurg 1971;34(4):488–93.

62. Guerra WK, Gaab MR, Dietz H, et al. Surgical decompression for traumatic brain swelling: indications and results. J Neurosurg 1999;90(2):187–96.

63. Tagliaferri F, Zani G, Iaccarino C, et al. Decompressive craniectomies, facts and fiction: a retrospective analysis of 526 cases. Acta Neurochir 2012; 154(5):919–26.
64. Li X, von Holst H, Kleiven S. Decompressive craniectomy causes a significant strain increase in axonal fiber tracts. J Clin Neurosci 2013;20(4): 509–13.
65. von Holst H, Li X, Kleiven S. Increased strain levels and water content in brain tissue after decompressive craniotomy. Acta Neurochir 2012;154(9): 1583–93.
66. Whitfield PC, Patel H, Hutchinson PJ, et al. Bifrontal decompressive craniectomy in the management of posttraumatic intracranial hypertension. Br J Neurosurg 2001;15(6):500–7.
67. Timofeev I, Hutchinson PJ. Outcome after surgical decompression of severe traumatic brain injury. Injury 2006;37(12):1125–32.
68. Guresir E, Vatter H, Schuss P, et al. Rapid closure technique in decompressive craniectomy. J Neurosurg 2011;114(4):954–60.
69. Timofeev I, Dahyot-Fizelier C, Keong N, et al. Ventriculostomy for control of raised ICP in acute traumatic brain injury. Acta Neurochir Suppl 2008;102: 99–104.
70. Hayhurst C, Byrne P, Eldridge PR, et al. Application of electromagnetic technology to neuronavigation: a revolution in image-guided neurosurgery. J Neurosurg 2009;111(6):1179–84.
71. Nwachuku EL, Puccio AM, Fetzick A, et al. Intermittent versus continuous cerebrospinal fluid drainage management in adult severe traumatic brain injury: assessment of intracranial pressure burden. Neurocrit Care 2014;20(1):49–53.
72. Cooper PR, Golfinos JG. Head injury. 4th edition. New York: McGraw-Hill, Medical Pub. Division; 2000.
73. Bullock MR, Chesnut R, Ghajar J, et al. Surgical management of depressed cranial fractures. Neurosurgery 2006;58(Suppl 3):S56–60 [discussion: Si–iv].
74. Marbacher S, Andres RH, Fathi AR, et al. Primary reconstruction of open depressed skull fractures with titanium mesh. J Craniofac Surg 2008;19(2): 490–5.
75. Ali B, Ghosh A. Antibiotics in compound depressed skull fractures. Emerg Med J 2002;19(6):552–3.
76. Ratilal BO, Costa J, Pappamikail L, et al. Antibiotic prophylaxis for preventing meningitis in patients with basilar skull fractures. Cochrane Database Syst Rev 2015;(4):CD004884.
77. Brodie HA, Thompson TC. Management of complications from 820 temporal bone fractures. Am J Otol 1997;18(2):188–97.
78. Mendizabal GR, Moreno BC, Flores CC. Cerebrospinal fluid fistula: frequency in head injuries. Rev Laryngol Otol Rhinol (Bord) 1992;113(5):423–5.
79. Friedman AJ, Ebersold JM, Quast ML. Post-traumatic cerebrospinal fluid leakage. World J Surg 2001;25(8):1062–6.
80. Ommaya A. Neurosurgery. 2nd edition. New York: McGraw-Hill; 1996.
81. Chandler JR. Traumatic cerebrospinal fluid leakage. Otolaryngol Clin North Am 1983;16(3):623–32.
82. McGuirt WF Jr, Stool SE. Cerebrospinal fluid fistula: the identification and management in pediatric temporal bone fractures. Laryngoscope 1995; 105(4 Pt 1):359–64.
83. Leech PJ, Paterson A. Conservative and operative management for cerebrospinal-fluid leakage after closed head injury. Lancet 1973;1(7811): 1013–6.
84. Savva A, Taylor MJ, Beatty CW. Management of cerebrospinal fluid leaks involving the temporal bone: report on 92 patients. Laryngoscope 2003;113(1): 50–6.
85. Mathias T, Levy J, Fatakia A, et al. Contemporary approach to the diagnosis and management of cerebrospinal fluid rhinorrhea. Ochsner J 2016;16(2): 136–42.
86. Nyquist GG, Rosen MR, Friedel M, et al. Management of cerebrospinal fluid leaks of the anterior and lateral skull base. J Neurol Surg B Skull Base 2013;74(Suppl 1):A046.
87. Spetzler RF, Wilson CB. Management of recurrent CSF rhinorrhea of the middle and posterior fossa. J Neurosurg 1978;49(3):393–7.
88. Shapiro SA, Scully T. Closed continuous drainage of cerebrospinal fluid via a lumbar subarachnoid catheter for treatment or prevention of cranial/spinal cerebrospinal fluid fistula. Neurosurgery 1992; 30(2):241–5.
89. Rimmer J, Belk C, Lund V, et al. Immunisations and antibiotics in patients with anterior skull base cerebrospinal fluid leaks. J Laryngol Otol 2014;128(7): 626–9.
90. Vaccines and Immunizations. Centers for Disease Control and Prevention. 2015. Available at: http://www.cdc.gov/vaccines/vpd-vac/pneumo/vacc-in-short.htm. Accessed February 1, 2016.
91. Guyot LL, Michael DB. Post-traumatic hydrocephalus. Neurol Res 2000;22(1):25–8.
92. Paoletti P, Pezzotta S, Spanu G. Diagnosis and treatment of post-traumatic hydrocephalus. J Neurosurg Sci 1983;27(3):171–5.
93. Tribl G, Oder W. Outcome after shunt implantation in severe head injury with post-traumatic hydrocephalus. Brain Inj 2000;14(4):345–54.
94. Low CY, Low YY, Lee KK, et al. Post-traumatic hydrocephalus after ventricular shunt placement in a Singaporean neurosurgical unit. J Clin Neurosci 2013;20(6):867–72.
95. Bontke CF, Boake C. Traumatic brain injury rehabilitation. Neurosurg Clin N Am 1991;2(2):473–82.

96. De Bonis P, Pompucci A, Mangiola A, et al. Post-traumatic hydrocephalus after decompressive craniectomy: an underestimated risk factor. J Neurotrauma 2010;27(11):1965–70.

97. Marmarou A, Foda MA, Bandoh K, et al. Posttraumatic ventriculomegaly: hydrocephalus or atrophy? A new approach for diagnosis using CSF dynamics. J Neurosurg 1996;85(6):1026–35.

98. Czosnyka Z, Czosnyka M, Owler B, et al. Clinical testing of CSF circulation in hydrocephalus. Acta Neurochir Suppl 2005;95:247–51.

99. Singh I, Haris M, Husain M, et al. Role of endoscopic third ventriculostomy in patients with communicating hydrocephalus: an evaluation by MR ventriculography. Neurosurg Rev 2008;31(3):319–25.

100. De Bonis P, Tamburrini G, Mangiola A, et al. Post-traumatic hydrocephalus is a contraindication for endoscopic third-ventriculostomy: isn't it? Clin Neurol Neurosurg 2013;115(1):9–12.

101. Rahme R, Weil AG, Sabbagh M, et al. Decompressive craniectomy is not an independent risk factor for communicating hydrocephalus in patients with increased intracranial pressure. Neurosurgery 2010;67(3):675–8 [discussion: 678].

102. Ding J, Guo Y, Tian H. The influence of decompressive craniectomy on the development of hydrocephalus: a review. Arq Neuropsiquiatr 2014;72(9):715–20.

103. Honeybul S, Janzen C, Kruger K, et al. The impact of cranioplasty on neurological function. Br J Neurosurg 2013;27(5):636–41.

104. Di Stefano C, Sturiale C, Trentini P, et al. Unexpected neuropsychological improvement after cranioplasty: a case series study. Br J Neurosurg 2012;26(6):827–31.

105. Segal DH, Oppenheim JS, Murovic JA. Neurological recovery after cranioplasty. Neurosurgery 1994;34(4):729–31.

106. Bender A, Heulin S, Röhrer S, et al. Early cranioplasty may improve outcome in neurological patients with decompressive craniectomy. Brain Inj 2013;27(9):1073–9.

107. Honeybul S, Ho KM. Long-term complications of decompressive craniectomy for head injury. J Neurotrauma 2011;28(6):929–35.

108. Gooch MR, Gin GE, Kenning TJ, et al. Complications of cranioplasty following decompressive craniectomy: analysis of 62 cases. Neurosurg Focus 2009;26(6):E9.

109. Wachter D, Reineke K, Behm T, et al. Cranioplasty after decompressive hemicraniectomy: underestimated surgery-associated complications? Clin Neurol Neurosurg 2013;115(8):1293–7.

110. Schuss P, Vatter H, Marquardt G, et al. Cranioplasty after decompressive craniectomy: the effect of timing on postoperative complications. J Neurotrauma 2012;29(6):1090–5.

111. Beauchamp KM, Kashuk J, Moore EE, et al. Cranioplasty after postinjury decompressive craniectomy: is timing of the essence? J Trauma Acute Care Surg 2010;69(2):270–4.

112. Liang W, Xiaofeng Y, Weiguo L, et al. Cranioplasty of large cranial defect at an early stage after decompressive craniectomy performed for severe head trauma. J Craniofac Surg 2007;18(3):526–32.

113. Klinger DR, Madden C, Beshay J, et al. Autologous and acrylic cranioplasty: a review of 10 years and 258 cases. World Neurosurg 2014;82(3):e525–30.

114. Glover LE, Tajiri N, Lau T, et al. Immediate, but not delayed, microsurgical skull reconstruction exacerbates brain damage in experimental traumatic brain injury model. PLoS One 2012;7(3):e33646.

115. Yadla S, Campbell PG, Chitale R, et al. Effect of early surgery, material, and method of flap preservation on cranioplasty infections: a systematic review. Neurosurgery 2011;68(4):1124–30.

Repetitive Head Impacts and Chronic Traumatic Encephalopathy

Ann C. McKee, MD[a,b,c,d,*], Michael L. Alosco, PhD[b,c],
Bertrand R. Huber, MD, PhD[a,b]

KEYWORDS

- Chronic traumatic encephalopathy • Repetitive head impacts • Traumatic brain injury
- Neurodegenerative disease • Tau protein • Subconcussion • Concussion

KEY POINTS

- A panel of expert neuropathologists recently defined chronic traumatic encephalopathy (CTE) as a unique neurodegenerative tauopathy characterized by a pathognomonic lesion. The pathognomonic lesion consists of a perivascular accumulation of abnormally hyperphosphorylated tau in neurons and astrocytes distributed in an irregular fashion with a propensity for sulcal depths of the cerebral cortex.
- The development of research criteria for the clinical diagnosis of CTE, known as traumatic encephalopathy syndrome, will facilitate clinical research in CTE.
- The number of years of exposure to contact sports, not the number of concussions, is significantly associated with more severe tau pathology in CTE, suggesting that repetitive head trauma, including subconcussive injury, is the primary stimulus for disease.
- Recent studies in neurodegenerative disease brain bank cohorts suggest that among amateur athletes, changes of CTE are more common than previously recognized.
- The development of in vivo biomarkers for CTE to facilitate the diagnosis of CTE during life and therapeutic strategies to help individuals with suspected CTE are critically needed.

INTRODUCTION

There are growing concerns that cumulative repetitive head impact exposure through routine participation in contact and collision sports is associated with increased risk of chronic neurologic and neuropsychiatric problems.[1,2] Among the issues associated with cumulative repetitive mild traumatic brain injury are persistent postconcussive symptoms and long-term problems in memory and cognition, including the development of chronic traumatic encephalopathy (CTE).[1–6]

CTE is a unique neurodegenerative disorder that occurs as a latent consequence of cumulative repetitive head impacts (RHIs), including concussion and subconcussion. CTE was first associated with the sport of boxing in 1928, when Harrison Stanford Martland described the clinical features of a neuropsychiatric syndrome that affected pugilists, a condition then known as "punch drunk" or "dementia pugilistica."[7] Over the following decades, it was gradually recognized that the condition affected men and women with a broad

Disclosures/Funding: See last page of article.
All authors report no financial conflicts.
[a] Department of Pathology and Laboratory Medicine, VA Boston Healthcare System, 150 South Huntington Avenue, Boston, MA 02130, USA; [b] Department of Neurology, Boston University School of Medicine, 72 East Concord Street, Boston, MA 02118, USA; [c] CTE Program, Alzheimer's Disease Center, Boston University School of Medicine, 72 East Concord Street, Boston, MA 02118, USA; [d] Department of Pathology, Boston University School of Medicine, 72 East Concord Street, Boston, MA 02118, USA
* Corresponding author. 72 East Concord Street, Robinson 7800, Boston, MA 02118.
E-mail address: amckee@bu.edu

range of exposure to repetitive brain trauma, including physical abuse,[8] head banging,[9,10] poorly controlled epilepsy, dwarf-throwing,[11] and rugby.[10] The term "chronic traumatic encephalopathy" or "CTE" was introduced by Critchley in his 1949 monograph "Punch drunk syndromes: the chronic traumatic encephalopathy of boxers,"[12] and has subsequently become the preferred designation. Recently, CTE has been described in athletes playing popular modern contact sports including American football, soccer, baseball, wrestling, ice hockey, as well as in military personnel exposed to RHI during military service, including explosive blast.[1,2,5,13–15] Currently, one of the great concerns to public heath is the identification of CTE in teens and amateur athletes at the high school and collegiate levels.[2,5,16] Although this past decade has seen a dramatic increase in public awareness of CTE and an equally dramatic rise in scientific research focused on the long-term effects of RHI, the science to identify the precise risks of RHI exposure and the development of CTE in amateur and professional athletes and military veterans lags behind. Like many neurodegenerative diseases, currently CTE can only be diagnosed after death by neuropathologic examination, and the precise incidence and prevalence of CTE remain unknown. Large-scale, longitudinal prospective studies are needed to directly address these public concerns and close the existing gaps in the basic and clinical science related to the natural history, evaluation and management, and long-term effects of RHI exposure.

NEUROPATHOLOGY OF CHRONIC TRAUMATIC ENCEPHALOPATHY
Microscopic Pathology

The neuropathology of CTE is increasingly well defined. In 2013, in the largest case series study to date, McKee and colleagues[2] reported the spectrum of p-tau pathology in 68 male subjects with a history of exposure to RHI with neuropathological evidence of CTE, ranging in age from 17 to 98 years (mean 59.5 years). In young subjects with the mildest forms of CTE, focal perivascular epicenters of hyperphosphorylated tau (p-tau) immunoreactive neurofibrillary tangles (NFTs) and astrocytic inclusions were found clustered at the depths of the cortical sulci; in subjects with severe disease, a profound tauopathy involved widespread brain regions. Other abnormalities encountered in advanced disease included abnormal deposits of phosphorylated TAR DNA-binding protein of 43 kDa (TDP-43) protein, neuroinflammation, varying amounts of beta amyloid plaques, neuronal loss, and white matter degeneration.

Based on these findings, preliminary criteria for the neuropathological diagnosis of CTE and a 4-tiered staging system for grading pathologic severity were proposed (**Fig. 1**).

In 2015, as the first part of a series of consensus panels funded by the National institute of neurological disorders and stroke/National institute of biomedical imaging and bioengineering (NINDS/NIBIB) to define the neuropathological criteria for CTE, these preliminary neuropathological criteria were used by 7 expert neuropathologists to blindly evaluate 25 cases of various tauopathies, including CTE, Alzheimer disease, progressive supranuclear palsy, argyrophilic grain disease, corticobasal degeneration, primary age-related tauopathy, and parkinsonism dementia complex of Guam without

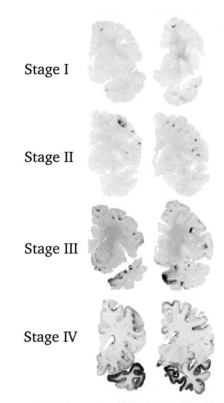

Stage I

Stage II

Stage III

Stage IV

Fig. 1. Stages of hyperphosphorylated tau pathology in CTE. In stage I CTE, p-tau pathology is restricted to isolated foci in the cerebral cortex; the focal lesions consist of perivascular accumulation of p-tau as neuronal and astrocytic inclusions, with NFTs and dot-like structures. In stage II CTE, there are multiple p-tau lesions typically found at the depths of the cerebral sulci. In stage III CTE, p-tau pathology is widespread in the cortex, and the amygdala, hippocampus and entorhinal cortex show neurofibrillary pathology. In stage IV CTE, there is widespread severe p-tau pathology affecting most regions of the cerebral cortex and the medial temporal lobe, with sparing of the calcarine crtex. All images, CP-13 immunostained 50 μm tissue sections.

any knowledge of the subjects age, sex, athletic history, clinical symptoms, or gross neuropathological findings. The results demonstrated that there was good agreement among the neuropathologists who reviewed the cases (Cohen kappa: 0.67) and even better agreement between reviewers and the diagnosis of CTE (Cohen kappa: 0.78) using the preliminary criteria. In addition, the panel refined the preliminary criteria and defined CTE as a distinctive disease with a pathognomonic lesion.[17] The pathognomonic lesion of CTE was defined as an accumulation of abnormal tau in neurons and astroglia distributed around small blood vessels at the depths of cortical sulci and in an irregular pattern (**Fig. 2**). The group also defined supportive but nonspecific features of CTE (**Box 1**)[17] and determined that the diagnostic features of CTE were distinct from the age-related astrocytic p-tau pathology (ARTAG) commonly found in the white matter of the temporal lobe and basal regions of the brain.[18] ARTAG is nonspecific and nondiagnostic, and may be found in a variety of conditions, including aging, CTE, and many others.

Using the NINDS criteria for CTE, Bieniek and colleagues[16] reviewed the clinical records and brains of 1721 cases donated to the Mayo Clinic Brain Bank over the past 18 years and found 32% of contact sport athletes had evidence of CTE pathology. No cases of CTE were found in 162 control brains without a history of brain trauma or in 33 cases with a history of a single traumatic brain injury (TBI). Of the 21 with CTE pathology, 19 had participated in football or boxing, and many were multiple-sport athletes including rugby, wrestling, basketball, and baseball. One athlete played only baseball, and another athlete only played basketball. Similarly, Ling and colleagues[19] screened 268 cases of neurodegenerative disease and controls in the Queen Square Brain Bank for Neurologic Disorders using the preliminary McKee criteria[2] and found changes of CTE in 11.9% of neurodegenerative disorders and 12.8% of elderly controls. Of the cases with changes of CTE, 93.8% had a history of TBIs; 34% had participated in high-risk sports including rugby, soccer, cricket, lacrosse, judo and squash; and 18.8% were military veterans.

Beta Amyloid Pathology in Chronic Traumatic Encephalopathy

Beta-amyloid (Aβ) plaques are found in 52% of individuals with CTE; Aβ plaques are significantly associated with age in CTE and have not been found before the age of 50 years.[20] Aβ plaques in CTE, when they occur, are typically less dense than in Alzheimer disease and predominantly diffuse.[1] Aβ plaques are also significantly associated with accelerated tauopathy, Lewy body formation, dementia, parkinsonism, and inheritance of the ApoE4 allele.[20]

Gross Pathology

Gross macroscopic alterations are usually found only in moderate-to-severe CTE. Common gross neuropathological changes include

1. Cavum septum pellucidum and septal fenestrations
2. Reduced brain weight and cerebral atrophy; the atrophy is typically bilateral and most severe in the frontal and medial temporal lobes, including the hippocampus, amygdala, and entorhinal cortex
3. Thalamic and hypothalamic atrophy, including the mammillary bodies
4. Thinning of the corpus callosum, particularly in the posterior isthmus
5. Ventricular dilation with disproportionate dilation of the third ventricle
6. Depigmentation of the locus coeruleus and substantia nigra

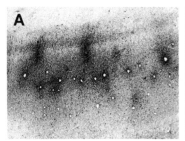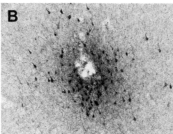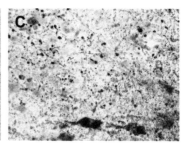

Fig. 2. The pathognomonic lesion of CTE. The pathognomonic lesion of CTE consists of an accumulation of abnormally phosphorylated tau in neurons and astroglia distributed around small blood vessels at the depths of cortical sulci and in an irregular pattern. There are typically neurofibrillary tangles, p-tau inclusions in thorned astrocytes as well as dot-like structures in the neuropil. (*A*) Magnification X40, (*B*) magnification X 200, (*C*) magnification X 600; all images, CP-13 immunostained 50 μg tissue sections, (*C*) counterstained with cresyl violet.

rage behaviors.[21–23] Cognitively, the most prominent deficits are memory, executive functioning, and impaired attention. Approximately 45% of subjects with CTE develop dementia; of subjects over the age of 60 years, 66% develop dementia. Complaints of chronic headaches occur in 30% of patients.[21] Motor symptoms, including dysarthria, dysphagia, coordination problems, and parkinsonism may also develop.

The age of symptom onset varies from as early as 19 to over 65 years of age. The precise factors that modulate clinical expression of disease are not known; cognitive reserve and lifestyle choices might play important roles. Typically, the clinical symptoms of the disease begin after a latency period of approximately 15 years. Most subjects have a history of concussions; however, 16% of CTE subjects with neuropathologically confrmed CTE have no history of concussion, suggesting that subconcussive hits and cumulative exposure to trauma are sufficient to lead to CTE. Overall, the number of years of RHI exposure, not the number of concussions, is significantly associated with hyperphosphorylated tau (p-tau) pathology in CTE.[2]

Stern and colleagues[21] reported that there are 2 distinct clinical presentations of CTE:

1. Younger age of onset (mean age of approximately 35 years) with initial behavioral (predominantly explosivity, impulsivity, and physical and verbal violence) and mood changes (depression, hopelessness, suicidality) that later progressed to deficits in cognition
2. Older age of onset (mean age of approximately 60 years), with initial cognitive impairment (most prevalent impairments in episodic memory, executive function, and attention); many subjects in this subgroup exhibit behavioral/mood changes throughout the course of the illness.

Members of the older subgroup that presents with cognitive symptoms are also more likely to exhibit more advanced neuropathology relative to the behavioral/mood subgroup (54.5% vs 27.3% stage IV CTE). Dementia is also prevalent in the cognitive subgroup, with an average interval of 8 years between dementia diagnosis and death.

CLINICAL ASPECTS OF CHRONIC TRAUMATIC ENCEPHALOPATHY
Clinical Presentation

The clinical presentation of CTE characteristically begins in 1 or more of 4 distinct domains: mood, behavior, cognitive, and motor. Early behavioral symptoms include explosivity, verbal and physical violence, loss of control, impulsivity, paranoia, and

Proposed Diagnostic Research Criteria

Recently, Montenigro and colleagues[22] conducted a systematic literature review of more than 200 published cases to develop diagnostic research criteria for the clinical manifestations of CTE, or traumatic encephalopathy syndrome (TES). TES refers to the clinical diagnosis of CTE, whereas CTE is used for cases with neuropathological verification. The diagnosis of TES requires 5 general criteria, 3 core clinical features, and 9 supportive features.

The general criteria for TES include:

1. A history of multiple impacts to the head (eg, via contact sports, military service, domestic violence, head banging, among others), including concussion and subconcussion
2. No other neurologic disorder that accounts for all of the clinical features, although it can be co-morbid with other psychiatric and neurodegenerative conditions
3. Presence of clinical features for at least 12 months.
4. At least 1 core clinical feature that is a change from baseline.
5. A minimum of 2 of supportive features.

The 3 core clinical features include

1. Behavioral symptoms primarily characterized by aggressive and explosive behaviors
2. Mood dysfunction characterized by depression and related symptoms (eg, hopelessness, depression)
3. Cognitive difficulties that involve cognitive decline and impaired cognitive test performance (ie, 1.5 standard deviations [SD] below the normative mean) in attention, executive function, and/or episodic memory.

Supportive features involve impulsivity, anxiety, apathy, paranoia, suicidality, headache, motor signs, documented decline, and delayed symptom onset (at least 2 years after RHI exposure). These core and supportive features are used to classify individuals into 1 of the 4 distinct diagnostic TES variants: TES behavioral/mood variant (TES-BMv), TES cognitive variant (TES-COGv), TES mixed variant (TES-MIXv), and TES dementia (TES-D) (**Table 1**).

Motor features are added as a modifier to the variant, if present, and the clinical course should also be described (eg, stable course, progressive course, or unknown/inconsistent), with the exception of TES-D, in which a progressive course is a requirement. Taken together, the development of TES has provided initial criteria to aid in the investigation of the pathophysiological mechanisms of CTE and assist in the designation of unlikely CTE, possible CTE, or probable CTE.

In Vivo Biomarkers

TES diagnostic criteria are meant to be used in conjunction with future biomarkers for in vivo

Table 1
Traumatic encephalopathy syndrome diagnostic variants

TES Variant	Symptoms
Behavioral/ mood	Only behavioral or mood core features (or both) • Aggression/explosivity • Impulsivity • Depression
Cognitive	Only cognitive core features • Impairments in attention, executive function, or episodic memory
Mixed	Both cognitive core features and behavioral or mood core features (or both)
Dementia	Progressive decline in cognitive core features with or without behavioral or mood core features, in addition to evidence of functional impairment

Data from Montenigro PH, Baugh CM, Daneshvar DH, et al. Clinical subtypes of chronic traumatic encephalopathy: literature review and proposed research diagnostic criteria for traumatic encephalopathy syndrome. Alzheimers Res Ther 2014;6(5–8):1–17.

diagnoses of possible or probable CTE (ie, an individual who meets criteria for TES and exhibits biomarker evidence of CTE [when they become available] would be diagnosed with probable CTE). Currently, there are no validated biomarkers for CTE, but there are several potential future biomarkers for probable CTE that remain to be validated:

1. Normal amyloid beta levels and elevated p-tau/ tau ratios in the cerebrospinal fluid[22]
2. Structural MRI-measured abnormalities of the septum pellucidum, and volumetric determination of cortical thinning, white matter reduction and cortical atrophy[22]
3. Advanced structural and functional neuroimaging modalities (eg, diffusion tensor imaging, magnetic resonance spectroscopy, functional MRI, susceptibility weight imaging, positron emission tomography [PET]).

PET imaging has enabled the study of cerebral protein pathology in Alzheimer disease and frontotemporal lobar degeneration and may become useful 1 day for the detection of p-tau pathology in subjects with suspected CTE. Young subjects with CTE would be expected to be Aβ negative using (11)C-Pittsburgh compound B ((11)C-PiB) or (18)F-florbetapir amyloid-β (Aβ)

PET radioligands,[24] whereas novel PHF-tau radioligands such as [F-18]-T807[25] would be expected to show uptake in the gray-white matter cortical junctions. In addition, PET radiolabelled probes to detect neuroinflammatory activity (eg, activated microglia) may potentially be useful to show neuroinflammatory changes characteristic of early and advanced CTE.[26]

Risk Factors

Among former football players, duration of football career, age at death, and years since football retirement all correlate with the pathologic severity of CTE.[2] Age of first exposure to RHI may also play a role in modulating the response to RHI. Former professional National Football League (NFL) players who played football before the age of 12 years had more severe cognitive loss on neuropsychiatric testing and increased microstructural abnormalities in the corpus callosum on diffusion tensor imaging compared with age-matched subjects who did not play football until after the age of 12 years.[27,28] Genes, most likely multiple genes, are also likely to modify CTE risk, including the inheritance of the apolipoprotein e4 (APoE e4) allele, MAPT H1 haplotype, and TMEM106B.[16] Lifestyle factors (eg, alcohol, substance abuse, performance-enhancing drugs, or obesity) might also influence susceptibility or disease progression, but have not yet been tested empirically.

SUMMARY

The past decade has seen a marked rise in scientific research on the long-term effects of RHI and the development of CTE, yet there remain many knowledge gaps that limit understanding of this disease. Although there is overwhelming evidence that CTE affects some professional football players, the risk for CTE in amateur contact sport athletes at the high school and collegiate levels remains to be determined. Larger, prospective studies are needed to address CTE risk for the general population and military veterans to define the parameters of RHI exposure, gender and genetics that influence susceptibility. Furthermore, prospective studies are needed to precisely define the clinical manifestations of the disease and the role of factors such as cognitive reserve, lifestyle choice, and co-morbid medical conditions in the clinical expression of the disease. In vivo biomarkers to facilitate the clinical diagnosis of CTE and monitor potential therapies are urgently needed. Given the millions of Americans involved in contact sports, as well as military personnel who experience RHI, CTE is clearly a public health concern. Although there is intense public pressure to address these concerns immediately and reduce the dangers of contact sports among amateur and professional athletes as well as to protect and improve care for military veterans, these solutions will require large-scale, longitudinal prospective studies as well as diligence and patience.

DISCLOSURES/FUNDING

The authors gratefully acknowledge the use of the resources and facilities at the Edith Nourse Rogers Memorial Veterans Hospital (Bedford, Massachusetts), the Boston VA Healthcare System, and the Boston University School of Medicine. They also gratefully acknowledge the help of all members of the Chronic Traumatic Encephalopathy Program at Boston University School of Medicine, the Boston VA, as well as the individuals and families whose participation and contributions made this work possible. This work was supported by the Department of Veterans Affairs, the Veterans Affairs Biorepository (CSP 501), National Institute of Neurological Disorders and Stroke (1U01NS086659-01), the National Institute of Aging Boston University Alzheimer's Disease Center (P30AG13846; supplement 0572063345–5), Department of Defense (W81XWH-13-2-0064, CENC award WXWH-13-2-0095), the National Operating Committee on Standards for Athletic Equipment and the Concussion Legacy Foundation. This work was also supported by unrestricted gifts from the Andlinger Foundation, the World Wrestling Entertainment and the National Football League. Michael Alosco is also supported by the T32-AG06697 post-doctoral fellowship and National Institutes of Health under grant (1F32NS096803-01).

REFERENCES

1. McKee AC, Cantu RC, Nowinski CJ, et al. Chronic traumatic encephalopathy in athletes: progressive tauopathy after repetitive head injury. J Neuropathol Exp Neurol 2009;68(7):709–35.

2. McKee AC, Stern RA, Nowinski CJ, et al. The spectrum of disease in chronic traumatic encephalopathy. Brain 2013;136(Pt 1):43–64.

3. McAllister T, Flashman L, Maerlender A, et al. Cognitive effects of one season of head impacts in a cohort of collegiate contact sport athletes. Neurology 2012; 78(22):1777–84.

4. Gavett BE, Stern RA, McKee AC. Chronic traumatic encephalopathy: a potential late effect of sport-related concussive and subconcussive head trauma. Clin Sports Med 2011;30(1):179–88.

5. McKee AC, Daneshvar DH, Alvarez VE, et al. The neuropathology of sport. Acta Neuropathol 2014; 127(1):29–51.

6. McKee AC, Stein TD, Kiernan PT, et al. The neuropathology of chronic traumatic encephalopathy. Brain Pathol 2015;25(3):350–64.

7. Martland HS. Punch drunk. J Am Med Assoc 1928; 91(15):1103–7.

8. Roberts G, Whitwell H, Acland PR, et al. Dementia in a punch-drunk wife. Lancet 1990;335(8694):918–9.

9. Hof P, Knabe R, Bovier P, et al. Neuropathological observations in a case of autism presenting with self-injury behavior. Acta Neuropathol 1991;82(4): 321–6.

10. Geddes J, Vowles G, Nicoll J, et al. Neuronal cytoskeletal changes are an early consequence of repetitive head injury. Acta Neuropathol 1999; 98(2):171–8.

11. Williams DJ, Tannenberg AE. Dementia pugilistica in an alcoholic achondroplastic dwarf. Pathology 1996; 28(1):102–4.

12. Critchley M. Punch-drunk syndromes: the chronic traumatic encephalopathy of boxers. In: Hommage a Clovis Vincent. Paris: Maloine; 1949.

13. Omalu BI, DeKosky ST, Minster RL, et al. Chronic traumatic encephalopathy in a National Football League player. Neurosurgery 2005;57(1):128–34.

14. Omalu BI, DeKosky ST, Hamilton RL, et al. Chronic traumatic encephalopathy in a national football league player: part II. Neurosurgery 2006;59(5): 1086–93.

15. Goldstein LE, Fisher AM, Tagge CA, et al. Chronic traumatic encephalopathy in blast-exposed military veterans and a blast neurotrauma mouse model. Sci Transl Med 2012;4(134):134ra160.

16. Bieniek KF, Ross OA, Cormier KA, et al. Chronic traumatic encephalopathy pathology in a neurodegenerative disorders brain bank. Acta Neuropathol 2015;130(6):877–89.

17. McKee AC, Cairns NJ, Dickson DW, et al. The first NINDS/NIBIB consensus meeting to define neuropathological criteria for the diagnosis of chronic traumatic encephalopathy. Acta Neuropathol 2016; 131(1):75–86.

18. Kovacs GG, Ferrer I, Grinberg LT, et al. Aging-related tau astrogliopathy (ARTAG): harmonized evaluation strategy. Acta Neuropathol 2016;131(1): 87–102.

19. Ling H, Holton JL, Shaw K, et al. Histological evidence of chronic traumatic encephalopathy in a large series of neurodegenerative diseases. Acta Neuropathol 2015;130(6):891–3.

20. Stein TD, Montenigro PH, Alvarez VE, et al. Beta-amyloid deposition in chronic traumatic encephalopathy. Acta Neuropathol 2015;130(1):21–34.

21. Stern RA, Daneshvar DH, Baugh CM, et al. Clinical presentation of chronic traumatic encephalopathy. Neurology 2013;81(13):1122–9.

22. Montenigro PH, Baugh CM, Daneshvar DH, et al. Clinical subtypes of chronic traumatic encephalopathy: literature review and proposed research diagnostic criteria for traumatic encephalopathy syndrome. Alzheimers Res Ther 2014;6(5–8):1–17.

23. Mez J, Solomon T, Daneshvar D, et al. Pathologically confirmed chronic traumatic encephalopathy in a 25 year old former college football player. JAMA Neurol 2016;73(3):353–5.

24. Landau SM, Breault C, Joshi AD, et al. Amyloid-β imaging with Pittsburgh compound B and florbetapir: comparing radiotracers and quantification methods. J Nucl Med 2013;54(1):70–7.

25. Chien DT, Bahri S, Szardenings AK, et al. Early clinical PET imaging results with the novel PHF-tau radioligand [F-18]-T807. J Alzheimers Dis 2013; 34(2):457–68.

26. Ramlackhansingh AF, Brooks DJ, Greenwood RJ, et al. Inflammation after trauma: microglial activation and traumatic brain injury. Ann Neurol 2011;70(3): 374–83.

27. Stamm JM, Bourlas AP, Baugh CM, et al. Age of first exposure to football and later-life cognitive impairment in former NFL players. Neurology 2015; 84(11):1114–20.

28. Stamm JM, Koerte IK, Muehlmann M, et al. Age at first exposure to football is associated with altered corpus callosum white matter microstructure in former professional football players. J Neurotrauma 2015;32(22):1768–76.

Index

Note: Page numbers of article titles are in **boldface** type.

Neurosurg Clin N Am 27 (2016) 537–543
http://dx.doi.org/10.1016/S1042-3680(16)30071-7
1042-3680/16/$ – see front matter

UNITED STATES POSTAL SERVICE®
Statement of Ownership, Management, and Circulation
(All Periodicals Publications Except Requester Publications)

1. Publication Title	2. Publication Number	3. Filing Date
NEUROSURGERY CLINICS OF NORTH AMERICA	010 – 548	9/18/2016

4. Issue Frequency	5. Number of Issues Published Annually	6. Annual Subscription Price
JAN, APR, JUL, OCT	4	$380.00

7. Complete Mailing Address of Known Office of Publication (Not printer) (Street, city, county, state, and ZIP+4®)

ELSEVIER INC.
360 PARK AVENUE SOUTH
NEW YORK, NY 10010-1710

Contact Person
STEPHEN R. BUSHING

Telephone (Include area code)
215-239-3688

8. Complete Mailing Address of Headquarters or General Business Office of Publisher (Not printer)

ELSEVIER INC.
360 PARK AVENUE SOUTH
NEW YORK, NY 10010-1710

9. Full Names and Complete Mailing Addresses of Publisher, Editor, and Managing Editor (Do not leave blank)

Publisher (Name and complete mailing address)

LINDA BELFUS, ELSEVIER INC.
1600 JOHN F KENNEDY BLVD. SUITE 1800
PHILADELPHIA, PA 19103-2899

Editor (Name and complete mailing address)

JENNIFER FLYNN-BRIGGS, ELSEVIER INC.
1600 JOHN F KENNEDY BLVD. SUITE 1800
PHILADELPHIA, PA 19103-2899

Managing Editor (Name and complete mailing address)

ADRIANNE BRIGIDO, ELSEVIER INC.
1600 JOHN F KENNEDY BLVD. SUITE 1800
PHILADELPHIA, PA 19103-2899

10. Owner (Do not leave blank. If the publication is owned by a corporation, give the name and address of the corporation immediately followed by the names and addresses of all stockholders owning or holding 1 percent or more of the total amount of stock. If not owned by a corporation, give the names and addresses of the individual owners. If owned by a partnership or other unincorporated firm, give its name and address as well as those of each individual owner. If the publication is published by a nonprofit organization, give its name and address.)

Full Name	Complete Mailing Address
WHOLLY OWNED SUBSIDIARY OF REED/ELSEVIER, US HOLDINGS	1600 JOHN F KENNEDY BLVD. SUITE 1800 PHILADELPHIA, PA 19103-2899

11. Known Bondholders, Mortgagees, and Other Security Holders Owning or Holding 1 Percent or More of Total Amount of Bonds, Mortgages, or Other Securities. If none, check box. ► ☐ None

Full Name	Complete Mailing Address
N/A	

12. Tax Status (For completion by nonprofit organizations authorized to mail at nonprofit rates) (Check one)
The purpose, function, and nonprofit status of this organization and the exempt status for federal income tax purposes:
☐ Has Not Changed During Preceding 12 Months
☐ Has Changed During Preceding 12 Months (Publisher must submit explanation of change with this statement)

PS Form 3526, July 2014 [Page 1 of 4 (see instructions page 4)]   PSN: 7530-01-000-9931   PRIVACY NOTICE: See our privacy policy on www.usps.com.

---

13. Publication Title
NEUROSURGERY CLINICS OF NORTH AMERICA

14. Issue Date for Circulation Data Below
JULY 2016

15. Extent and Nature of Circulation		Average No. Copies Each Issue During Preceding 12 Months	No. Copies of Single Issue Published Nearest to Filing Date
a. Total Number of Copies (Net press run)		360	456
b. Paid Circulation (By Mail and Outside the Mail)	(1) Mailed Outside-County Paid Subscriptions Stated on PS Form 3541 (Include paid distribution above nominal rate, advertiser's proof copies, and exchange copies)	94	115
	(2) Mailed In-County Paid Subscriptions Stated on PS Form 3541 (Include paid distribution above nominal rate, advertiser's proof copies, and exchange copies)	0	0
	(3) Paid Distribution Outside the Mails Including Sales Through Dealers and Carriers, Street Vendors, Counter Sales, and Other Paid Distribution Outside USPS®	55	75
	(4) Paid Distribution by Other Classes of Mail Through the USPS (e.g., First-Class Mail®)	0	0
c. Total Paid Distribution (Sum of 15b (1), (2), (3), and (4))		149	190
d. Free or Nominal Rate Distribution (By Mail and Outside the Mail)	(1) Free or Nominal Rate Outside-County Copies Included on PS Form 3541	48	66
	(2) Free or Nominal Rate In-County Copies Included on PS Form 3541	0	0
	(3) Free or Nominal Rate Copies Mailed at Other Classes Through the Mail (e.g., First-Class Mail)	0	0
	(4) Free or Nominal Rate Distribution Outside the Mail (Carriers or other means)	0	0
e. Total Free or Nominal Rate Distribution (Sum of 15d (1), (2), (3) and (4))		48	66
f. Total Distribution (Sum of 15c and 15e)		197	256
g. Copies not Distributed (See Instructions to Publishers #4 (page 83))		163	200
h. Total (Sum of 15f and g)		360	456
i. Percent Paid (15c divided by 15f times 100)		76%	74%

* If you are claiming electronic copies, go to line 16 on page 3. If you are not claiming electronic copies, skip to line 17 on page 3.

16. Electronic Copy Circulation	Average No. Copies Each Issue During Preceding 12 Months	No. Copies of Single Issue Published Nearest to Filing Date
a. Paid Electronic Copies	0	0
b. Total Paid Print Copies (Line 15c) + Paid Electronic Copies (Line 16a)	149	190
c. Total Print Distribution (Line 15f) + Paid Electronic Copies (Line 16a)	197	256
d. Percent Paid (Both Print & Electronic Copies) (16b divided by 16c × 100)	76%	74%

☒ I certify that 50% of all my distributed copies (electronic and print) are paid above a nominal price.

17. Publication of Statement of Ownership

☒ If the publication is a general publication, publication of this statement is required. Will be printed
in the OCTOBER 2016 issue of this publication. ☐ Publication not required.

18. Signature and Title of Editor, Publisher, Business Manager, or Owner

STEPHEN R. BUSHING - INVENTORY DISTRIBUTION CONTROL MANAGER   Date 9/18/2016

I certify that all information furnished on this form is true and complete. I understand that anyone who furnishes false or misleading information on this form or who omits material or information requested on the form may be subject to criminal sanctions (including fines and imprisonment) and/or civil sanctions (including civil penalties).

PS Form 3526, July 2014 (Page 3 of 4)   PRIVACY NOTICE: See our privacy policy on www.usps.com.

Moving?

Make sure your subscription moves with you!

To notify us of your new address, find your **Clinics Account Number** (located on your mailing label above your name), and contact customer service at:

Email: journalscustomerservice-usa@elsevier.com

800-654-2452 (subscribers in the U.S. & Canada)
314-447-8871 (subscribers outside of the U.S. & Canada)

Fax number: 314-447-8029

Elsevier Health Sciences Division
Subscription Customer Service
3251 Riverport Lane
Maryland Heights, MO 63043

ELSEVIER

Printed and bound by CPI Group (UK) Ltd, Croydon, CR0 4YY

08/05/2025

01864686-0016